Fundamentals of Veterinary
Microbiology

Fundamentals of Veterinary Microbiology

Andrew N. Rycroft, BSc, PhD, FRCPath
Professor of Veterinary Microbiology
Royal Veterinary College
University of London, London, UK

WILEY Blackwell

This edition first published 2024
© 2024 John Wiley & Sons Ltd

The right of Andrew N. Rycroft to be identified as the author of this work has been asserted in accordance with law.

Registered Offices
John Wiley & Sons, Inc., 111 River Street, Hoboken, NJ 07030, USA
John Wiley & Sons Ltd, The Atrium, Southern Gate, Chichester, West Sussex, PO19 8SQ, UK

For details of our global editorial offices, customer services, and more information about Wiley products visit us at www.wiley.com.

Wiley also publishes its books in a variety of electronic formats and by print-on-demand. Some content that appears in standard print versions of this book may not be available in other formats.

Library of Congress Cataloging-in-Publication Data applied for

PB: 9780470659472
ePDF: 9781119908371
epub: 9781119908364

Cover Design: Wiley
Cover Image: © Andrew N. Rycroft

Set in 9.5/12.5pt STIXTwoText by Straive, Pondicherry, India
Printed and bound by CPI Group (UK) Ltd, Croydon, CR0 4YY

C9780470659472_171123

For the four amigos, Simon, Frances, Jennifer and Edward, and for

Genny Moran whose kindness, encouragement and support were always there.

Contents

Preface

This book is based on my lectures and the lecture notes for the veterinary microbiology and infectious disease of animals developed at the RVC since 1992. It is intended to focus on pathogenicity and what we know of the host–pathogen relationship. However, it has also been necessary to keep in mind what is relevant for veterinary practitioners (in the widest sense) and the need to give background detail for those wanting to explore further.

Not all the chapters cover the same type of material. Not all the chapters have the same level of detail. The format is deliberately not formulaic, so that each chapter has different sections for different groups of microorganisms, and I hope that is recognised as positive. That is because the level of knowledge differs between diseases, as does the breadth of research and understanding we have on a given pathogen. A part of our knowledge of veterinary pathogens has been inferred from research into human pathogens for which the research funding has always been much better. For example, much of what we know about *Bordetella bronchiseptica* arises from work on *B. pertussis* because of its importance as the cause of childhood whooping cough. We have an inferior understanding of some animal pathogens such as *Pasteurella multocida* or *Erysipelothrix rhusiopathiae* even though they can have a minor role in human infection. Some pathogens, exclusively seen in animals, have long been neglected.

I have tried to simplify the taxonomic issues of bacteria of veterinary importance. Remembering names is hard enough without them changing every few years and I know how it infuriates veterinary students when names change! Modern analysis of whole-genome sequences has allowed a further proliferation of bacterial species names. We don't need that for most practical purposes and so I have attempted to walk the line in taxonomy between being correct yet not complicating the subject with dozens of new names for minor pathogens.

I have also tried to refer to human disease agents that are related to the animal pathogens. So much of the quality research that has informed us of the pathogenic mechanisms in human pathogens has been relevant to pathogens of animals. Of course, the medical pathogens attract the research funding. Nevertheless, there have also been good opportunities to investigate animal pathogens that have translated into better understanding of human pathogens. It is also interesting and useful to understand the relationship of the human disease agents to those causing disease in animals.

While I have included antimicrobial drugs and discussed bacterial resistance mechanisms, I have generally not attempted to give suggestions for antimicrobial treatments. That is another subject area altogether and it is open to very different views, pressures, geographical factors and ideas. Only occasionally, where it is relevant to the microbiology or history, have I ventured into mentioning antimicrobial treatment.

There are very many people who should be thanked for their contribution to this book through their careful research into the pathogens of animals. There are others I wish to thank, particularly the pathologists (Hal Thompson, Lawson Macartney, Irene McCandlish, Os Jarrett, Sonja Jeckel), geneticists (Simon Baumberg), bacteriologists (Peter Kite, Peter Taylor, Steve Hammond, Harry Smith, David Taylor, John Smith, Werner Goebel, Niels Friis) and mycologists (Glyn Evans, Christine Dawson) who kindly taught or unknowingly inspired me over the years.

Finally, I must offer my gratitude to the many undergraduate, postgraduate and doctoral students of microbial pathogenicity and veterinary medicine who were obliged to spend time exploring aspects of microbiology with me in their research projects. These addressed so many research questions and led to discussions that forced me to strive to become *au fait* with the stream of new ideas, pathogens and techniques.

I hope you find the book helpful.

Andrew N. Rycroft
Northaw, February 2023

About the Companion Website

This book is accompanied by a companion website:

www.wiley.com/go/veterinarymicrobiology

The website includes:

- Figures
- Case studies

1

The Bacterial Cell

Bacterial Structure

Bacteria are prokaryotic cells. The term 'prokaryote' includes the bacteria, the Archaea and blue-green algae. The distinguishing feature of a prokaryote is that its nucleus is not surrounded by a nuclear membrane, but the nuclear material (DNA) is free in the cytoplasm of the cell. In addition, there is no nucleolus, mitotic spindle or (usually) any separate chromosomes. Bacterial cells are distinctively smaller in size than eukaryotic cells of plants, animals and fungi (Figures 1.1 and 1.2).

Shape

Individual bacteria have characteristic shapes. The cells may be spherical (coccus), rod shaped (bacillus), comma shaped (curved rod), spiral (spirochaete) or filamentous. Bacterial shape differs to some degree with the growth conditions (e.g. whether in the body or artificial medium of one kind or another). In some species, therefore, a bacterium may appear as long rods in lab culture, but as short rods or coccobacilli in the body when causing disease. Nevertheless, the shape of most bacteria can be seen in the light microscope and is an important clue to their identity (Figure 1.3).

Anatomy of the Bacterial Cell

The bacterial cell consists of the protoplast containing numerous organelles, which is bounded by a thin, elastic, semi-permeable cytoplasmic membrane supported by the porous, relatively permeable rigid cell wall which bears a number of other structures (Figure 1.4).

Cytoplasmic Structures: Ribosomes, Nuclear Body

The cytoplasm is a gel containing organic and inorganic solutes, enzymes, ribosomes and the nucleic acids DNA and RNA. The ribosomes of prokaryotic cells are smaller than those of eukaryotic cells (plants, animals, fungi). They are known as 70S rather than the 80S ribosomes found in eukaryotic cells. This reflects a size difference because the Svedberg unit (S) is a unit of sedimentation and 80S ribosomes have a greater sedimentation rate than 70S. Both prokaryotic and eukaryotic ribosomes function to synthesise peptides (proteins), but they are sufficiently different organelles in the two groups for them to respond differently to inhibitors of protein synthesis such as some antibiotics which selectively disrupt the function of the ribosome.

The nuclear material (the DNA) is not a true nucleus. It is sometimes referred to as the nuclear body in bacteria because it is effectively free-floating in the cytoplasm. Bacterial cells are haploid (one copy of each gene) and the DNA is arranged in a single closed circular molecule of about 1000 µm in length. The bacterial chromosome is not bound to protein histones

Fundamentals of Veterinary Microbiology, First Edition. Andrew N. Rycroft.
© 2024 John Wiley & Sons Ltd. Published 2024 by John Wiley & Sons Ltd.
Companion website: www.wiley.com/go/veterinarymicrobiology

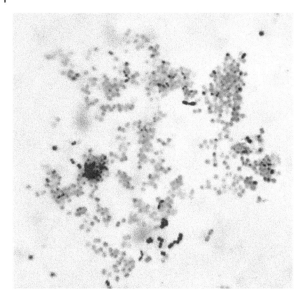

Figure 1.1 Bacterial cells stained by Gram stain and seen by light microscopy. The shape and arrangement are clear, but the resolution of the cells is limited by the light microscope.

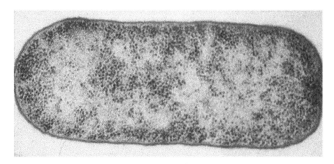

Figure 1.2 Transmission electron microscope picture of a bacterial cell. The small granular organelles scattered throughout the cell are ribosomes; lighter regions are due to nuclear material.

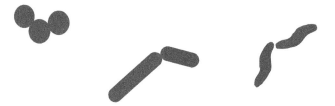

Figure 1.3 Bacteria show different shapes: cocci, rods and curved rods.

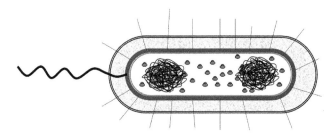

Figure 1.4 Prototypic bacterial cell to show the common subcellular features.

as it is in eukaryotic cells, and it does not stain like a mammalian chromosome. In a section through a bacterial cell in the electron microscope, it appears as complex folds. Two or even four nuclear bodies may be seen in a bacterial cell as DNA replication and segregation occurs before cell division.

Multiplication of bacteria is by simple growth and fission, not by mitosis. It is now recognised that bacteria have a cytoskeleton, which is needed for successful cell division. When a bacterial cell grows to sufficient size, the FtsZ protein forms a ring structure in the middle of the cell, known as the Z-ring. This apparently constricts or contracts to make a pinch point or septum for cell division. FtsZ also acts to organise other cell division proteins at the site of septum formation, so it is likely to have a complex role. Other cytoskeletal proteins are necessary for positioning of the septum, involved in the shape of the bacterial cell and in the successful partitioning of the daughter chromosomes into separate ends of the cell following DNA replication (Egan et al. 2020).

The cytoplasmic membrane (or plasma membrane) limits the cytoplasm. It is a typical fluid-mosaic model lipid bilayer about 9 nm across. It is composed of phospholipid and protein. The phospholipids are primarily phosphatidyl ethanolamine, with smaller proportions of phosphatidyl glycerol and cardiolipin (Figure 1.5).

Sterols are absent in almost all bacteria, but some *Mycoplasma* species, which have no cell wall, require sterols for growth and incorporate these into their membrane where they are essential for membrane stability. The membrane is flexible and is usually supported by a cell wall to maintain its integrity. The cytoplasmic membrane is the site of active transport via specific permease proteins. Its integrity is also essential for the maintenance of the proton gradient which is the driving force of electron transport and hence oxidative phosphorylation. Electron carriers of the respiratory chain, and ATPase, are located on the cytoplasmic membrane.

The Bacterial Cell Wall

The structures external to the cytoplasmic membrane constitute the bacterial envelope. One of these, the bacterial cell wall, provides the characteristic shape of the organism and prevents osmotic lysis of the cytoplasmic membrane. If the wall is ruptured, the cytoplasm expands through the gap and the cytoplasmic membrane bursts, killing the organism. This breakdown process is called lysis and can be caused by a number of agents: the enzyme lysozyme, some antibiotics, enzymes produced by bacteriophages (bacterial viruses) or enzymes produced by bacteria themselves (Figure 1.6).

Figure 1.5 The cytoplasmic membrane: phospholipid bilayer embedded with protein molecules.

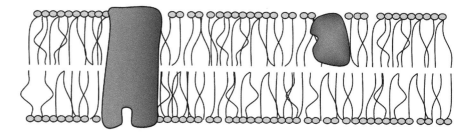

Figure 1.5 The cytoplasmic membrane: phospholipid bilayer embedded with protein molecules.

When the cell wall is weakened or lost due to one of these agents in a situation where osmotic lysis does not occur (hypertonic solution), the shape of the organism may change. Spheroplasts (from Gram-negatives) and protoplasts (from Gram-positives) are formed. If bacteria lose their cell wall *in vivo* (in the body of an animal), they are known as L-forms which may be a means by which some bacteria persist in the body during infection.

The cell wall of bacteria is a crucial structure as it is the site of action of some important groups of antimicrobials and the location of certain important antigens utilised both in identification of bacteria and in the immune response of the body to bacterial infection.

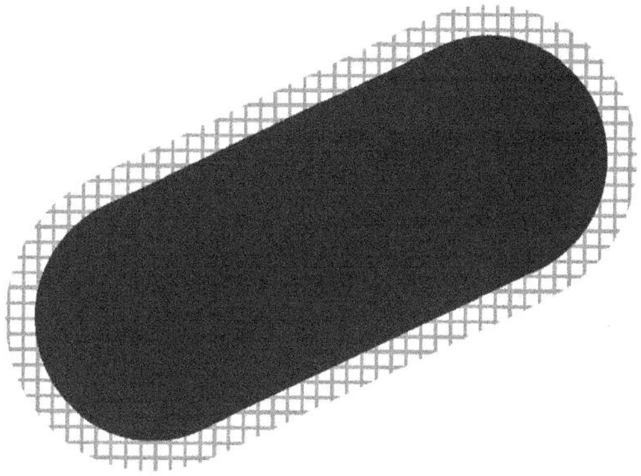

Peptidoglycan

Bacterial cell walls are quite different from those of eukaryotic cells, and they contain substances unique to bacteria. Peptidoglycan, formerly known as mucopeptide or murein, is the most important component of the cell wall. It is common to both Gram-positive and Gram-negative cells. It surrounds the cell, external to the cytoplasmic membrane, as a single bag-like molecule. It is composed of linear glycan chains of alternating residues of *N*-acetylglucosamine and *N*-acetyl muramic acid. These are linked together by short peptide bridges to form a cross-linked insoluble polymer (Rohs and Bernhardt 2021).

The peptide bridges vary between different organisms, but they are known to contain biologically exotic substances including meso-diaminopimelic acid, D-alanine and D-glutamic acid. The peptidoglycan is a rigid structure which gives shape and strength to the bacterial cell wall.

Peptidoglycan forms the basic structure of the bacterial cell wall and similar peptidoglycan is found in the unconventional, obligate intracellular bacteria: *Chlamydia* and *Rickettsia* (Figure 1.7).

Figure 1.6 The cell wall peptidoglycan surrounds the cytoplasmic membrane as a tough sack-like structure.

Figure 1.7 Peptidoglycan: long, linear glycan chains cross-linked by short peptide bridges to form the tough cell wall polymer.

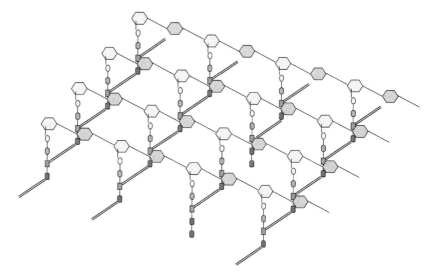

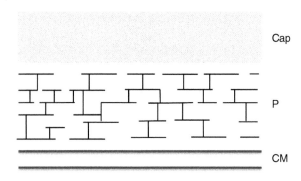

Cap

P

CM

Figure 1.8 Simplified Gram-positive cell envelope structure: thick peptidoglycan layer.

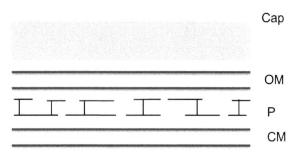

Cap

OM

P

CM

Figure 1.9 Simplified Gram-negative cell envelope structure: thin peptidoglycan and a second membrane – the outer membrane.

In addition, other accessory polymers are also found in most bacteria. Gram-positive organisms, such as staphylococci, contain teichoic acids composed of either poly-glycerol phosphate or poly-ribitol phosphate. These occur both within and on the surface of the cell wall and may account for 20–50% of the dry mass of the cell wall. On the streptococci, teichoic acids are sometimes the Lancefield group 'carbohydrate' antigens used in their classification and identification (Figure 1.8).

In Gram-negative cells, the peptidoglycan is much thinner than in Gram-positive organisms. Outside the peptidoglycan lies a second lipid bilayer membrane, the outer membrane (OM). This is a similar membrane to the inner, cytoplasmic membrane but it contains different proteins and, in addition to the phospholipids of the cytoplasmic membrane, a component unique to Gram-negative bacteria: lipopolysaccharide (LPS). This is located in the outer leaflet of the outer membrane. The outer membrane functions to protect Gram-negative bacteria against a harsh environment. It acts as a barrier and yet it allows molecules through via general porins (outer membrane proteins which act as a diffusion pore for small molecules) and substrate-specific porins (Figure 1.9).

Lipopolysaccharide

Lipopolysaccharide has three regions to the molecule. The lipid region (lipid A) is relatively invariable and contains 3-hydroxy fatty acids linked to a diglucosamine backbone. These fatty acids are hydrophobic and intercalate into the phospholipid bilayer of the OM (Putker et al. 2015) (Figure 1.10).

Linked to the lipid A is a short oligosaccharide which is variable between bacterial types, and which contains very unusual sugar residues. This is known as the LPS core region that protrudes into the environment. In some bacteria, the LPS stops at this point, and they are known as R-form or 'rough' bacteria. Such bacteria will auto-agglutinate in saline (unless other polysaccharides are external to the LPS) and these bacteria are often of low virulence. However, in many bacteria there is a third region, the O-side chain. This is a repeating oligosaccharide (perhaps five or six sugars linked together in the same pattern) with as many as 50 or 80 repeat units of this extending into the external environment of the bacterium. This makes the surface of the bacterium hydrophilic, and the O-side chain is highly antigenic, being the O or somatic antigen of Gram-negative bacteria. With a full O-side chain, bacteria are termed S-form or "smooth", and virulent bacteria are often of this type.

The LPS also has biological properties. The lipid A part of the molecule was thought to disrupt mammalian cell membranes. It is now known to act in a more subtle way to cause a host of biological effects upon the body, including pyrogenicity (raised body temperature) and the manifestations of Gram-negative septicaemia and circulatory collapse. The LPS is therefore also termed 'endotoxin' because it is toxic and yet a part of the bacterial cell and not secreted. In fact, we can think of the LPS as a signal, alerting the body to the presence a foreign invader. LPS becomes associated with the LPS binding protein. It then interacts with tissue macrophages through the CD14 protein, Toll-like receptor 4 (TLR4) and an associated protein called MD-2. Through cell signalling pathways, this leads to the release of potent cytokines such as IL-1

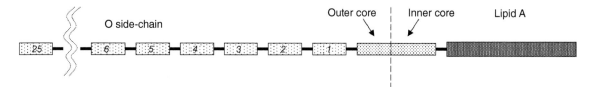

O side-chain   Outer core   Inner core   Lipid A

25   6   5   4   3   2   1

Figure 1.10 Lipopolysaccharide structure.

and TNF-α. In turn, these act on the hypothalamus to cause increased body temperature (fever) and other pro-inflammatory biological effects including vasodilation and hypotension.

In mycobacteria, which are Gram-positive organisms, wax-like mycolic acids are covalently linked to the peptidoglycan. These make the bacteria 'acid fast', resistant to desiccation, some disinfectants and most of the body's immune defence mechanisms.

Capsule

Many bacteria are surrounded with a layer of polysaccharide material known as the capsule (Figure 1.11).

Capsules may be either homopolysaccharide, being composed of a polymeric form of a single sugar type, or heteropolysaccharide, having two or sometimes more sugar residues. Very unusual sugar residues may be found quite often. In some cases, the capsule may be thick and visible in the light microscope (using special stains) and makes the bacterial colony viscous and slimy. In others, only a very thin layer, known as a microcapsule, is present. This means that the polysaccharide can be detected only by chemical or serological means or by electron microscopy (Orskov et al. 1977).

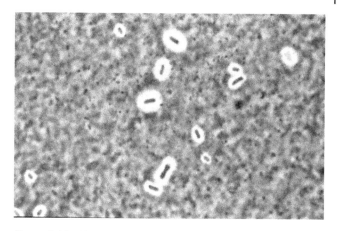

Figure 1.11 Negatively stained image of capsules of *E. coli*. Particles of India ink are excluded from the clear polysaccharide capsule which shows up as a bright area surrounding the dark bacteria.

Most capsules are antigenic but some are relatively non-antigenic, presenting a surface which the body and the biochemical components of the immune system fail to recognise as foreign. Furthermore, the capsular antigen may mask other, deeper antigens in the cell envelope such as the teichoic acids or LPS which are easily 'seen' as foreign.

The function of capsules, at least in the body, is to evade phagocytosis and some of the most important pathogens have capsules which are essential for their ability to cause disease. One such organism is *Bacillus anthracis*. This has a most unusual capsule in that it is not polysaccharide but poly-amino acid: poly D-glutamic acid. This capsule is essential for *B. anthracis* to survive in the body and cause the disease anthrax. It is also important in the identification of *B. anthracis* in the blood of a fallen animal. The capsule shows a characteristic pink or mauve colour surrounding the bacterial cell (M'Fadyean reaction) when stained with polychrome methylene blue. This is diagnostic. It is also an important statutory examination before the removal and disposal of the carcass of a sudden death case in a large animal can be carried out.

Flagellae

Bacteria also carry surface appendages. Flagellae are protein structures which function in the movement of bacteria – motility (Figure 1.12).

They are composed of protein subunits (flagellin), and these are important antigens in the identification of some bacteria (e.g. the H antigens of *Salmonella*). Bacterial flagellae are carried as a polar flagellum at the end of the cell (such as on *Pseudomonas aeruginosa*) or they may be present over the surface of the bacterium which are referred to as peritrichous flagellae (such as on *Proteus mirabilis*). The flagellae of spirochaetes are specialised in being located not externally, but within the periplasmic space (between the inner and outer membranes). Here, they are termed 'axial filaments' but serve the same function.

Flagellae cause bacteria to be motile by rotating (Bardy et al. 2003). Because it is curved, the filament of a flagellum acts as a propeller driving the organism through the

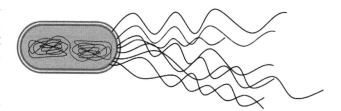

Figure 1.12 Bacterial flagellae are spiral structures attached at the cell envelope.

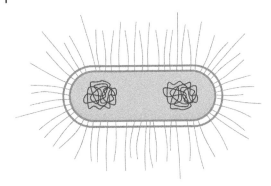

medium. The energy for this rotation is derived from the proton motive force (PMF) or proton gradient at the cytoplasmic membrane by a molecular electric motor. In this, protons pass through the mechanism across the membrane and bring about a part turn of the flagellum.

Many bacteria are chemotactic, reacting positively to some chemical stimuli by moving towards them and/or negatively to others.

Fimbriae

Fimbriae are also protein surface appendages. They are sometimes referred to as pili and are composed of subunits of pilin. They are thinner and shorter than flagellae and can only be seen by electron microscopy (Figure 1.13).

Figure 1.13 Bacterial fimbriae. Very fine surface appendages.

With a few exceptions, fimbriae are only present on Gram-negative bacteria. Their function in nature is to adhere to surfaces but different bacteria carry different fimbriae that adhere to different surfaces – some through extremely specific interactions. In some cases, this is a mucosal surface such as the small intestine or the urinary tract of an animal. Fimbriae in pathogenic bacteria may function as colonisation factors without which they would not cause disease. Antibody to fimbrial antigens can be protective in preventing attachment of the pathogen. Thus, fimbrial protein is the basis for a number of new or experimental vaccines against a surprising variety of diseases.

Sex pili are specialised fimbriae involved in the process of conjugation or transfer of plasmid genes between bacterial cells.

Spores

Bacterial spores are produced by only two genera: *Bacillus* and *Clostridium*. They are correctly known as endospores and are formed inside the mother cell in response to adverse conditions. They are not reproductive, only one spore being produced per bacterium and only one bacterium being produced by the germination of a spore. Spores are able to tolerate heat, desiccation, cold, radiation and chemical treatments that vegetative bacteria cannot survive (Nicholson et al. 2000).

Bacterial spores comprise the genomic DNA of the cell, surrounded by the cytoplasmic membrane and a layer of 'normal' peptidoglycan. External to this is the cortex, a specialised thick layer of peptidoglycan that has a much looser, less cross-linked structure. It is known to be responsible for the dehydration of the spore's core and is probably the structure which confers resistance to heat, desiccation and radiation. The coat protein is a keratin-like, very thick, highly resistant protein stabilised by disulfide (—S—S—) bonds. It probably confers chemical resistance on the spore (Figure 1.14).

Bacterial spores may remain viable for many years. They are reawakened by favourable environmental conditions. However, some spores require an activation step such as heat-shock or boiling to trigger germination. Germination is the

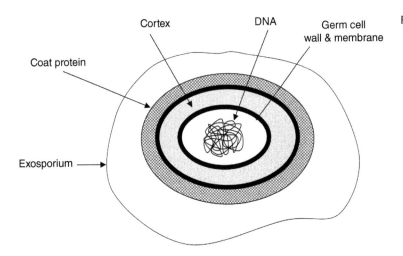

Coat protein

Cortex   DNA   Germ cell wall & membrane

Figure 1.14 Bacterial endospore structure.

Exosporium

resynthesis of metabolic enzymes, and the degradation and removal of spore-specific components and outgrowth is the return to life as a vegetative bacterial cell.

Spores are important because they are the microorganisms that are most difficult to destroy and because they are formed by a number of very important veterinary bacterial pathogens. These include the agents of clostridial diseases of sheep, tetanus, botulism, blackleg of cattle and also anthrax.

The position of a spore within the mother cell tends to be characteristic of a particular species. Spores are produced at the end of a bacterium (terminal spore), as by *Clostridium tetani*, or within the centre of the cell (central spore). Similarly, a clostridial spore will bulge the mother cell and distend it considerably outside the normal bounds of the bacterium; the spores of *Bacillus* are more confined to the bounds of the bacterial wall (Figures 1.15 and 1.16).

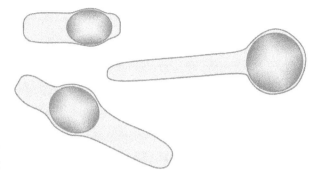

Figure 1.15 Morphology of bacterial endospores formed within a 'mother' cell. These vary according to the species of bacteria producing them.

Other Forms of Bacteria

L-forms of bacteria are sometimes generated during infection by adaptation of pathogens such as streptococci. These are produced during treatment with antibiotics which damage cell walls. They lose their cell wall peptidoglycan and remain viable in protected areas of the body. This may allow infection to persist in spite of antibiotic treatment, and by reverting to the normal (cell-walled) form of the pathogen they can produce relapses of infection. While L-forms may be responsible for some cases of chronic or unexplained recurrent infection, in practice they are rarely detected in veterinary infections.

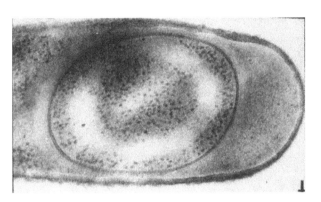

Figure 1.16 Transmission electron microscopic image of an endospore formed within a vegetative 'mother' cell.

References

Bardy, S.L., Ng, S.Y.M., and Jarrell, K.F. (2003). Prokaryotic motility structures. *Microbiology* 149: 295–304.

Egan, A.J.F., Errington, J., and Vollmer, W. (2020). Regulation of peptidoglycan synthesis and remodelling. *Nature Reviews Microbiology* 18: 446–460.

Nicholson, W.L., Munakata, N., Horneck, G. et al. (2000). Resistance of Bacillus endospores to extreme terrestrial and extraterrestrial environments. *Microbiology and Molecular Biology Reviews* 64: 548–572.

Ørskov, I., Ørskov, F., Jann, B., and Jann, K. (1977). Serology, chemistry, and genetics of O and K antigens of *Escherichia coli*. *Bacteriological Reviews* 41: 667–710.

Putker, F., Bos, M.P., and Tommassen, J. (2015). Transport of lipopolysaccharide to the gram-negative bacterial cell surface. *FEMS Microbiology Reviews* 39: 985–1002.

Rohs, P.D.A. and Bernhard, T.G. (2021). Growth and division of the peptidoglycan matrix. *Annual Review of Microbiology* 75: 315–336.

2

Metabolism, Growth and Culture of Bacteria

Multiplication of bacteria is by binary fission. As the bacterial cell grows in size, the bacterial chromosome replicates by the semi-conservative replication of DNA, beginning at a site known as the origin. New cell wall forms at the poles of the cell and at the septum or cross-wall where the cell will divide. If separation of the daughter cells is delayed after cell division, then the characteristic arrangements of bacteria (chains of streptococci, bunches of staphylococci) are produced, depending on the plane of cleavage.

Although bacteria do not have a sexual cycle, the exchange of genetic material may occur naturally between individuals of the same or related genus by the process of conjugation: self-directed transfer of plasmid DNA (see Chapter 4).

The speed of bacterial growth is measured as the generation time. The generation time is the interval from completion of septum formation to septum formation, or from one bacterial cell to two cells at the same stage. This may be as short as 20 minutes for *Escherichia coli* and as long as 16 hours (even under optimised conditions) for *Mycobacterium bovis*. The generation time for bacteria growing in the body may be quite long as they may be deprived of certain important nutrients.

A starting culture of bacteria in a fixed quantity of culture fluid is termed a 'batch culture' and it goes through a predictable series of growth phases. The first of these is lag phase when the organism is adjusting to the new environment and synthesising new enzymes. No increase in bacterial numbers takes place during this time. The bacteria then enter log (or exponential) phase in which a period of sustained growth and division takes place. With bacteria dividing to become 2, 4, 8, 16, 32 and so on, the increase in numbers or turbidity (cloudiness) is exponential. When a nutrient is exhausted or a toxic metabolite begins to inhibit growth, the bacteria enter stationary phase. No further increase in numbers then occurs. Decline phase is the final stage in which bacteria die at an exponential rate (exponential decay) (Figure 2.1).

In industrial culture, batch culture is often used for the production of antibiotics. Secondary metabolites are only formed in late exponential or stationary phase. Some processes use continuous culture, in which a population is grown by constantly supplying fresh medium to the culture and removing culture at the same rate. This allows a controlled steady state to be achieved whose growth rate can be manipulated at will. Growth in the body is closer to continuous culture than batch culture, but the analogy is not simple.

Atmospheric Requirements of Bacteria

Many bacteria grow well in air. Some, such as *Bordetella bronchiseptica* and *M. bovis*, cannot do without the oxygen present in air. They are said to be obligate aerobes.

Others that grow in air can tolerate conditions in which there is no O_2. These, such as *E coli*, are termed 'facultative anaerobes': they have the capacity to metabolise anaerobically but they prefer to utilise molecular oxygen as the terminal electron acceptor, when it is available, for respiratory metabolism. This is because respiratory metabolism generates a far greater amount of energy in terms of ATP than does fermentation.

Microaerophilic bacteria prefer a reduced oxygen tension. They will not grow or grow very poorly in the absence of O_2 or in the open atmosphere. *Campylobacter* species are microaerophilic.

Other organisms are unable to tolerate molecular O_2. They are termed 'obligate anaerobes'. The degree of 'strictness' varies between organisms such that some clostridia will tolerate and grow in a few per cent O_2 (aerotolerant anaerobes) while others will be killed by even brief exposure to oxygen. Strict anaerobes are thought to be sensitive to O_2 because they

Fundamentals of Veterinary Microbiology, First Edition. Andrew N. Rycroft.
© 2024 John Wiley & Sons Ltd. Published 2024 by John Wiley & Sons Ltd.
Companion website: www.wiley.com/go/veterinarymicrobiology

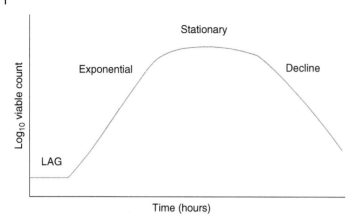

Figure 2.1 The phases of bacterial growth in batch culture.

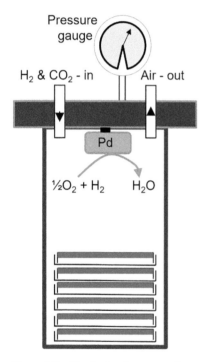

Figure 2.2 The basis of an anaerobe jar to provide an atmosphere free of O_2.

possess a respiratory chain (electron transport chain) which, through partial reduction of O_2, generates free radicals such as superoxide (O_2^-) and hydrogen peroxide (H_2O_2). These highly reactive compounds are normally decomposed very rapidly by enzymes (superoxide dismutase and catalase) and cause no harm. Strict anaerobes do not possess these enzymes and are damaged by them. For example, when O_2^- and H_2O_2 are allowed to combine, they yield the extremely toxic hydroxyl radical ($^.OH$). Strict anaerobes include *Dichelobacter nodosus* (the agent of ovine foot rot) and *Brachyspira hyodysenteriae* (swine dysentery).

To have an anaerobic environment in the clinical laboratory and enable the culture of anaerobic bacteria, an anaerobic jar has been traditionally used. This was an airtight sealable jar, with pressure gauge and valves to allow gas in and gas out. Culture plates or broths were placed in the jar and the lid closed. Part of the air was removed with a vacuum pump and then hydrogen gas (often mixed with CO_2 for safety) was run into the jar. Using the accelerating effect of the palladium catalyst attached to the inside of the lid, the H_2 combines with the residual O_2 until all the O_2 is consumed and the atmosphere is free of any oxygen. This was incubated in the 37 °C incubator (Figure 2.2).

To replace gas cylinders, gas packs able to generate H_2 were introduced. More recently, gas packs with their own catalyst have become popular and, for large numbers of clinical cultures or for research, an anaerobic cabinet is used. An indicator system, often just some methylene blue solution to indicate a chemically reduced atmosphere, is used to verify that anaerobic conditions have been achieved.

Despite their sensitivity to O_2, some strict anaerobes such as *Clostridium* species can still respire but they use elements other than oxygen as a terminal electron acceptor. Some use NO_3^- and release NO_2^- or N_2. These are denitrifying bacteria, and the process is anaerobic respiration.

Bacteria which do not have the oxygen-detoxifying enzymes but possess no respiratory chain to generate free radicals are aerotolerant. This includes the lactobacilli (usually harmless commensals and also used to make yoghurt) and many of the streptococci which include species that are important animal pathogens. These organisms are indifferent to the presence or absence of oxygen and generate their energy solely by non-respiratory metabolism (fermentations).

Nutritional Requirements

Bacteria may be autotrophic, making their own nutrients from carbon dioxide and inorganic salts together with a source of nitrogen, iron, calcium, phosphorus and other mineral nutrients. Other organisms, which require a source of preformed organic nutrients, are heterotrophic and these include all the pathogens of man and animals. Some, such as *E. coli*, will grow in a solution of glucose in phosphate buffer and ammonium sulfate together with a minimal source of inorganic metal salts. Others, such as streptococci, require complex preformed organic compounds as nutrients and building blocks together with co-factors and vitamins which they are unable to synthesise themselves (Markey et al. 2013).

Bacteriological media, for the routine isolation of pathogens in a clinical laboratory, reflect the complex requirements of pathogens in general. This is so that one or two standard complex media can be used which will be expected to grow the majority of cultivable pathogens when the population of bacteria in a clinical sample is not known. They are therefore prepared from digested meat and extracts of yeast, etc. These complex preparations are then supplemented where necessary with blood, serum, etc. to further enrich them.

pH Requirements

Most of the bacteria of veterinary importance grow best in the pH range 7.2–7.6, but many can tolerate conditions outside this range and still grow satisfactorily.

Among the acidophiles (growing under relatively acid conditions) are the lactobacilli; the alkophiles include *Vibrio* spp. including *V. cholerae*, the cause of the human disease cholera.

Temperature Requirements

Most pathogenic bacteria produce optimum growth at approximately 37 °C. Some can grow at temperatures between 15 °C and 45 °C. Those only able to grow at low temperature (less than 20 °C) are called psychrophiles and those only able to grow at high temperature are called thermophiles. Because these are so far from the body temperature of mammals, they are not pathogens of animals. Growth at low temperature (10–15 °C) is a characteristic of *Listeria* spp. This is known as a psychrotroph because it can also grow at normal body temperature.

Culture Media

All bacteria that may cause disease or live on a body are heterotrophic. They require a preformed source of carbon for building new molecules and for energy. Among these, some have very diverse metabolic capability. They can degrade complex organic molecules and build complex molecules from nothing more than glucose, inorganic nitrogen, inorganic phosphate and some trace elements. *E. coli* is one such species that will grow on a solution of ammonium salts, phosphate buffer and glucose.

Defined media are a mixture of substances whose chemical properties can be exactly reproduced and defined. Nevertheless, many bacteria of veterinary and medical importance have evolved to require preformed complex organic molecules for their nutrition, and these cannot be exactly defined.

Media for routine use are prepared from digested meat (e.g. peptone or brain heart infusion) together with extracts of yeast, and often supplemented with blood or serum. These are known as complex media. The basic material for bacteriological medium is prepared as freeze-dried powder to be reconstituted with water and sterilised by heating (Figure 2.3).

A complex liquid medium is termed a broth, e.g. nutrient broth or tryptone soya broth. In order to be able to grow colonies separated from each other on the surface of a medium, the broth must be solidified. For this purpose, agar is used at a concentration of 1.0–1.5%. In the past, gelatine was used to solidify a medium but at temperatures much above 28 °C, gelatine melts so it was unsuitable for cultures incubated at 37 °C. Also, some bacteria digest gelatine and liquify it. Instead, agar, an inert complex galactan polysaccharide extracted from seaweed, melts at 95 °C and then re-solidifies at 45 °C. This is perfect: it allows the addition of heat-labile substances to different growth media before they are allowed to solidify and yet there is no chance of the agar melting when incubated even at temperatures above 37 °C. Agar is not digested by bacteria, nor used as a nutrient.

Common complex media used for routine clinical microbiology include blood agar (a rich meat extract and peptone base supplemented with 7% horse, sheep or calf blood when cooled to 55 °C) and heated blood agar (known as

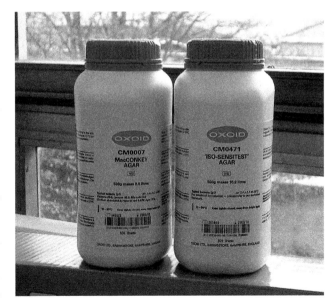

Figure 2.3 Bottles of commercial bacteriological medium for reconstituting.

chocolate agar) which is prepared as blood agar but heated to 85 °C to coagulate and denature blood proteins before allowing to cool. The characteristic colour provides the trivial name. These are poured into petri dishes at about 50 °C.

Selective and Differential Media

Some complex media contain substances which deliberately inhibit the growth of particular organisms while allowing others to grow. MacConkey's agar is the most widely used of these. It contains peptone as the main nutrient, bile salts (a mild detergent) which have a weak suppressive effect on non-intestinal bacteria, and lactose and neutral red which together detect lactose fermentation. Because it differentiates lactose fermenters (pink colonies) from non-lactose fermenters (yellow colonies), it is also a differential medium. Other selective media, which often have a similar differential system incorporated, include XLD (xylose, lysine, desoxycholate) medium and DCA (desoxycholate citrate agar) although there are many others that have been devised for the selective isolation and recognition of specific pathogens (Markey et al. 2013).

Enrichment Broths

Enrichment broths increase the number of the organism sought relative to the normal bacteria present. These are used primarily in the isolation of salmonellae from faecal material where a very large number of commensal organisms are present compared with the pathogen. The most important examples are selenite F broth and tetrathionate broth for the enrichment of *Salmonella*. After incubation, samples are taken from the cultured enrichment broth and plated onto a suitable selective, differential medium which will allow salmonellae to be distinguished.

Culture of Bacteria on a Solid Medium

Bacterial growth appears as a haze in liquid medium and as discrete colonies on solid media. Each bacterial colony is the descendant of one bacterial cell. If the inoculating material contains many bacteria, colonies will develop closely to give confluent growth. If separated or diluted, this inoculum can give rise to discrete colonies. To achieve single colonies from a mixture or a large number of bacteria, material is diluted on a plate; the process is called 'streaking' or 'plating out' (Figure 2.4).

Dilution of an inoculum can also be done by serial 10-fold dilution in tubes of saline. A pure culture must be obtained before the properties of a bacterial isolate can be investigated, and this is normally done by selecting a single colony and subculturing it.

Each stage (set of streaks) is a further dilution because the loop should be sterilised by flaming. In this way, the bacteria in the inoculum are reduced in number until they become separated enough to form individual colonies and the components of a mixture (e.g. a mixed infection) can be seen. When the properties of a bacterial isolate are investigated, perhaps to identify it, one colony is selected and subcultured. The properties of the clone of cells derived from it are then studied as a pure culture.

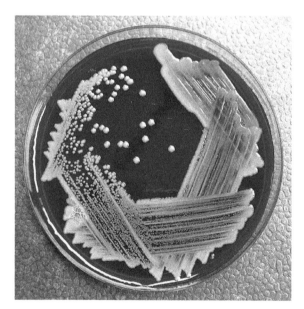

Figure 2.4 A culture after plating out and overnight incubation shows separated colonies (each is a clone derived from a single bacterial cell). The colonies all look the same so this is likely to be a pure culture.

Identifying Bacteria in Culture

Bacterial cultures are identified by comparing the morphological, cultural, biochemical and antigenic properties of an unknown isolate with those of known bacterial species (Barrow and Feltham 2009). Many of the bacteria regularly isolated from disease in animals can be identified provisionally by an experienced bacteriologist from their appearance on standard media supplemented by the use of one or two appropriate tests.

The growth medium is important in determining the characteristics of a bacterial colony. Bacterial isolation is usually carried out on a rich medium which allows the growth of most bacteria (e.g. blood agar) together with a selective medium (MacConkey's medium) which inhibits some bacteria while allowing growth of others and distinguishing lactose fermenters from non-lactose fermenters.

Once isolated in pure culture and the basic growth characteristics recognised, a pathogen is identified by a variety of directed tests and investigations. The skill of taking an unknown isolate in culture and applying the correct tests to identify it take some time to develop. In recent years, methods based on matrix-assisted laser desorption/ionisation-time of flight (MALDI-TOF) mass spectrometry (MS) have become widely used for the rapid and accurate identification of bacterial and fungal pathogens in clinical microbiology (Clark et al. 2013; Angeletti 2017). Nevertheless, well-prepared cultures are still needed to separate and provisionally categorise bacterial pathogens from a clinical sample.

References

Angeletti, S. (2017). Matrix assisted laser desorption time of flight mass spectrometry (MALDI-TOF MS) in clinical microbiology. *Journal of Microbiological Methods* 138: 20–29.

Barrow, G.I. and Feltham, R.K.A. (2009). *Cowan and Steel's Manual for the Identification of Medical Bacteria*, 3e. Cambridge: Cambridge University Press.

Clark, A.E., Kaleta, E.J., Arora, A., and Wolk, D.M. (2013). Matrix-assisted laser desorption ionization-time of flight mass spectrometry: a fundamental shift in the routine practice of clinical microbiology. *Clinical Microbiology Reviews* 26: 547–603.

Markey, B.K., Leonard, F.C., Archambault, M. et al. (2013). *Clinical Veterinary Microbiology*, 2e. Edinburgh: Mosby Elsevier.

3

Sterilisation and Disinfection

Both sterilisation and disinfection are needed to control microorganisms. Firstly, in medicine and surgery it is essential that we can prevent pathogenic organisms, particularly bacteria but also viruses, fungi and parasites, from entering the body and causing disease. It is vital that injectable drugs, dressings and instruments can be guaranteed sterile. We also need to be able to control microorganisms in microbiology. It is necessary to have sterile culture medium which is free of environmental contaminants but also to ensure cultures of pathogens can be destroyed when they are no longer needed and thereby protect personnel. Finally, in the food industry, hygiene is important but the canning and bottling industry requires foodstuff to be sterile, to prevent both spoilage and the disease botulism.

Some years ago, we could be certain in our use of the term 'sterilisation'; it was an absolute process. The sterilisation of an object or liquid implies the complete destruction of all microorganisms on or in that material. However, it is now not so clear. In 1983, bacteria were discovered in deep-sea hydrothermal vents called black smokers. In these hydrothermal vents, super-heated water passes through the Earth's crust into the cold water of the deep ocean floor. Such bacteria were reported to survive and grow in a titanium chamber at high pressure and at temperatures of at least 250 °C. This has since been revised downwards but bacteria are known that can double their numbers in an autoclave operating for 24 hours. The hyperthermophile *Methanopyrus kandleri* will grow at 122 °C.

This has meant that our fundamental ideas of heat sensitivity of biological processes had to be revised. Nevertheless, in practical terms the chance that extreme thermophilic bacteria could cause harm to animals, humans or plants is negligible since the organisms cannot grow at ambient temperatures. They are so outside their natural habitat that they would simply die in an animal body.

Similarly, the recognition of the agents of transmissible spongiform encephalopathies (TSE) such as new-variant CJD, bovine spongiform encephalopathy (BSE) and scrapie has altered our perception of the certainty of sterilisation. The TSE agent (known as a prion) is not destroyed by autoclaving or indeed by many of the chemical methods used to kill bacteria, viruses and even bacterial spores. Whether these agents are a form of life is debatable and most biologists would view them as heat-stable proteins or self-replicating toxins. Nevertheless, surgical materials contaminated with small quantities of TSE agent represent a hazard to human and animal health and the infectivity of TSE agents is not removed or destroyed by the methods we have come to depend upon as providing reliable sterilisation.

Wet Heat

In the laboratory, veterinary surgery or hospital, autoclaving is the most widely used and effective means of sterilisation. Autoclaving is the heating of an object or liquid with saturated steam to 121 °C for 15 minutes. Dry heat or unsaturated moist heat is less effective at killing than saturated steam.

The simplest form of autoclave is the domestic pressure cooker. Water is boiled under pressure of 15 lb per square inch. At this pressure above normal atmospheric pressure, water will not boil until it reaches 121 °C. As it heats to 100 °C, boiling begins and steam is generated. This increases the pressure inside the vessel and suppresses the boiling until the required pressure is reached. At this pressure, the water and steam are at 121 °C. At this temperature, foodstuffs cook much quicker. Similarly, microorganisms, including the most resistant spores, are killed in the water-saturated atmosphere after 15 minutes

Fundamentals of Veterinary Microbiology, First Edition. Andrew N. Rycroft.
© 2024 John Wiley & Sons Ltd. Published 2024 by John Wiley & Sons Ltd.
Companion website: www.wiley.com/go/veterinarymicrobiology

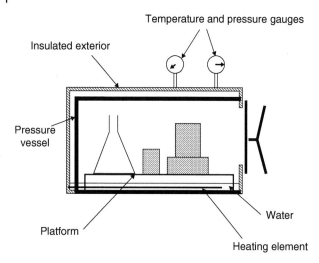

Figure 3.1 The basic components of a simple autoclave.

of this treatment. Higher pressure, leading to higher temperature, can be used in some equipment for a shorter sterilisation time (Denyer 1987a) (Figure 3.1).

Practical Precautions When Autoclaving

When autoclaving, it is necessary to recognise two important details which seem obvious but are often overlooked or ignored. First, time must be allowed for the whole of an object to reach 121 °C. For a bottle of 500 ml of liquid, this may be 30–45 minutes. Similarly, a pack of dressings may remain insulated from the moisture and heat deep inside them, and therefore fail to sterilise unless time is allowed for the material to heat up. This is seen on occasions when bottles of agar culture media are taken out of the autoclave without having melted entirely and therefore having failed to reach even 100 °C.

Second, it is essential that steam is allowed access to all the surfaces of a solid object. If dressings are wrapped tightly so that access for the steam is not possible, only dry heat will be applied to the dressings. Furthermore, air must be removed from the object because the temperature of a 50% air/steam mixture at the same pressure is only 112 °C. Under these conditions, materials may remain contaminated, and it is the endospores of *Clostridium* which may survive to infect wounds over which the dressings are used.

Modern autoclaves are used in all hospitals and many surgeries. They may have an electric element to heat water inside the autoclave or a separate steam generator. Additionally, they have devices to ensure the removal of air from the steaming chamber and timing devices and sensors to monitor the heating, sterilising and cooling parts of the cycle.

Controls of the Efficiency of Sterilisation

In addition to the use of thermocouples to monitor temperature in modern autoclaves, there are three types of control used to ensure efficient sterilisation by the autoclave. The first of these is autoclave tape. This can be attached to any object to be sterilised, and the tape changes to show black stripes when heating has occurred. However, this is less than satisfactory because exposure to hot steam for a few seconds will change the tape and this is only useful to confirm that an object has been put through the autoclave.

Indicator strips are also available commercially. They change colour when the correct temperature has been applied for the necessary period. They can be placed in the most inaccessible part of the load or within a bottle of liquid of similar volume to those being sterilised and are an excellent quality control measure.

Finally, the use of a standard spore suspension of *Bacillus stearothermophilus* can be used to monitor sterilisation. This organism is non-pathogenic but yields spores of the highest heat resistance. They are produced on strips of paper for convenience. If these spores (produced under controlled conditions to ensure heat resistance) are killed, it may be safely assumed that other spores are also killed. The one disadvantage of this method is that the result is not available immediately but requires time for culture of the spore strip to be pronounced sterile – perhaps 48 hours (Denyer 1987b).

Boiling

Boiling is not a means of sterilisation, but it can be very useful for disinfection: the removal of infectious material. Boiling water is commonly used in veterinary practice for decontaminating glassware, metal surgical tools, etc. Vegetative bacteria are killed rapidly, as are viruses and fungi. However, bacterial spores will survive.

If we ask the question, what might survive boiling that could be harmful, it reveals how valuable boiling can be. The spore formers are *Clostridium* and *Bacillus* species. Pathogenic clostridia such as *Clostridium tetani* or *C. perfringens* can be present wherever there is any possibility of soil or faecal contamination. However, if the material is known to be clean, with no likelihood of faecal material, or it will never be exposed to an anaerobic environment, we can discount *Clostridium*. In the case of *Bacillus* species, while they are ubiquitous in the environment and even the air we breathe, very few are able to cause disease. The one exception is *B. anthracis* but the possibility that this pathogen might be present in a surgery or even intestinal contents is so remote as to be irrelevant. Other *Bacillus* species are occasionally implicated in disease: *B. cereus* in mastitis and food poisoning, *B. licheniformis* in bovine abortion. Both of these are soil organisms in the environment and therefore rarely occur in a surgery. Otherwise, *Bacillus* species are of such low disease potential that we can discount them as pathogens except in severely immunocompromised individuals such as those undergoing cancer chemotherapy. In the absence of an autoclave, boiling can be a quick and effective means of disinfecting clean materials such as surgical instruments.

Tyndallisation

Tyndallisation is an old-fashioned method. It is the process of steaming at 100 °C on three consecutive days. It is used to sterilise substances which are heat labile and would be damaged or destroyed by autoclaving. On the first steaming, vegetative bacteria are killed, and spores are activated (woken up by the heat shock). Steaming on the second day kills vegetative bacteria formed from the germinated spores. The third steaming is considered precautionary, to kill any remaining germinated spores. The spores must be contained in a nutrient medium for germination to occur and therefore this method is of no use for solid objects.

Pasteurisation

This is similarly not a method of sterilisation but of disinfection by heating. It is used to remove the majority of vegetative organisms from milk. This helps to preserve milk which would otherwise deteriorate through microbial spoilage. More particularly, a temperature is used which is known to kill the important pathogens which are carried in milk: *Brucella abortus* and *Mycobacterium bovis*. This is either 72 °C for 15 seconds or 63 °C for 30 minutes. However, it also destroys other vegetative pathogenic bacteria, the list of which could be long but certainly includes *Salmonella*, *Campylobacter*, *Staphylococcus aureus*, *Coxiella*, *Listeria* and many others that may contaminate cows', goats' or ewes' milk. Some bacteria survive the pasteurisation process.

Higher temperatures can be used to enhance keeping qualities but do not really improve safety and can compromise the taste and quality of the milk beyond what is usually acceptable. Ultra-heat-treated (UHT) milk is heated to 140 °C for a few seconds which effectively sterilises the milk and allows it to be stored at room temperature for months. While eventual deterioration of the milk occurs, this is from the action of residual heat-stable enzymes such as lipases rather than microbial growth.

Dry Heat

Dry heat sterilisation is usually found in the laboratory rather than the clinic. Flaming the bacteriological loop is one example of dry heat sterilisation. The hot air oven is another. Because dry heat is less efficient at killing than wet heat, a higher temperature for a longer period is required. This is usually considered to be 160 °C for 45 minutes. Higher temperatures for a shorter time can be used. This is not suitable for liquids or plastics but is used to sterilise glassware and metal objects.

Radiation

Ultraviolet light kills viruses and bacteria and, at high enough dose, it is sporicidal. UV lamps are used in decontaminating rooms used for surgery and microbiological hoods. The destructive action of UV light is on the DNA of the cell. Thymine dimers are formed in the DNA which interfere with subsequent replication and transcription of the DNA. Repair of UV damage can take place naturally and overcome the effects of the radiation. UV light is not very penetrating and therefore only clean surfaces in direct exposure to the radiation will be sterilised (Kuo 2018).

Ionising radiation (γ-radiation) from a cobalt-60 source is used to sterilise heat-labile materials on an industrial scale. The ^{60}Co has a half-life of about 5.25 years. It is much more penetrating than UV because of its higher energy (frequency). The source requires a reinforced concrete building with 2 m-thick walls and is kept in a water-filled tank from which it is raised

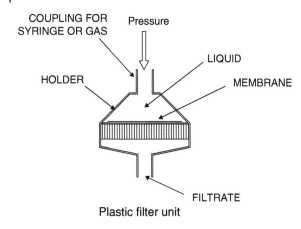

COUPLING FOR SYRINGE OR GAS
Pressure
LIQUID
HOLDER
MEMBRANE
FILTRATE

Plastic filter unit

Figure 3.2 A simple membrane filter unit for removing microorganisms from liquids.

when in use. Sources of γ-radiation are uncommon and are restricted to producers of sterile plastics and surgical apparatus such as plastic syringes, needles, dressings and catheters. Sterilisation takes place by passing the materials through the irradiation chamber on a conveyor. The radiation dose is regulated by the speed of the conveyor and materials may require several hours of exposure to ensure sterility (Denyer 1987a).

Filtration

This is used to remove bacteria and bacterial spores from solution. It is not a form of sterilisation because viruses and in some cases mycoplasmas (bacteria without cell walls) may pass through the filter. However, it is useful in being applicable to heat-labile solutions such as injectable drugs.

In the past, elaborate apparatus was used with asbestos pads, unglazed porcelain or sintered glass as the filtering medium. These have been superseded by membrane filters which are simple to handle, can be sterilised before use by autoclaving, are disposable and available in a variety of pore sizes and materials of different properties (Figure 3.2).

Modern membranes for filtration are made from cellulose acetate, polyvinylidene fluoride (PVDF) and nylon. They are used in some kind of holder and either positive or negative pressure is applied to speed the passage of fluid through the membrane. To prevent bacteria entering the filtrate, a pore size of 0.22 μm is normally considered acceptable.

While filtration is not a form of sterilisation because viruses will pass through, it can be effectively used as a means of sterilisation if the material being filtered is not likely to contain any virus of animal origin. For example, solutions of injectable drugs produced by chemical methods that never come in contact with animal cells would never contain animal viruses. The concern with such material is to remove viable bacteria and fungi, and filtration would adequately serve that purpose.

Chemicals

Chemicals which kill microorganisms are generally referred to as disinfectants or biocides. They vary widely in their action, potency for microorganisms and toxicity for the host. Those known to be non-toxic to tissues are used as antiseptics. However, some chemical agents are clearly potent enough to be considered as sterilising agents.

Sterilising Agents

Those reactive chemicals which are able to sterilise include hypochlorite (HOCl), 10% ethylene oxide ($CH_2.O.CH_2$) and 4% formaldehyde (HCHO). They will kill all groups of microorganisms including vegetative bacteria, endospores, viruses, mycobacteria and fungi. Their activity is subject to concentration, temperature, time and the presence of organic material, and for this reason their ability to sterilise is difficult to define. The concentration and conditions for sterilisation by chemicals are therefore determined for a given set of circumstances by experiment.

Hypochlorite

Hypochlorite is formed by dissolving chlorine gas in water.

$$Cl_2 + H_2O \rightarrow HCl + HOCl$$

Undissociated hypochlorous acid is a potent oxidising agent at 200 ppm, but its antimicrobial activity depends on pH. Under acid conditions (pH 5.0), the HOCl is favoured and it is effective as a microbial killing agent.

$$OCl^- + H^+ \rightarrow HOCl$$

Undissociated HOCl is 100-fold more potent as a bactericidal agent compared to OCl^-. However, the solution is relatively unstable under acid conditions and chlorine gas will be evolved. It is therefore stored under alkaline conditions until needed and then diluted to retrieve its potency.

$$NaOH + HOCl \rightarrow NaOCl + H_2O$$

Hypochlorite is widely used for disinfection of clean materials and surfaces and in the dairy industry to ensure milking equipment is free of viable microorganisms (Scott and Gorman 1987).

Ethylene Oxide

Ethylene oxide is explosive when mixed with air. It is also considered carcinogenic. Therefore, for sterilisation, it is usually mixed with CO_2 in a leak-proof, explosion-proof steriliser chamber and is used within a strict protocol to ensure the safety of operators. This obviously means it cannot be used for sterilisation in an open space such as a veterinary practice. All this might suggest it is impractical but there are some real advantages and practical value with ethylene oxide. In particular, the method sterilises heat-labile disposable plastic ware which could not be autoclaved before use; it is an alternative to γ-radiation.

Aldehydes

Formaldehyde gas (HCHO) is used to fumigate and sterilise rooms. More regularly, it is used as an aqueous solution. Formaldehyde dissolves in water to a concentration of about 37% w/v. This is formalin. A 10% solution of this, usually buffered and with physiological saline, is the fixative used to preserve tissue material for histopathology. Tissue fixed like this will be rapidly sterilised as the formaldehyde penetrates the tissues. Formaldehyde is also sometimes used for low-temperature (75 °C) steam and formaldehyde sterilisation using specially designed apparatus. Like ethylene oxide, formaldehyde is toxic and carcinogenic. Glutaraldehyde solution $[CH_2(CH_2CHO)_2]$, like formalin, may also be used as both a tissue fixative, particularly for electron microscopy, and a sterilising agent.

Disinfectants (for Decontamination)

Disinfection, by whatever means, is the removal of the majority of infectious material. Chemical disinfectants are those chemicals which can be safely used to decontaminate and kill infectious agents. Some are considered sufficiently harmless, with a good selective toxicity that they may be used on the skin, broken skin or mucous membranes (such as mouthwash). These would fall into the category of antiseptics but there is no clear cut-off between antiseptic and disinfectant: some are suitable for use on tissues and some are less suitable. There are a wide range of disinfectant products but most fall into about six basic chemical groups.

Alcohols

Ethanol (CH_3CH_2OH) and isopropanol ($CH_3.CHOH.CH_3$) are used to kill vegetative bacteria. At a concentration of 70%, ethanol will kill bacteria, mycobacteria, enveloped and non-enveloped viruses. Isopropanol is also used but is considered less effective against viruses. Neither is able to kill bacterial spores.

Phenolics

The phenolics are a wide range of related chemicals based on phenol. Phenol itself (C_6H_5OH) is hepatotoxic and has a rapid caustic effect on skin. It has the historic significance of being the first 'antiseptic' deliberately used in surgery by Lister in 1867. It was also the standard disinfectant to which the potency of others was compared in the phenol coefficient. Phenol itself is no longer used as a disinfectant or antiseptic.

Phenol derivatives, substituted with a variety of chemical groups, are often less toxic but also less potent in their microbicidal activity. Cresols (methyl phenol) are solubilised with soap and known as Lysol®. Others, based on xylenol (dimethyl phenol), include Hycolin® and Stericol®.

While these phenolics were considered highly effective against mycobacteria, the agent of tuberculosis, from 2001 they were not supported as part of the EU Biocidal Products Directive Review.

Some literature states that the phenolics are sporicidal; other information suggests that they are only slowly active against endospores at best. Certainly, they are effective against vegetative bacteria, mycobacteria, fungi and viruses but they cannot be considered with the sterilising agents without having undisputed sporicidal activity.

Coal tar derivatives emulsified in water (traditional black or white disinfectants) are prepared by solubilising the high boiling point tar acids. They are used as disinfectants on farms in highly contaminated areas and as foot dips, etc.

Chloroxylenol, marketed as Dettol®, is para-chloro-meta-xylenol. This is mild enough in toxicity to be used on skin, mucous membranes and open wounds in animals except cats and pigs, for whom it is toxic. It has relatively weak antibacterial activity, being most effective against Gram-positive bacteria but this activity is reduced further in the presence of organic matter. It is solubilised in a soap solution and mainly used because of its lack of toxicity for humans (Scott and Gorman 1987).

Bisphenols are chemicals composed of two phenol groups which may be linked in different ways. Hydroxy halogenated derivatives such as hexachlorophene and triclosan are the most active of these and have been widely used. Their action again is primarily against Gram-positive bacteria; they have the limitation of being bacteriostatic and with little or no activity against *Pseudomonas*. Hexachlorophene is also known to be neurotoxic. It was used at one time in baby bath preparations but was withdrawn following deaths associated with brain damage. However, after the removal of the products in 1971 there was a documented four-month outbreak of staphylococcal disease in hospital nurseries in the US.

Biguanides

The most well-known biguanide disinfectant is chlorhexidine, used under the trade names Hibitane® and Hibiscrub®. They are generally considered to have low toxicity but can be ototoxic. Chlorhexidine is most effective against Gram-positive bacteria, less so against Gram-negatives, and biguanides have no action against endospores. Their value against non-enveloped viruses is variable and they are only active against mycobacteria when in alcoholic solution: the ethanol is assumed to aid penetration.

At physiological pH, chlorhexidine is a dissociated cation. This interacts with the negatively charged bacterial surface leading to membrane perturbation and cell death through loss of membrane integrity and thence the proton gradient conferring the proton-motive force.

Quaternary Ammonium Compounds

These are cationic detergents, such as cetrimide (hexadecyltrimethylammonium bromide), having a polar group at one end and a lipophilic component at the other. Like biguanides, when dissociated, the ammonium group acquires a positive charge and interacts with the negatively charged bacterial surface, causing disruption of the cytoplasmic membrane. Vegetative Gram-positive bacteria are sensitive while Gram-negatives are less so. When cetrimide is combined with chlorhexidine, the two act synergistically and this combination is marketed as Savlon®.

Pseudomonas aeruginosa is intrinsically resistant to cationic detergents, perhaps because of the outer membrane structure, such that 0.03% w/v cetrimide is used as a selective agent in culture medium for *P. aeruginosa*. Enveloped viruses are sensitive while non-enveloped viruses, mycobacteria, many fungi and all endospores are unaffected by cationic detergents.

Another example of a cationic detergent is benzalkonium chloride, used widely in household products, medicines and supermarket disinfectants.

Oxidising Agents

Disinfectants in this group include hydrogen peroxide (H_2O_2), peracetic acid (CH_3CO_3H) and Virkon® S (potassium peroxymonosulfate). Diluted H_2O_2 (<3% w/v) can be used for cleaning surfaces and has been used as an oral and skin antiseptic.

It is effective in inactivation of virus and killing vegetative bacteria, some fungi, mycobacteria and some endospores. It is environmentally acceptable since it decomposes to water and oxygen. Peracetic acid is a broadly active microbicidal agent. It is used in agriculture, maintaining hygiene in the food industry (such as cheese making and brewing) and as a water purifier and disinfectant. It is, however, a potent oxidising agent and a severe irritant to eyes, skin and the respiratory tract.

Virkon is now a widely used product. It is again broadly effective against a wide range of bacteria, viruses and fungi. It is used in places where control of pathogens is needed such as veterinary surgeries, hospitals, laboratories and animal care facilities.

Halogens

Chlorine is discussed above. It is also used at very low concentration in the treatment of drinking water to ensure it cannot carry pathogens and as a widely used, cheap, household disinfectant.

Iodine is used more widely as a skin disinfectant for preparation before surgery and in application to wounds. This is particularly when mixed with the water-soluble polymer povidone for a slow release known as an iodophor: povidone-iodine.

References

Denyer, S.P. (1987a). Principles and practice of sterilisation. In: *Pharmaceutical Microbiology*, 4e (ed. W.B. Hugo and A.D. Russell). Oxford: Blackwell Scientific Publications.

Denyer, S.P. (1987b). Sterilisation control and sterility testing. In: *Pharmaceutical Microbiology*, 4e (ed. W.B. Hugo and A.D. Russell). Oxford: Blackwell Scientific Publications.

Kuo, J. (2018). Disinfection processes. *Water Environment Research* 90: 947–977.

Scott, E.M. and Gorman, S.P. (1987). Chemical disinfectants, antiseptics and preservatives. In: *Pharmaceutical Microbiology*, 4e (ed. W.B. Hugo and A.D. Russell). Oxford: Blackwell Scientific Publications.

4

Bacterial Genes and Gene Transfer

The Bacterial Genome

The bacterial chromosome is usually a single closed circle of double-stranded DNA. Occasionally, microorganisms have been shown to have their chromosome in two separate closed circles or in linear form. The chromosome is haploid (only one copy of each gene) and is about 4×10^6 base pairs (4000 kb) long in *E. coli*. It carries all the genes required for the life of the cell (Krawiec and Riley 1990).

Plasmids are found in many (but not all) bacteria. They are additional circular pieces of DNA. Some are small (as little as 1 kb) while others are large (up to 300 kb) and are carried in a range of copy numbers from 1 to 50 copies per chromosome. They carry non-essential functions such as pathogenicity factors, extra catabolic pathways, bacteriocins, antibiotic resistance genes and self-transmissibility. Several different plasmids may be carried by a bacterial strain (Salyers and Whitt 1994).

Mutation and Phenotypic Adaptation

Mutation is a change in the nucleotide sequence of the DNA of an individual which is permanently inherited by the progeny of that individual. In bacteria, a mutation is often dominant because the organism is haploid. Mutations can be a change in a single nucleotide or much larger changes such as a deletion, insertion or inversion of a piece of DNA. Some mutations are silent while others can cause important changes or loss of function and in some cases can be lethal. Mutants in a population of bacteria are usually lost because they are unable to compete with the wild-type organism. While usually detrimental to the individual, occasionally a mutational change will be of some positive help to the organism. For the approximately 1 in 10 000 million (1 in 10^{10}) *E. coli* with the correct single nucleotide change in the *rpsL* gene, there will be an advantage if the bacteria are then exposed to the antimicrobial drug streptomycin because this individual will be relatively resistant to streptomycin. The single nucleotide change in the small subunit of the ribosome protein L prevents the effect streptomycin would normally have on protein synthesis. Mutation of bacteria to drug resistance is significant in veterinary and human medicine but is less important in reality than resistance due to additional antibiotic resistance genes entering the cell.

Phenotypic adaptation, in contrast, is a metabolic adjustment of the entire population in response to a change in the environment. This effect is reversible when the environmental change is reversed. There are now known to be many two-component detection systems in bacteria that operate to sense the environment and cause modification of the expression of genes and the metabolism they control (Lewin 1994).

Other Important Aspects of Mutation

Mutations are also important in live vaccines. This is particularly so in viral vaccines, but attenuated strains of *Salmonella enterica*, *Bacillus anthracis* and *Bordetella bronchiseptica* are used as veterinary vaccines. They carry mutations which decrease their virulence but do not directly affect the antigenicity of the bacteria. Mutations are also important in the

Fundamentals of Veterinary Microbiology, First Edition. Andrew N. Rycroft.
© 2024 John Wiley & Sons Ltd. Published 2024 by John Wiley & Sons Ltd.
Companion website: www.wiley.com/go/veterinarymicrobiology

evolution of all organisms. In the long term, gene alteration and rearrangement is responsible for the antigenic diversity of bacteria and the observed subtle changes in the specificity of important bacterial antigens such as the subtypes of K88 fimbrial antigen of porcine *E. coli* strains.

Gene Transfer in Bacteria

Apart from mutation and selection, other processes which promote variation in bacterial populations are known to operate. Genetic material may be transferred from one individual to another and may be stably inherited. There are three processes by which bacteria can naturally acquire exogenous genetic material: conjugation, transduction and transformation (Lewin 1994).

Conjugation

Conjugation is the plasmid-mediated process whereby a copy of a plasmid is transferred from a donor bacterium into a recipient which does not possess that plasmid. It is perhaps the closest analogy to sexual reproduction that is seen in bacteria. It is particularly important in the enterobacteria (*Escherichia coli/Salmonella/Proteus* group), *Pseudomonas* and *Staphylococcus* (Figure 4.1).

Transduction

Generalised transduction is the accidental mispackaging of bacterial chromosome or plasmid DNA into the progeny of a bacteriophage particle which has infected the bacterium. Normally, bacteriophages (bacterial viruses) only package exact copies of their own genome. Occasionally, residual bacterial DNA will take its place by mistake and the particle is then non-infective. However, the particle can still inject that DNA into a further, recipient bacterium which may inherit the bacterial DNA without harm (Figure 4.2).

Transformation

Transformation is the uptake, by some bacteria, of exogenous naked DNA. Some bacteria, such as the human pathogen *Haemophilus influenzae*, some other members of the *Pasteurellaceae* family and *Bacillus* spp., are naturally transformable (Redfield et al. 2006). Many others, such as *E. coli*, are not 'competent to transformation' unless treated with chemicals, such as cold $CaCl_2$ solution, followed by a heat shock. Transformation may be important for acquiring new DNA in the natural world, but it is also the means by which DNA is introduced into organisms following its manipulation *in vitro* (for genetic engineering) (Figure 4.3).

Natural transformation is thought to involve a multicomponent DNA uptake system and appears to be the same in both Gram-positive and Gram-negative bacteria. Being in the condition to allow transformation, bacteria are said to be 'competent to transformation'. This requires the production of a type IV pilus for exposure on the cell surface. A protein known as ComEA then binds DS DNA in the periplasm. This converts the DNA into SS DNA for carriage across the cytoplasmic membrane, probably via a channel formed by another protein, ComEC. The DNA must then be protected from nucleases before integration into the genome. Some species require short, specific nucleotide sequences known as uptake sequences within the DNA to enable its uptake. An example is *Actinobacillus pleuropneumoniae*, a veterinary pathogenic organism considered very difficult to transform until uptake sequences were discovered and utilised for efficient natural transformation.

Electroporation is a newer method of transformation that uses a high-voltage pulse of electrical energy to persuade bacteria (or other cell types) to take up DNA. It is thought that this opens pores in the cell membrane which allow bacteria to take up exogenous DNA.

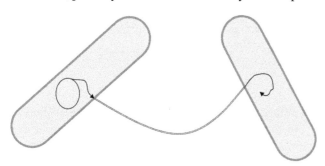

Figure 4.1 Bacterial gene transfer by conjugation through the sex pilus.

Figure 4.2 Generalised transduction.

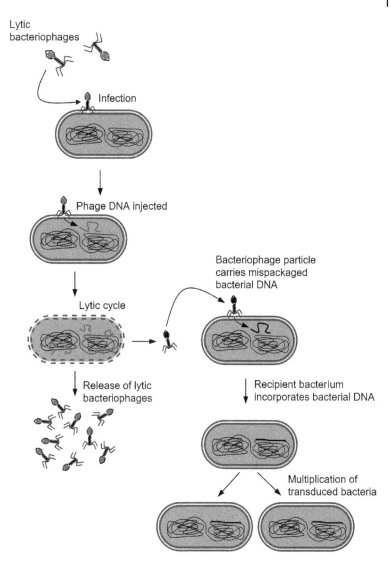

Figure 4.3 Bacterial transformation.

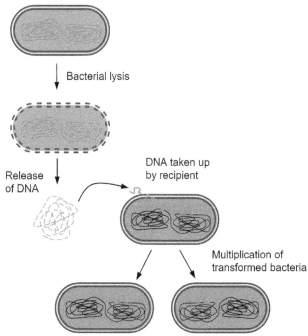

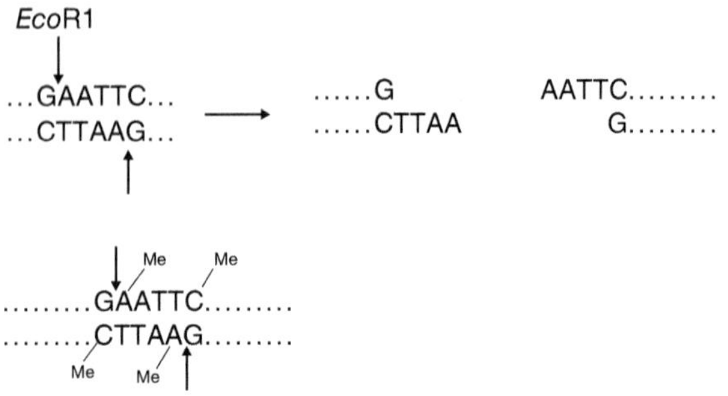

EcoR1
↓

...GAATTC...   ......G   AATTC.........
...CTTAAG...   ⟶   ......CTTAA   G.........
          ↑

          ↓ Me   Me
.........GAATTC.........
.........CTTAAG.........
      Me   Me ↑

Figure 4.4   Restriction endonuclease *Eco*R1 recognition sequence and cutting site. The endonuclease cuts the DNA. When adenine or cytosine is methylated, the DNA is not cut.

Restriction and Modification

Transfer of DNA to a bacterial cell by any mechanism may be prevented by endonuclease enzymes within the recipient bacterium. Unless the DNA is methylated at certain base sequences, it may be recognised as foreign and digested by restriction endonuclease (Bickle and Kruger 1993) (Figure 4.4).

Restriction can be an important barrier to genetic exchange between bacterial cells. This is an effective means by which bacteria prevent infection by bacteriophages (bacterial viruses). It is effectively an immune system for bacteria. The term 'restriction' arises from the restricted efficiency of infection by a bacteriophage that would normally cause lysis and death of the bacterial cell. When a restriction system is operating in a bacterial strain, the bacteriophage is restricted (prevented from causing that lytic infection) because the incoming DNA is degraded and lost. Occasionally, perhaps one in a thousand infection events will be successful. The bacteriophage will have introduced its DNA and this will become methylated by the methylase enzyme associated with the restriction endonuclease. Why should this happen? If there was no methylase, to cause methylation of specific sites in the host bacterial DNA, that too would be degraded by the restriction enzyme (Figure 4.5).

So, methylation at specific sequences is a means of protecting the host DNA. Sometimes, the methylase wins the race with the endonuclease and incoming bacteriophage DNA would then be protected. In such an event, the progeny bacteriophages are released from the host bacterium with modified (methylated) DNA. The bacteriophage DNA is effectively protected against that specific restriction system and the bacteriophage can then cause unrestricted infection of identical members of the same population.

Transposable Elements and Insertion Sequences

These are genetic elements able to transfer a copy of themselves from one genetic element to another. This is by so-called illegitimate (non-homologous) recombination. They appear to 'jump' from plasmid to plasmid, or plasmid to chromosome (Figure 4.6).

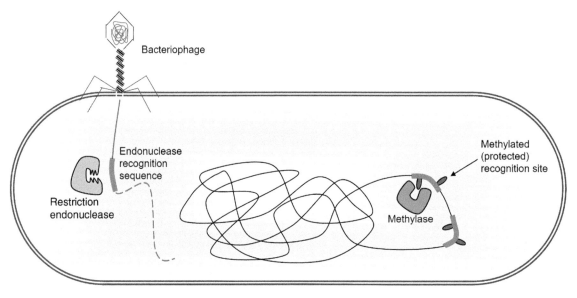

Figure 4.5   Restriction and methylation. The restriction endonuclease recognises the specific sequence on incoming DNA and cuts it. Methylases methylate the same sequence on the bacterial genome to prevent self-destruction (cutting) of its own DNA.

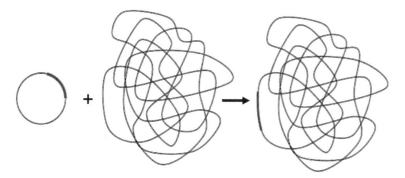

Figure 4.6 Transposition. An insertion sequence transfers from a plasmid to a chromosome.

Transposons (Tn) and insertion sequences (Is) are found in eukaryotes as well as prokaryotes. They enable the permanent addition of genes to plasmids and so help to build multiantibiotic-resistant plasmids. They also enhance the rearrangement, reassortment and evolution of genes in the biological world. Furthermore, they clearly promote the spread of genes such as antimicrobial resistance genes among bacteria although they require other genetic elements (a replicon such as a plasmid or chromosome) to carry them into another organism because the transposon cannot exist and replicate alone.

A transposon or insertion element consists of two inverted repeat sequences of DNA, between which is carried structural genes, usually including a gene for the transposase and sometimes specific marker genes such as one conferring antimicrobial resistance.

An inverted repeat sequence is a nucleotide sequence which is repeated elsewhere by its reverse complement, for example the 10 base pair inverted repeat shown in Figure 4.7.

5′-A-G-C-T-T-A-G-G-C-A..........................T-G-C-C-T-A-A-G-C-T-3′

3′-T-C-G-A-A-T-C-C-G-T..........................A-C-G-G-A-T-T-C-G-A-5′

Figure 4.7 Inverted repeat sequence in DNA.

References

Bickle, T.A. and Kruger, A.D. (1993). Biology of DNA restriction. *Microbiological Reviews* 57: 434–450.

Krawiec, S. and Riley, M. (1990). Organization of the bacterial chromosome. *Microbiological Reviews* 54: 502–539.

Lewin, B. (1994). *Genes V*. Oxford: Oxford University Press.

Redfield, R.J., Findlay, W.A., Bossé, J. et al. (2006). Evolution of competence and DNA uptake specificity in the *Pasteurellaceae*. *BMC Evolutionary Biology* 6: 82.

Salyers, A.A. and Whitt, D.D. (1994). *Bacterial Pathogenesis: A Molecular Approach*. Washington DC: American Society for Microbiology.

5

Bacterial Pathogenicity

Most bacteria are not pathogens. Most are free-living saprophytes or innocuous parasites. So, the vast majority of bacteria in and on the body are harmless to an animal and are known as the commensal flora, more recently termed the microbiota in a particular habitat or microbiome (Berg et al. 2020).

Pathogens are bacteria which are able to cause disease in animals, plants or human beings. They are the exceptions, even perhaps aberrations, among the microbial kingdom that have occurred by accident, such as through acquisition of new genetic material or even by deletion of DNA. Alternatively, they may have been transferred from one animal species to another and started a disease situation that was not present in the original host.

What advantage is there to being a pathogen? Probably, in most cases, very little compared to being a harmless commensal and living 'quietly'. Being a pathogen is just another way of living: surviving, reproducing and transmitting in a suitable environment.

Some bacteria have become very successful as pathogens. Take, for example, the pathogenic mycobacteria that have very successfully exploited animals and caused a great amount of disease globally. However, it could be argued that this is not a good example. Most *Mycobacterium* species live successfully in the environment and those few that are pathogenic – *M. bovis*, *M. tuberculosis*, *M. avium-paratuberculosis*, etc. – only cause overt disease after a long process of quiescence in the body: latent infection without pathological changes. Instead, take the example of *Streptococcus equi*, the cause of strangles in the horse. This transmits from horse to horse and assists its own transmission by setting up a disease state that results in the generation of a large quantity of highly infective secretion from the upper respiratory tract. This seems to allow *S. equi* to be successful in surviving, reproducing and transmitting. It has an advantage over the ancestors of *S. equi*; it does not usually kill the equine host but uses it as an effective tool for living.

Others might be considered purely accidental pathogens. These gain nothing from being a pathogen and it is a casualty of fate that tetanospasmin is produced in an anaerobic wound and that neurotoxin is effective at interfering with the release of neurotransmitters in the inhibitory synapses of a wide range of mammals. *Clostridium tetani* lives in the hindgut of animals and the enzyme that we know as a neurotoxin serves a useful function in garnering nutrients for the bacteria in its natural environment. No useful assistance is gained for the life and survival of the bacterium by it causing such a hideous paralysis in unfortunate animals.

Every pathogen appears to have its own unique specialisation and balance between harmless colonisation of a given host animal and ability to cause disease. In most cases, this confers an advantage to survival, reproduction and transmission.

Intracellular and Extracellular Pathogens

Those bacteria that cause disease may be extracellular pathogens such as streptococci and *Escherichia coli*, they may be obligate intracellular pathogens such as *Chlamydia* and *Coxiella*, or they may fall into the third group, the facultative intracellular pathogens. This latter group includes bacteria which do not normally reside intracellularly, but which may survive there as part of the infective or survival process, e.g. *Salmonella*, *Listeria*, *Mycobacterium*, *Brucella* and several others. The number of bacteria recognised as having this capability has steadily increased recently and a surprising proportion that were thought only to have an extracellular existence have since been shown to be capable of transient intracellular behaviour.

Pathogenicity

Pathogenicity is the ability of an infectious agent to cause disease. It is a property conferred by characteristics and attributes of the bacteria. Virulence, a term often used interchangeably with pathogenicity, is the measure or degree of that pathogenic ability.

Invasion is the process of microorganisms entering the tissues or host cells and spreading in the body.

An opportunistic pathogen is an agent capable of causing disease only when the host's resistance to infection is impaired or the natural bacteria changed or removed. While it is easier to think of bacteria as pathogens or commensals, in reality there is a very blurred overlap of the two. Pathogens can live as saprophytes in the environment or as commensals on the body. Bacteria that we consider commensals can sometimes turn pathogenic when circumstances allow. While very many bacteria are never recorded (with meaningful evidence) as causing disease in animals, occasional case reports of species that were thought of as harmless do appear. This has been highlighted by the immunosuppressive conditions that have become commonplace in human and animal medicine (Salyers and Whitt 1994).

To be pathogenic, an organism must usually be able to fulfil all the five steps below.

1) Gain access to the host.
2) Survive and multiply.
3) Acquire nutrients.
4) Resist or avoid the host defences.
5) Damage host tissues.

Access to the Host

Bacteria may enter the host from an external source (exogenous) or be already present on or in the body (endogenous). Organisms enter the host animal using different routes: injured skin or mucous membrane, the urinary tract, reproductive tract, gastrointestinal tract, respiratory route, etc.

Avoiding Removal

In order colonise the host, pathogens often need to avoid or resist the flushing actions of fluids and mucus. For example, in the gut and on the urinary and respiratory tract mucosa, there are flushing, peristaltic and cilial mechanisms to remove particles including bacteria. The beating cilia of the trachea, viewed by microscope, is an amazing sight in which the tiny hair-like cilia beat perhaps five times a second, in synchrony, to propel mucus and trapped particles out of the respiratory tract. Non-harmful bacteria will be removed. That is why they are not harmful at that site. But adherence factors on pathogens cause specific attachment to receptors on the surface of host cells. Many of these adherence factors are fimbriae (sometimes called pili) but other bacterial components such as outer membrane proteins may also assist with sticking to mucosal surfaces (Finlay and Falkow 1989).

The first fimbriae to be discovered were termed type 1 fimbriae. It had been known that bacteria such as *Shigella flexneri* carried small, numerous filamentous appendages that could only be seen using electron microscopy. It was speculated that these might be organs of attachment. It was also noticed that bacteria such as *E. coli*, grown in culture, would cause the clumping (haemagglutination) of erythrocytes from the blood of a number of animals. This phenomenon was easy to recognise and study and it was found that this agglutination could sometimes be prevented by addition of the sugar mannose (mannose-sensitive agglutination), but the meaning of this was unclear. In 1955, it was shown by John Duguid that *E. coli* strains that carried fimbriae also agglutinated erythrocytes while those without fimbriae usually could not cause the clumping. In fact, these fimbriae are present on most enterobacteria. These are said to be mannose sensitive in their action if their binding to erythrocytes is inhibited by mannose and therefore recognises mannose as their receptor on the cell. These are not usually implicated in pathogenicity. However, those fimbriae whose haemagglutination or adherence to cells is not inhibited by mannose (mannose-resistant [MR] fimbriae) *are* considered to be pathogenicity characters. They include such fimbriae as K88 (now known as F4), K99 (F5), F41, 987P and others of enterotoxigenic *E. coli* which attach the bacteria to the small intestinal mucosa of animal species, e.g. pig. Other fimbriae, such as S-type and P-type, are found on strains able to colonise the urinary tract (Figure 5.1).

Fimbriae can be rather specific in the receptor they recognise. Those fimbriae such as K88 that are essential for attachment of *E. coli* strains to the small intestinal mucosa of calves and piglets do not attach to the cells of the human or canine small intestine. Hence, the strains of *E. coli* causing watery diarrhoea in farm animals do not cause the same effect in people or dogs. Enterotoxigenic strains able to cause traveller's diarrhoea in humans elaborate fimbriae with specificity for human cells: colonisation factor antigen (CFA)-1 and -2, for example.

Acquiring Nutrients

Securing limiting nutrients, particularly iron, in the face of powerful physiological Fe chelators (transferrin, haemoglobin, lactoferrin) is a property of some pathogens. Most nutrients, such as amino acids and sugars, are readily available in tissue fluids or mucosal surfaces. Some complex biological molecules can either be synthesised in the bacteria or are obtained from the body of the animal. However, almost all bacteria need iron for key metabolic processes. Yet it is so tightly held in the body of mammals that this is an effective bacteriostatic mechanism. The concentration of free iron in the mammalian body is around 10^{-18} M. This

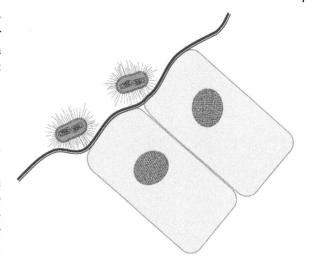

Figure 5.1 Specific adhesion of bacteria to a mucosal surface by fimbriae.

is one billionth of a nanomole per litre of body fluid and far too low to sustain the growth of bacteria. Pathogens use one of two means to secure iron. The first to be recognised was the production, by bacteria, of siderophores (Crosa 1989) (Figure 5.2).

These small molecules, such as enterobactin and aerobactin, are produced in the environment of the bacteria. They have a very high affinity for the free iron and so any free iron ions are chelated to the siderophore molecules. These are then taken in by the bacterial cell to satisfy the need for iron. Bacteria, such as members of the enterobacteria, bind the complexed siderophores to outer membrane proteins which are synthesised under iron-limiting conditions.

Secondly, some pathogens were found to acquire iron from the bound state in the body using transferrin-binding proteins. In an energy-dependent process, a protein complex on the surface of the bacteria (transferrin-binding protein A and B) binds transferrin and causes the iron to be 'snatched' and transferred from the transferrin across the outer membrane (Figure 5.3).

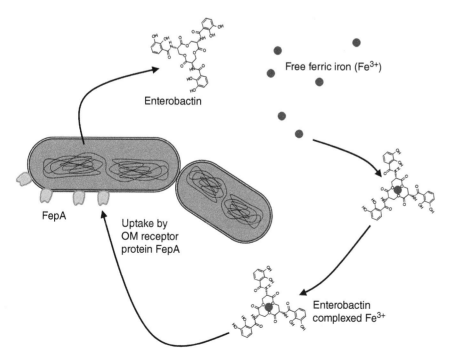

Enterobactin

Free ferric iron (Fe^{3+})

FepA

Uptake by OM receptor protein FepA

Enterobactin complexed Fe^{3+}

Figure 5.2 Chelation of iron by siderophores.

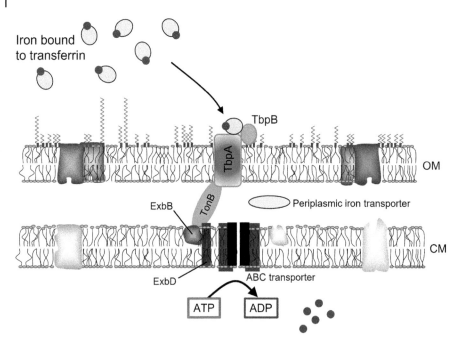

Figure 5.3 Transferrin binding activity found in many pathogens. The pathogen carries surface proteins able to bind transferrin and actively remove the iron in an energy-dependent process.

This is a very abundant source of iron available only to those that carry this mechanism, common among members of the *Pasteurellaceae* family of Gram-negatives. Similar mechanisms operate in Gram-positive pathogens and there are perhaps further undiscovered mechanisms allowing bacteria to obtain their essential iron.

Evading the Host Defences

The primary defence of the body of animals is uptake and killing by phagocytic cells. Phagocytic ingestion is evaded by extracellular pathogens while intracellular pathogens either hide inside relatively harmless cells or resist the killing mechanisms of professional phagocytic cells.

Harmless bacteria, or at least those lacking a specific antiphagocytic mechanism, are destroyed by macrophages and neutrophils (or the equivalent cells such as heterophils in avian species). The term 'surface phagocytosis' was coined by Barry Wood to describe the process of phagocytic cells trapping bacteria against a surface such as a fibrin clot and engulfing them (Figure 5.4).

When bacteria produce a polysaccharide capsule, surface phagocytosis is still able to operate, at least with some bacteria. However, the hydrophilicity conferred by this hydrated polysaccharide gel is thought to prevent the phagocytic cells from recognising the bacteria as foreign. Capsule is probably masking those molecules on the bacterial surface that would be recognised as inherently foreign by Toll-like receptors (Finlay and Falkow 1989).

To overcome this and allow engulfment to proceed, the body utilises complement. This is a complex series of proteins present naturally in blood plasma that can recognise bacteria as foreign and marks them for destruction. It is a catalytic system that amplifies through the sequential enzymic cleavage of the next components in the system. Fortunately, the complement proteins recognise most capsular polysaccharides as foreign. Complement is constantly being activated, or ticking over, but not allowed to run away. Initial

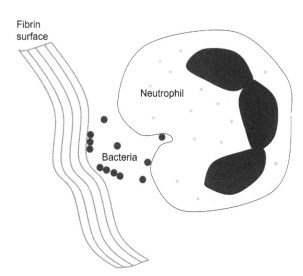

Figure 5.4 Surface phagocytosis.

recognition of the capsule as foreign allows the early components of complement to form a stable C3 convertase on the bacterial surface. This is known as activation of complement by the alternative pathway in which C3 is cleaved to C3b and C3a. This leads to the deposition of component C3b on the bacterial surface. C3b is a very potent opsonin. It signals to the neutrophils to ingest the particle and attempt to destroy it in a process known as opsonophagocytosis, which is part of the innate immune system (Figure 5.5).

Some surfaces are not recognised by complement. Capsules are chemically (and antigenically) highly variable. Some bacteria have evolved to produce capsules that fail to stabilise the C3 convertase. In this case, opsonophagocytosis instigated by the alternative pathway does not function, or does not function well, and neutrophils do not engage

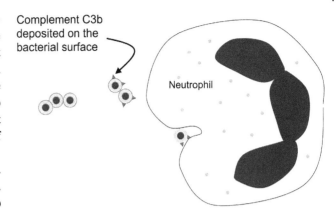

Figure 5.5   Complement-enhanced opsonophagocytosis.

with the infecting microorganisms. Here, the adaptive immune response is needed. Antigen, such as capsular polysaccharide, is sometimes referred to as a B-cell antigen. It is not processed but recognised directly by surface immunoglobulin on B-lymphocytes. Interaction with a large area of an intact antigenic component such as a capsule (polymers of simple repeating structural units) will cross-link B-cell receptors and trigger B-cell activation in a thymus-independent mechanism. In as little as five days, an animal will produce detectable quantities of antibody, particularly IgM. Thymus-dependent mechanisms also operate but these require antigen processing and presentation, interactions between B-lymphocytes and T-helper lymphocytes, together with co-stimulatory cytokines. These interactions inevitably take longer than direct B-cell activation.

As antibody appears in the animal, this will bind to that capsule polysaccharide to which the innate immune system was effectively blind. Now, complement can be activated, this time by the classical (antibody-dependent) pathway, and C3b is deposited on the bacterial surface. IgM is particularly effective at activation of complement via the classical pathway. Once this happens, the microorganisms will be recognised by the neutrophils and the infection attacked with the full weight of the phagocytic system (Figure 5.6).

Polysaccharide capsules are the most important structures in bacteria resisting phagocytosis. The O-antigen component of lipopolysaccharide (LPS) is considered to play a similar role. In addition, there are a wide range of other surface and secreted components that carry out a similar function or contribute to phagocytic resistance. Such components include M protein of streptococci and protein A of staphylococci. Soluble factors such as anti-chemotaxins of *Bordetella* spp. prevent phagocytic cells being directed to the site of infection at an early stage and some bacterial toxins destroy the phagocytic cells.

Bacteria also resist the humoral defences of the body. These include the antibacterial effects of β-lysin and the direct bactericidal activity of complement against Gram-negative bacteria. Further activities include enzymes such as proteases and lysozyme. Resistance to these is conferred by capsules and the outer membrane barrier.

Bacteria may also hide from the host defences by assuming an intracellular habitat. While some organisms such as *Listeria* will stimulate epithelial cells to take them in, others are phagocytosed by professional phagocytic cells.

Figure 5.6   Antibody-directed complement-mediated opsonophagocytosis.

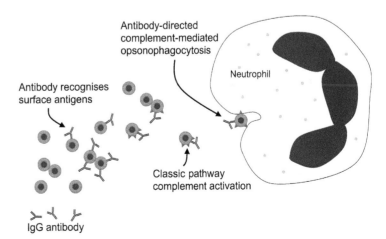

Different mechanisms are used by bacteria to enter and survive the hostile intracellular environment. Some bacteria, such as *Mycobacterium bovis* and *Salmonella enterica* serovar Typhimurium, are known to inhibit the maturation of the phagosome (containing the ingested bacteria) and prevent fusion of the phagosome with the lysosome (carrying the bactericidal chemicals). Others, such as *Listeria monocytogenes*, lyse the phagosomal membrane and escape into the cytoplasm. Still others, such as *Mycobacterium lepraemurium*, are able to resist inactivation by the potent lysosomal factors (Schaible and Kaufmann 2004). The strategy of many other bacteria, such as staphylococci, for intracellular survival is not yet fully known.

Damaging the Host

Bacteria which have not been removed by the immune defences of a host will damage that host, either through the production of extracellular or cell-associated toxins or through provoking the immune system to cause damaging effects (Finlay and Falkow 1989).

Exotoxins

Exotoxins were originally considered to be produced only by Gram-positive organisms such as clostridia, staphylococci and streptococci. They are protein and heat-labile, e.g. collagenase, haemolysins, leucocidins, proteases, diphtheria toxin, tetanospasmin and anthrax toxin. Since 1980, it has become apparent that many Gram-negatives also produce extracellular toxins and the number recognised is increasing all the time. These include cholera toxin, *E. coli* enterotoxins, haemolysins, *Pseudomonas* exotoxin A, RTX cytolysins, *Pasteurella* osteolytic toxin, *Mannheimia* leukotoxin and *Bordetella* dermonecrotic toxin (Gopalakrishnakone et al. 2018).

There are six categories of bacterial exotoxins. These are usually released during bacterial growth.

- Cytolytic toxins
- Enzymes
- Enterotoxins/ADP-ribosylation toxins
- Neurotoxins
- Superantigens
- Type III secretion systems

Cytolytic Toxins

The cytolytic toxins are sometimes, but not always, haemolysins. Haemolysins are often recognised and discussed as a property of bacteria because they are easily seen around colonies on blood agar; they are easy to study. Haemolysin production is used to describe and identify bacterial colonies. Haemolysins are also sometimes associated with pathogenic species. However, they are also produced by entirely non-pathogenic bacteria such as *Bacillus* species readily isolated from the normal air. Conversely, other bacteria produce cytolysins that contribute to pathogenicity, yet these have no haemolytic effect.

An example of a haemolytic and cytolytic toxin is streptolysin S. This toxin is, like many, most extensively studied in the exclusively human pathogen *Streptococcus pyogenes* (or Lancefield Group A streptococcus), but very closely related cytolysins are found in β-haemolytic strains of *S. equi*, *S. equisimilis* and Group G streptococci and indeed a number of other bacterial pathogens (Figure 5.7).

Streptolysin S is a small, yet potent cytolytic toxin. It is a 2.7 kDa peptide that can only be cytotoxic when associated

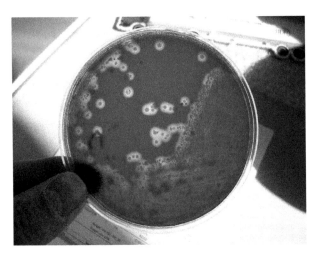

Figure 5.7 The effect of streptolysin S around colonies of *Streptococcus equi*.

with the bacterial cell surface or when specific carrier molecules are present. It has a broad spectrum of cytolytic activity against mammalian cells, including erythrocytes, platelets and leucocytes. The mechanism of cell damage is not yet understood but is thought to form pores through the cell membrane and disruption of the cell contents.

In contrast, the cytolytic toxin ApxIII produced by many strains of the pig pathogen *Actinobacillus pleuropneumoniae* is not haemolytic. It is a large protein which, by aggregation into a ring form, makes a very large pore in the cell membrane of macrophages and neutrophils. The consequence of rapid cytolysis of neutrophils is not only the removal of the most effective defence against these and similar pathogens, but the release of all the neutrophil cell contents including those lysosomal chemicals intended for the destruction of ingested bacteria. Closely related pore-forming cytolysins are produced by *Mannheimia haemolytica* (calf pneumonia), *Bordetella bronchiseptica* and the α-haemolysin of *E. coli*. The α-toxin of *Staphylococcus aureus* is an unrelated pore-forming cytolysin.

The Enzymes

Many of the secreted enzymes of pathogens, particularly Gram-positive bacteria, have been recognised as having toxic effects on tissues. Some of the earliest recognised toxins were enzymes and haemolysins. As was considered scholarly at the time, many of these were given Greek letters of the alphabet: α, β, μ, λ and so on. As further species of bacteria were studied, the burgeoning number of toxins they produced were, in turn, also given letters of the Greek alphabet. Yet the α-toxin of one organism usually bore no relationship to the protein or enzyme activity of the α-toxin of another species, even from the same bacterial genus. Unsurprisingly, this has caused confusion for those of us not intimately familiar with the different toxins yet trying to make sense of them.

Common enzyme activities secreted by bacteria include phospholipase C of *Clostridium perfringens* (α-toxin), hyaluronidase, collagenase, protease, lipase and others. These digest tissues in the living host as a means of releasing nutrients for the growing bacteria. Some will be considered in more detail with the specific pathogens where they contribute to disease and where they have been very effectively utilised as the basis for toxoid vaccines used widely to prevent bacterial disease in farm animals.

ADP-Ribosylation Toxins

These toxins are ADP-ribosyl transferases. These are enzymes that catalyse the addition of one or more ADP-ribose moieties to a protein. They can be highly specific in their action because ADP-ribosylation of proteins is a means of cell signalling and gene regulation in mammalian tissues (Figure 5.8).

Examples include toxins such as the heat-labile enterotoxin (LT) of *E. coli*. This comprises five B subunits carrying one A subunit in a complex 88 kDa protein. Once delivered to the cell surface, part of the A subunit enters the cell. This carries the ribosyl transferase activity that causes an ADP-ribose to be transferred to the guanine nucleotide-binding protein (G-protein) on the inside of the cell membrane. This causes the G-protein to be switched off so that it no longer controls the production of cAMP. As a result, the intracellular concentration of cAMP increases. This activates the chloride channel in the cell membrane to actively transport chloride and sodium out of the cell into the lumen of the gut. Water follows the Na$^+$ and Cl$^-$ and this is seen as a watery diarrhoea (secretory diarrhoea) leading to dehydration, electrolyte loss and metabolic acidosis.

ADP-ribosylation toxins are also recognised in some important human pathogens including pertussis toxin of *Bordetella pertussis*, diphtheria toxin of *Corynebacterium diphtheriae* and cholera toxin of *Vibrio cholerae*.

The Neurotoxins

If we did not now know better, the bacterial neurotoxins and the diseases they generate could be considered as a purposeful malevolence on the part of some bacteria. The truth, of course, is that these toxins (like many others)

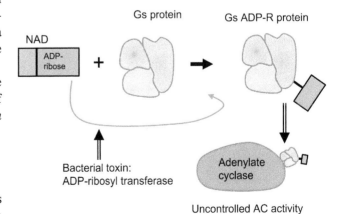

Figure 5.8 Action of ADP ribosylation of host cell Gs by bacterial toxin causes uncontrolled adenylate cyclase activity.

serve a useful purpose for the bacteria. They are often enzymes needed for an aspect of metabolism. Damage to animal tissues or production of paralysis is simply an extremely undesirable accident.

An example neurotoxin is botulinum toxin. In reality, there are several related but antigenically distinct botulinum toxins with subtle differences in activity. They are the most poisonous proteins known. They act at the neuromuscular junction by blocking the release of acetylcholine from the synaptic vesicle to the acetylcholine receptor. The active botulinum toxins are zinc metalloprotease enzymes that cleave the SNARE proteins that are essential for the fusion of the synaptic vesicle with the membrane at the synaptic cleft. This prevents membrane fusion and release of the acetylcholine causing a flaccid paralysis and, usually, death. Tetanus toxin (tetanospasmin) is another neurotoxin with potent effects which acts on inhibitory neurons with different neurotransmitters (GABA and glycine) to cause uncontrolled excitation of the motor neurons and an unrelieved muscle-tensing paralysis.

Superantigens

The first superantigen toxin was found causing cases of toxic shock in women in the late 1970s. It was associated with staphylococcal infection of the genital tract and the use of tampons for extended times. The toxin, named TSST-1, was found to cause non-regulated activation of a high proportion of T-lymphocytes so that their proliferation led to massive release of cytokines and the pathological effects of those chemicals on the body. The superantigen toxin TSST-1 from *S. aureus* is a protein of 22 kDa. The protein binds to the invariable regions on the MHC Class II molecules on antigen-presenting cells such as dendritic cells and cross-bridges to the receptor on the T-cell. Instead of the interaction requiring an antigen to bridge the MHC and T-cell receptor, which would be a rare event in immune recognition during infection, the process of T-cell activation is short-circuited (Figure 5.9).

TSST-1 is one of many superantigens now recognised. These contribute to disease through pathophysiological effects and shock, but also contribute to the progress of infection by interfering with the normal immunological processes needed to generate acquired immunity and combat bacterial infections.

Type III Secretion Systems

Surprisingly, as late as the 1980s, the means by which *Salmonella* damaged enterocytes and caused degeneration of the enteric villi was not known. It was known that *Salmonella* entered cells of the host gut, but toxin damage was also strongly suspected. Substantial efforts were made to find and purify the soluble toxin that (it was thought) must be causing the damage from *S. enterica* infection. There was no soluble toxin.

By careful study of the genes of the *Salmonella* chromosome and plasmid, and analysis of many mutants lacking those gene functions, it was recognised that a key step in *Salmonella* pathogenicity and damage to enterocytes is close association of the organism with the enterocyte. This requires a type 3 secretion system (T3SS). This is a needle-like structure at the submicroscopic level, used as a sensory probe to detect eukaryotic cells of the right type (Figure 5.10). Once interaction with the host cell has been established, the needle apparatus (known as the injectosome) enables the secretion of proteins that permit the bacteria to infect

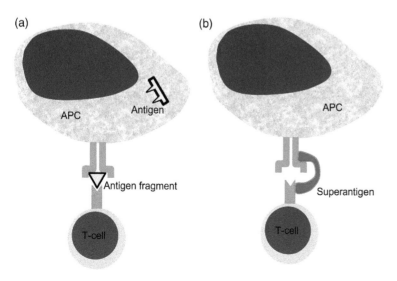

Figure 5.9 (a) Normal antigen presentation; (b) bacterial superantigen cross-bridging the T-cell receptor and the MHC Class II complex without the need for a specific antigen fragment.

those cells (see Chapter 9). Effector proteins are transferred directly from the bacteria into the enterocyte. This leads to stimulated endocytosis so that the bacteria are engulfed by the cell. Ultimately, this allows the pathogen to survive and escape an immune response.

Endotoxin

Endotoxin is different. This is LPS – in fact the lipid A portion of LPS. It is part of the outer membrane of Gram-negatives and therefore is never found in Gram-positive bacteria. It has numerous systemic pathophysiological effects when able to interact with the host, e.g. fever following injection of endotoxin into an animal. However, its release in the body during infection is still an ill-defined process. LPS is an amphipathic molecule: it has both hydrophilic and hydrophobic ends and dissolves poorly in aqueous solution. Instead, it forms micelles in which many LPS molecules aggregate at the hydrophobic end with the hydrophilic polysaccharide component projecting outwards. It is released from bacteria as outer membrane 'blebs' or as a result of the breakdown of dying bacteria (Figures 5.11 and 5.12).

Salmonella enterica

Enterocyte

Figure 5.10 The type 3 secretion system of bacteria such as *Salmonella enterica* injects effector proteins into the host cell.

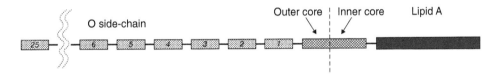

Figure 5.11 Lipopolysaccharide (LPS) is composed of lipid A linked through the core oligosaccharide to the repeating O-antigen units.

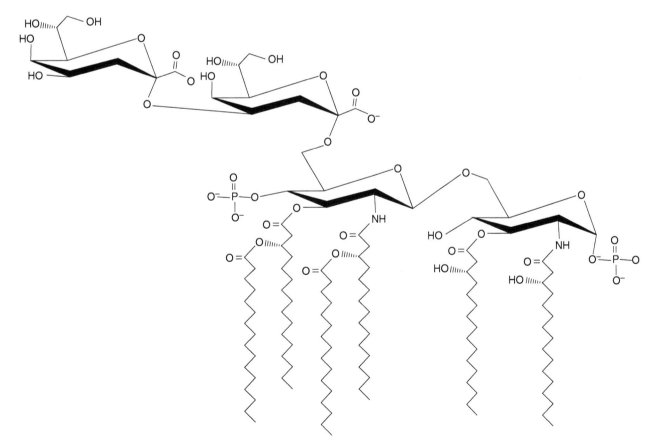

Figure 5.12 Structure of lipid A. The minimal Re chemotype lipopolysaccharide of *Salmonella*, sometimes known as KDO2-lipid A. Two KDO residues are linked to the acetylated glucosamine disaccharide (lipid A). Linkage of the KDO to the glucosamine disaccharide involves the product of the *kdtA* gene.

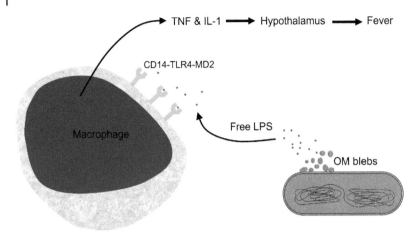

Figure 5.13 LPS interaction with macrophage.

The effects of endotoxin are thought to result from interaction of the lipid A with a receptor complex on the macrophage membrane CD14-TLR4-MD2. This stimulates the cell to produce and release tumour necrosis factor (TNF-α) and then interleukin (IL)-1. IL-1 acts on the hypothalamus to modulate temperature regulation and decrease peripheral blood flow via the conversion of arachidonic acid to prostaglandin (PG)-E2 which is active on the neural pathways of the hypothalamus. It is reasonable to consider that the body is reacting to common bacterial substances that are recognised as foreign using primitive mechanisms. This is supported by the fact that the host will also react to certain proteins (endotoxin proteins) and peptidoglycan in a very similar way (Figure 5.13).

Pathophysiological effects of endotoxin include fever, leucopaenia, hypotension, impaired organ perfusion, acidosis, activation of complement, intravascular coagulation, hypovolaemic shock and death.

Immunopathological Effects

Damage to body tissues may be the result of the body responding to the invading pathogen rather than the action of toxins. For example, an animal infected with bovine tuberculosis acquires a delayed hypersensitivity to the antigens of *Mycobacterium bovis*. It is this immune response itself, rather than the direct effects of the pathogen, which leads to tissue damage – an ill-defined process known as immunopathology in which the response by the immune system to tuberculous infection causes worsening pathology and wasting (see Chapter 22). This destruction occurs as a result of the action of proinflammatory cytokines, chemokines, immune cells and lipids that mediate TB-associated necrosis in the lung. As more is understood about the pathogenesis of tuberculosis, it is becoming apparent that the microorganism actively manipulates the immune system of the host. In so doing, it enables transmission of itself over a long period of time.

References

Berg, G., Rybakova, D., Fischer, D. et al. (2020). Microbiome definition re-visited: old concepts and new challenges. *Microbiome* 8: 103.

Crosa, J.H. (1989). Genetics and molecular biology of siderophore-mediated iron transport in bacteria. *Microbiological Reviews* 53: 517–530.

Finlay, B.B. and Falkow, S. (1989). Common themes in microbial pathogenicity. *Microbiological Reviews* 53: 210–230.

Gopalakrishnakone, P., Alape-Girón, A., Dubreuil, J.D. et al. (ed.) (2018). *Microbial Toxins*. Netherlands: Springer.

Salyers, A.A. and Whitt, D.D. (1994). *Bacterial Pathogenesis: A Molecular Approach*. Washington DC: American Society for Microbiology.

Schaible, U.E. and Kaufmann, S.H.E. (2004). Iron and microbial infection. *Nature Reviews Microbiology* 2: 946–954.

6

Bacterial Veterinary Vaccines

Prophylactic immunisation has been immensely successful in combatting infectious disease. Some of those successes have been in preventing or controlling bacterial disease. Indeed, many of the early vaccines from the late nineteenth century onwards were effective against toxigenic bacterial pathogens of humans: *Corynebacterium diphtheriae*, *Clostridium tetani* and *Bacillus anthracis*. However, the greater successes in vaccination since the mid-twentieth century have been against virus disease; it has proven very difficult to achieve the same against bacterial disease.

Perhaps this is due to the availability of antibacterial drugs such that prevention was not needed when cure was so easily available. However, despite persistent research to understand the detailed pathogenic mechanisms of bacteria and sustained efforts to test experimental vaccines, the results have often been less than was needed to justify producing and licensing products for preventing bacterial disease in animals.

There have been some wonderful successes in human medicine. The vaccines to prevent disease from the most common strains of *Haemophilus influenzae* (HIB vaccine) and *Neisseria meningitidis* have been very successful. But this type of conjugate vaccine is simply too expensive for use in farmed animals and even most companion animals. Immunising a chicken with three doses of vaccine costing even £10, $10 or €10 per dose would have too little uptake in the veterinary market to justify licensing the product. Hence, preventing animal disease by vaccination is constrained by the degree of efficacy that can be achieved, safety of the product and the cost of a vaccine in relation to the value of the animal.

Different types of bacterial vaccines are used in control and prevention of animal disease. These have different advantages and limitations.

Inactivated Vaccines

The majority of bacterial vaccines that have been developed for animal use are whole, killed bacteria. These are sometimes referred to as bacterins or inactivated vaccines. These are often cheap to produce because they involve careful growth of a known pure culture followed by harvesting and killing of the organisms. The method of killing can be through heat although this sometimes denatures important protein antigens. Alternatively, formalin solution (HCHO) is used over a period of time, often at low temperature, and then removed by washing (centrifugation). An alternative chemical agent widely used in virus inactivation is β-propiolactone. However, this compound is more expensive than formaldehyde and is a mild carcinogen.

Once the vaccine has been tested to ensure there are no live organisms remaining, the antigen might be tested for potency and checked to show that the expected immune response is achieved in a group of animals. In general, the response achieved is proportional to the amount of antigen used and this is improved by addition of adjuvant. Traditionally, antigen for animal vaccines has been mixed with aluminium hydroxide gel to which the antigen can adsorb for more effective presentation to the cells of the immune system. In this case, whole antigen will bind to B-lymphocyte receptors and this stimulates clonal expansion of B-cells to produce large quantities of the specific immunoglobulin molecule that the B-cell is primed to produce. Killed vaccines tend to cause a predominantly T-helper-2 (T_H2) response that help B-cells make antibody. At least two doses of an inactivated vaccine are administered to give a priming and an anamnestic response (Meeusen et al. 2007).

Fundamentals of Veterinary Microbiology, First Edition. Andrew N. Rycroft.
© 2024 John Wiley & Sons Ltd. Published 2024 by John Wiley & Sons Ltd.
Companion website: www.wiley.com/go/veterinarymicrobiology

Examples of inactivated vaccines used in animals include the *Leptospira interrogans* component of canine vaccines, *Salmonella* vaccine in cattle and erysipelas vaccine in pigs. They stimulate antibody, which may be protective or partially protective against infection, but this antibody usually declines rapidly after peaking. They are also serotype specific. Unless the serotype antigen is the same as that required for protection, the vaccine may have little value. Serotype specificity is a complex subject. Whole bacteria are a mixture of many antigens and the potency, influence and protective value of a range of antigens can affect the effect of a given vaccination (Day 2017).

Notably, a number of inactivated vaccines are directed at protection of very young animals, immediately after birth, via passive (colostral) antibody from the dam. The dam must therefore be vaccinated at the optimum time in advance of parturition in order to allow for the development of the antibody response. Young animals suckling colostrum become immunised because the intestine in many neonatal animals is permeable to immunoglobulin. The antibody therefore reaches the circulation. It has also been shown that lymphocytes transferred with colostrum may also remain viable and contribute to the immunological protection. Vaccines protecting against disease such as colisepticaemia are widely used in this way.

Live-attenuated Vaccines

Live bacterial vaccine strains have advantages and disadvantages compared with killed vaccines. They must be attenuated sufficiently to be unable to cause disease yet, it seems, not so attenuated that they fail to 'knock on the door' of the immune system. They have the advantage that they multiply within the host, creating a strong antigenic stimulus. Only a single dose may be required and no adjuvant is needed. Furthermore, live vaccines can give a sustained immune response with good immunological memory, a predominantly T-helper-1 (T_H1) response with a cell-mediated immune component, and sometimes an immune response directed to the mucosal surface.

Several live vaccines have been used to prevent bacterial disease in animals. Among these, the Sterne strain of *Bacillus anthracis*, a strain of *Salmonella* serovar Dublin (Mellavax®), the S19 strain of *Brucella abortus* and S55 (Intrac) strain of *Bordetella bronchiseptica* for kennel cough. All of these were derived empirically rather than by rational attenuation. There has been concern that mutations could revert and the vaccine become fully virulent. Some live vaccines caused a degree of disease, some caused anaphylaxis and some failed to protect as intended, and all have now been removed from use in most of the world. One exception is the poultry vaccines against *Mycoplasma gallisepticum* and *M. synoviae* infection (Barbour et al. 2000). These are temperature-sensitive mutants for delivery as eye drops or inhalation vaccines and are in widespread use.

With the advent of genetic manipulation, genome sequencing, directed mutagenesis and improved understanding of pathogenicity mechanisms, it has become realistic to design rationally derived live vaccine strains. However, few of these have yet become commercially available because of concerns that genetically manipulated organisms could be released into the wider environment.

An exception to this is the *aroA* mutants. Mutants of *Salmonella*, deficient in the common aromatic biosynthesis pathway caused by a transposon-generated deletion mutation of the *aroA* gene, were shown in 1981 to be avirulent (Hoiseth and Stocker 1981). They were also shown to be capable of generating a protective immune response by oral inoculation of calves. The paradigm was extended to other pathogens by deliberate mutagenesis of the *aroA* gene and other mutations in related and unrelated genes. A current intranasal vaccine for kennel cough and *Bordetella* infection in the cat is an *aroA* mutant of *B. bronchiseptica*. Another *aroA*-based vaccine was the equine strangles vaccine (Meeusen et al. 2007). Unfortunately, in the field this was shown to cause strangles-like disease and was withdrawn.

Other defined attenuated mutants of pathogens may become commercially useful vaccines in the future. However, there is a dilemma. It is logical to discover the virulence determinant and attenuate the pathogen by mutation of the gene for that determinant. However, such mutants may then lack the key antigen needed for a protective immune response. Instead, subtle changes to the gene encoding a key virulence determinant can eliminate pathogenicity while allowing that antigen to stimulate the animal to make a protective immune response. This has been shown to work in a number of cases as typified by deletion of the phospholipase D (PLD) of *Corynebacterium pseudotuberculosis* and re-expression of a genetically detoxified PLD from the same strain to achieve protection against caseous lymphadenitis in sheep (Hodgson et al. 1994).

Toxoid Vaccines

Toxoids are inactivated toxins. Bacterial toxoid vaccines are among the most effective and widespread vaccines and have been available for use in humans and animals for nearly 100 years. Toxoids are produced by treating preparations of toxin or toxin mixture with formalin. This destroys the toxigenic property of the protein, usually by inactivation of the specific enzymatic activity. The material is then mixed with an adjuvant to promote the immunological effect of the antigen before being safely delivered to the animal. Although the toxic property is no longer active, the immunological properties are still present, and the toxoid is able to generate an immune response to the protein that is able to neutralise the same toxin if it is encountered in a future infection.

Examples of vaccines of this type are tetanus toxoid used in horses (and widely in humans) and the multivalent vaccines used to protect farm animals against clostridial diseases such as black quarter in cattle and struck and pulpy kidney disease in sheep.

Subunit Vaccines

Subunit vaccines are composed of a limited range of specific antigens prepared with adjuvant. Relatively few subunit vaccines have been developed for control of bacterial disease. However, the logic of using only the key protective antigens as vaccine components is rational. Many viral vaccines, such as the hepatitis B vaccine, make use of key subunits but virus proteins do not necessarily have a function in the survival of the pathogen or damage to the host. Bacterial vaccines of this type usually include components known to be needed for pathogenicity (Meeusen et al. 2007).

One situation in which they have been developed is for control of neonatal diarrhoea (scours) in farm animals. Enterotoxigenic *E. coli* (ETEC) relies on fimbrial adhesins and enterotoxin and so vaccines contain the B subunit of the heat-labile enterotoxin (LT) coupled with known fimbrial proteins, K88, K99, 987P. These are administered to the sow or cow so that protective antibody is developed and secreted in the colostrum. This antibody bathes the surface mucosa of the intestine of the newborn animal to prevent attachment of ETEC and neutralise its enterotoxin.

Vaccines against contagious porcine pleuropneumonia have also been of this type. One vaccine used a combination of a 42 kDa outer membrane protein and the three Apx toxins produced in varying combinations by all the strains of *Actinobacillus pleuropneumoniae*. These protein molecules naturally lose potency as toxins, probably by aggregation, and so no detoxification was necessary. The vaccine reduced lung lesions and clinical disease but suffered the drawback of inducing fever in vaccinated piglets. This was because lipopolysaccharide (endotoxin) was co-purified with the Apx vaccine antigens.

A different vaccine against the same disease was composed of five recombinant antigens prepared in *E. coli*. This did not suffer the side-effect because the R-form lipopolysaccharide of a laboratory strain of *E. coli* does not so readily co-purify with the Apx toxin. In any case, ApxII was only one of the recombinant antigens used.

Addition of more antigens into a vaccine does not always improve the protective efficacy of a subunit vaccine and can have unexpected consequences. This was demonstrated in experiments to improve the multi-Apx vaccine by addition of another common surface antigen, peptidoglycan binding protein (PalA). Pigs immunised with the two cytotoxins ApxI and ApxII were protected against challenge with *A. pleuropneumoniae*. However, pigs immunised with PalA showed more severe respiratory signs and had a higher mortality. They also displayed much more severe lung lesions after necropsy than animals not immunised with PalA. This correlated with the immune response: pigs that developed antibody titers against PalA after immunisation were more significantly affected by challenge with *A. pleuropneumoniae* serotype 1. The protective efficacy of the ApxI and ApxII vaccine was completely lost when it was supplemented with PalA (van den Bosch and Frey 2003).

Autogenous or 'On-Farm' Vaccines

When there is an outbreak of disease on a farm, but no commercial vaccine is available to control the outbreak, a licence may be granted for production of a vaccine for use on that farm. The causative organism must be isolated and identified on the premises and that strain used to make the vaccine as a simple, whole bacterial inactivated vaccine. These vaccines are then prepared by veterinary laboratories or specialised companies, checked for purity and sterility, prepared to the right concentration, mixed with adjuvant and administered under veterinary advice. Many examples have been used: some (such as *Glaesserella parasuis*) with great success and some (such as *Actinobacillus pleuropneumoniae*) without.

References

Barbour, E.K., Hamadeh, S.K., and Eidt, A. (2000). Infection and immunity in broiler chicken breeders vaccinated with a temperature-sensitive mutant of *Mycoplasma gallisepticum* and impact on performance of offspring. *Poultry Science* 79: 1730–1735.

Day, M.J. (2017). Small animal vaccination: a practical guide for vets in the UK. *In Practice* 39: 110–118.

Hodgson, A.L., Tachedjian, M., Corner, L.A., and Radford, A.J. (1994). Protection of sheep against caseous lymphadenitis by use of a single oral dose of live recombinant *Corynebacterium pseudotuberculosis*. *Infection and Immunity* 62: 5275–5280.

Hoiseth, S.K. and Stocker, B.A.D. (1981). Aromatic-dependent *Salmonella typhimurium* are non-virulent and effective as live vaccines. *Nature* 291: 238.

Meeusen, E.N.T., Walker, J., Peters, A. et al. (2007). Current status of veterinary vaccines. *Clinical Microbiology Reviews* 20: 489–510.

Van den Bosch, H. and Frey, J. (2003). Interference of outer membrane protein PalA with protective immunity against *Actinobacillus pleuropneumoniae* infections in vaccinated pigs. *Vaccine* 21: 3601–3607.

7

Antimicrobials: Action, Dynamics and Resistance

Targets of Antimicrobial Drugs

Antimicrobial drugs are required to have selective toxicity. That is, the bacterial target must be sufficiently different from any similar target that might be present in the host, otherwise the drug would harm the host. Different antimicrobial agents target different components in the bacterial cell. Depending on how these are viewed, six different target sites can be recognised. These targets vary considerably in the degree of selective toxicity offered by drugs engaging with them.

Peptidoglycan Synthesis

The cell wall component of bacterial cells is unique to bacteria and so the enzyme systems involved in its synthesis are not found in mammalian cells. All β-lactam drugs, penicillins, cephalosporins, monobactams and carbapenems act to inhibit the transpeptidase enzymes (known as penicillin-binding proteins) at the final cross-linking stage.

Other drugs also interfere with peptidoglycan synthesis but at an earlier stage in the pathway. Vancomycin and teicoplanin inhibit transfer of the preformed units of peptidoglycan to the glycan chains. Bacitracin targets the recycling of the carrier molecule responsible for transferring the units of peptidoglycan across the cytoplasmic membrane.

Protein Synthesis at the Bacterial Ribosome

The bacterial (70S) ribosome has fundamental differences from the eukaryotic (80S) ribosome. Some antimicrobials interfere with protein synthesis at the bacterial ribosome and selective toxicity usually comes from those differences. Antimicrobial drugs acting at the ribosome include the aminoglycosides: streptomycin, gentamicin, amikacin, kanamycin and others. Others include chloramphenicol and florfenicol, the macrolides (erythromycin, tulathromycin, azithromycin, tylosin and others), the lincosamides (lincomycin and clindamycin), the streptogramins (streptogramin and virginiamycin) and the steroidal antimicrobial fusidic acid.

One antimicrobial group, the tetracyclines (oxytetracycline, doxycycline and others) act effectively against both prokaryotic and eukaryotic ribosomes. Why are these drugs not toxic to mammalian cell ribosomes? It seems that selective toxicity is due to the reversible effect of tetracycline on the ribosome and the fact that it is concentrated inside bacterial cells to the stage where it is inhibitory to bacteria. Remarkably, this happens even within eukaryotic cells so that tetracyclines can be used against obligate intracellular bacterial pathogens such as *Chlamydia*.

Bacterial Folate Synthesis and Conversion

Folic acid is synthesised by most bacteria. It is then reduced to tetrahydrofolic acid and this is an essential co-factor in transfer of one-carbon units ($-CHO$ and $-CH_3$), particularly used in nucleic acid synthesis. The bacterial enzyme dihydropteroate synthase is competitively inhibited by sulfonamides (a structural analogue of para-aminobenzoic acid) while the final reduction step by dihydrofolate reductase is inhibited by trimethoprim. Selective toxicity for these agents arises because animals do not have this synthetic pathway and must obtain folic acid in their diet.

Fundamentals of Veterinary Microbiology, First Edition. Andrew N. Rycroft.
© 2024 John Wiley & Sons Ltd. Published 2024 by John Wiley & Sons Ltd.
Companion website: www.wiley.com/go/veterinarymicrobiology

DNA Metabolism

In order to replicate, or for it to be transcribed to mRNA, DNA must unwind the supercoils (using topoisomerase IV) and open the two base-paired strands of the double helix (using DNA gyrase – topoisomerase II). A synthetic quinolone carboxylic acid, nalidixic acid, was the original drug found to interfere with these functions. In the 1990s, new versions of quinolones, with a fluorine atom at the four position, were found to be much more potent. These drugs include enrofloxacin, norfloxacin and others. The rifamycins also interfere with transcription by inhibiting DNA-dependent RNA polymerase.

Cytoplasmic Membrane

The cytoplasmic membrane of bacteria is similar to the membrane around mammalian cells. Therefore, the selective toxicity of antimicrobials acting at the bacterial membrane is limited and many are not widely used. The bacterial cytoplasmic membrane must be intact so that the H^+ gradient can be used to generate energy through the proton motive force. Any damage to the membrane causes a short-circuit in the bacterial energy system. Polymyxins B and E form pores in the membrane; the ionophores monensin and valinomycin shuttle ions across the membrane and dissipate the ion gradient.

Metabolic Pathways

The action of some antimicrobials on aspects of bacterial metabolism is not always clear. Nitroimidazoles are prodrugs that are reductively activated (the nitro group is reduced) under low oxygen tension. Metronidazole is almost exclusively active against strictly anaerobic bacteria. Despite 60 years of research, the cytotoxic action of metronidazole is not definitively characterised. It has also been suggested that the target of this drug is DNA synthesis and repair of existing DNA (Dingsdag and Hunter 2018). The target of nitrofuran drugs is also unclear. Bacterial enzymes convert nitrofurantoin to reactive electrophilic intermediates known to attack bacterial ribosomal proteins and interfere with cellular processes and protein synthesis, and cause single-strand breaks in DNA (Komp Lindgren et al. 2015).

Antimicrobial Sensitivity

Determining whether a bacterial isolate is sensitive or resistant to a given antimicrobial can be important in successful treatment of disease and preventing unnecessary use of antimicrobials. The traditional method of antimicrobial sensitivity testing is the Kirby-Bauer disc diffusion test. Paper discs, impregnated with a fixed mass of antimicrobial, are placed on a lawn of bacteria seeded onto the surface of a suitable solid growth medium. This is then incubated at a suitable temperature (usually 37 °C) for an appropriate time (often 18 hours). Areas around each disc where bacterial growth has been inhibited indicate sensitivity of the seed organism to that drug (Allerton and Nuttall 2021). Superficially, this test seems very straightforward. In reality, the test needs careful standardisation of medium, preparation of inoculum and interpretation of the inhibition zone size. Even when these are carefully controlled, the test is still an *in vitro* test that is only reflecting part of the interaction between microorganism and drug in the body.

Minimum Inhibitory Concentration

A recognised measure of sensitivity is the minimum inhibitory concentration (MIC). Each drug–bacterial strain combination has a unique MIC value in µg/ml. The basic tube test uses a series of increasingly diluted antimicrobial dissolved in liquid culture medium. A small quantity of a pure suspension of the isolate under test is added to each dilution, incubated and examined for growth. The highest dilution (lowest concentration) showing no turbidity (no growth) is the concentration that is the MIC.

Minimum Bactericidal Concentration

If each tube showing no growth is sampled and the number of viable bacteria counted, the minimum bactericidal concentration (MBC) can be determined. The highest dilution showing a 3-log (1000-fold) reduction of the original inoculum is the MBC.

Clinical Breakpoints

Even when the correct disc diffusion procedures are followed, how do we determine whether a drug is likely to be effective in treating an infection? What MIC value or zone of inhibition can be considered sensitive and what is resistant? The clinical breakpoint is the criterion used to relate the *in vitro* values to a likely clinical outcome. This depends on clinical, pharmacological, microbiological and pharmacodynamic considerations. It is potentially different for every drug, every site of infection, every microorganism and every animal species. Ultimately, this is an educated guess, determined by committee.

Once an MIC value is agreed upon, below which a drug is likely to be effective, this can be translated into a minimum inhibition zone diameter in a Kirby-Bauer disc diffusion test. Some labs routinely offer automated MIC measurements and so these can be interpreted as likely to be sensitive (MIC below a given set value) or resistant (above a given agreed value).

Many clinical breakpoints are agreed for human treatments. However, these values are not fixed. Different committees recommend different MIC values for specific pathogens and different antimicrobial drugs. Far fewer breakpoints are established for veterinary pathogens and different animal species.

Unpredictability of Antimicrobial Action

In addition to these considerations, the effect of antimicrobials in the body can be unpredictable. The earliest example of this was the dye prontosil red discovered in 1932, which was active against streptococcal disease in mice but had no antibacterial activity *in vitro*. This is because the active drug, sulfanilamide, is only released by enzyme activity in the body of the animal.

Other drugs, such as clindamycin, may also show clinical efficacy while appearing ineffective *in vitro*. Conversely, drugs such as nitrofurantoin may show clear inhibition of a pathogen *in vitro* while failing to fulfil expectations in combatting urinary tract infection. It is necessary to recognise that the *in vitro* environment is quite different from the surface of a sensitivity test medium, and an immune system is operating in the body.

Attempts have been made to find or design drugs which interfere with the virulence mechanisms of a pathogen. Rather than simply inhibit its growth, a drug might remove an essential component for survival and so facilitate destruction of the pathogen by the innate or acquired immune response.

Genetic Detection of Antimicrobial Resistance

Although phenotypic sensitivity testing is valuable in checking sensitivity or resistance, increasingly this will be done through genetic means. The correlation of genetic elements with expressed resistance, or potential for resistance, is high. Future developments will see whole-genome sequencing (WGS) for detection and identification of pathogens in a mixture, and for determining resistance elements within those organisms. However, this does require computing power and large investment and cannot yet substitute for detecting living organisms, showing their relevance to disease and demonstrating the expression of antimicrobial resistance within the pathogen.

Bacterial Resistance to Antimicrobials

Bacterial resistance to an antibacterial agent may be either innate or acquired.

Innate Resistance

Not all bacteria are naturally sensitive to all antibiotics. For example, *Escherichia coli* is never sensitive to penicillin G or erythromycin. This is because the outer membrane acts as a molecular sieve excluding hydrophobic and large hydrophilic molecules. Penicillin G is hydrophobic; erythromycin is a large molecule (mass 734). Therefore, *E. coli* is naturally insensitive to these agents. Similarly, mycoplasmas are not sensitive to any of the peptidoglycan inhibitors as they possess no cell wall.

To overcome this innate resistance to penicillin G in Gram-negative bacteria such as *E. coli*, the molecule was slightly altered. The H on the side group was altered to NH_2. The NH_2 ionises to NH_3^+ at physiological pH and so the +ve charge makes the molecule polar and hence more hydrophilic. This is ampicillin and it readily enters through the porins and across the outer membrane to the site of action in the periplasm (Figure 7.1).

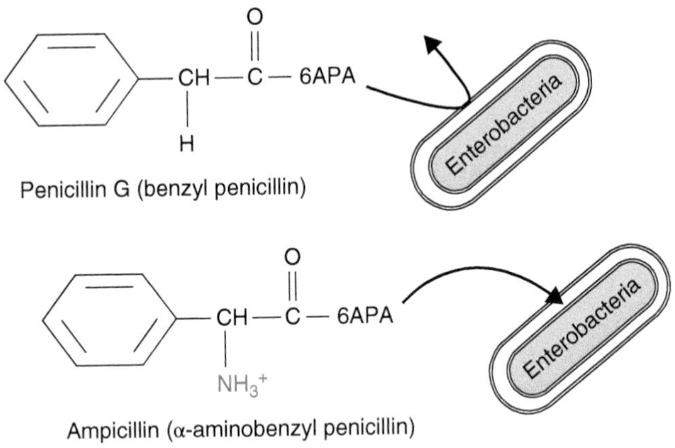

Figure 7.1 *Enterobacteriaceae* are intrinsically resistant to penicillin G. Altering the molecule to carry a positively charged amino group causes the molecule to be polar and hydrophilic.

Acquired Resistance

Bacteria which are naturally sensitive to a drug may become resistant to it. This is by either mutational change or acquisition of resistance genes.

Mutation

Spontaneous mutations in a given gene occur in bacterial cultures with a frequency of approximately 1 per 10^7 bacteria per cell division. In the presence of antibacterial agents, that frequency does not change but drug resistant mutants may be selected from the population of otherwise sensitive individuals. Mutation to antibiotic resistance occurs to an important degree with some agents but is not found with others. For example, streptomycin-resistant mutants of *E. coli* can be reproducibly found but chloramphenicol-resistant *E. coli* are not produced by mutation. In order to be easily selectable, a mutation to increase antibiotic resistance must take place in a single step. Sometimes, combinations of mutations are cumulatively acquired but this is unusual. Mutational changes causing antimicrobial resistance are sometimes detrimental to the microorganism and in the absence of the selection pressure, mutants are lost.

Examples of mutational change leading to antimicrobial resistance are many and diverse.

- Altering ribosomal structural proteins or rRNA, e.g. streptomycin resistance. Alteration of the small ribosomal protein L, encoded by the *rpsL* gene, prevents the binding of streptomycin to the bacterial ribosome. In this case, streptomycin fails to distort the ribosome and cause the misreading of mRNA and so in the mutant, normal protein synthesis continues in the presence of this antimicrobial.
- Decreased permeability of the outer membrane may cause resistance to β-lactams in some Gram-negatives. Alteration to outer membrane porins such as OmpF and OmpC may restrict access of the drug into the bacterial cell and reduced concentrations translate to a raised MIC (Fernández and Hancock 2012).
- Alteration of a target enzyme can bring about resistance. Resistance to rifampicin can be conferred by mutational alteration of the DNA-dependent RNA polymerase: transcription is no longer inhibited by rifampicin.

Acquisition of Resistance Genes

In addition to mutational events, bacteria may become resistant to antibacterials by acquiring new genetic information (DNA). Genetic determinants specifying drug resistance are usually encoded on plasmids, on integrative conjugative elements or sometimes on transposons. New genetic information brings about antimicrobial resistance in different ways.

Inactivating Enzymes A prime example of an inactivating enzyme is the ability of *Staphylococcus aureus* to produce β-lactamase (penicillinase enzymes) which are sometimes inducible in the presence of β-lactam antimicrobials. β-lactamases hydrolyse penicillins to penicilloic acid which is inactive; some cephalosporins are also hydrolysed.

Another plasmid-encoded, antibiotic-inactivating enzyme is chloramphenicol acetyltransferase which converts chloramphenicol to 3-acetoxy-chloramphenicol. The latter compound no longer binds to the bacterial ribosome and so is inactive.

Aminoglycoside antibiotics (neomycin, streptomycin, gentamicin) are inactivated by the aminoglycoside modifying enzymes: aminoglycoside *O*-phosphotransferase, *O*-nucleotidyltransferase and *N*-acetyltransferase. Again, the modified antibiotics no longer bind to the bacterial ribosome.

AmpC β-lactamases are chromosomally determined enzymes naturally found in many bacteria such as *Enterobacteriaceae* (Jacoby 2009). They may be upregulated through mutation and overexpressed to give significant resistance to some penicillins and some cephalosporins.

Bypass Mechanisms   Some resistance genes encode alternative enzymes so that a new, less sensitive enzyme pathway takes the place of the inhibited one. This is known with both sulfonamide and trimethoprim resistance in which an alternative dihydropteroic acid synthetase enables resistance to sulfonamide and an alternative dihydrofolate reductase enables microorganisms to evade the inhibitory effects of trimethoprim.

A similar bypass system is the cause of MRSA. *Staphylococcus aureus* can be resistant to β-lactamase stable penicillins by producing the alternative transpeptidase, a low-affinity penicillin-binding protein (PBP2a), encoded by the *mecA* gene or the more recently identified *mecC* gene. The *mecA* gene is carried on a 'resistance island' on the chromosome of *S. aureus*.

Methicillin-resistant *S. aureus* or *S. pseudintermedius* in the dog are significant because strains having this resistance are not susceptible to the β-lactam drugs used commonly to treat these infections. Strains of MRSA and MRSP are often resistant to a wide range of other agents due to other, independent mechanisms.

Efflux Pumps   Another common acquired resistance mechanism is the efflux system, a pumping system that actively ejects the molecule from the bacterial cell before it accumulates (Piddock 2006). Tetracycline resistance was the first efflux resistance mechanism to be recognised in 1980 (Ball et al. 1980). Efflux pumps are now known to be ubiquitous throughout nature in all types of eukaryotic and prokaryotic cells.

Multiple efflux systems can operate in a bacterial cell at any one time. Those that are highly specific are usually acquired on plasmids, transposons or other horizontally acquired genetic elements. Others, known as multidrug efflux systems, are broad in the choice of substrate. These are usually native to the bacterium and found encoded on the chromosome. They are activated or upregulated through increase in expression of the efflux pump protein, or from one or more amino acid substitutions that cause the protein to be more efficient at exporting solutes (Poole 2005).

An example of a multidrug efflux transporter is NorA of *Staphylococcus aureus*. This is a multidrug transporter that confers low-level resistance to several antibiotics, including fluoroquinolones. It can be upregulated, by mutational changes in regulatory functions, to increase the rate of efflux and increase the MIC for these drugs. When coupled with mutations in the target sites on the components of DNA gyrase (*gyrA*) or topoisomerase IV (*grlA* or *parC*), this leads to high-level, clinically relevant resistance to fluoroquinolones. In fact, the natural function of the NorA efflux pump is probably the secretion of siderophores needed for the acquisition of iron.

Transposons   Resistance genes on plasmids or the chromosome may be located within transposable elements. These are genetic elements able to transfer a copy of themselves to another replicon by so-called illegitimate (non-homologous) recombination. They appear to jump from plasmid to plasmid and plasmid to chromosome. They enable the accumulation of multiple resistance plasmids and enhance the spread of resistance genes in the biological world.

Multiple Antimicrobial Resistance

It has been known since the 1970s that plasmids may carry several resistance determinants and be self-transmissible. Such plasmids were termed R-factors. We now recognise that different mobile genetic elements are able to move within or between DNA molecules. These include insertion sequences, transposons, gene cassettes/integrons and integrative conjugative elements. Together, these genetic elements enable horizontal genetic exchange and therefore promote the acquisition and spread of resistance genes (Partridge et al. 2018). Selection for one resistance element may indirectly select for a cluster of unrelated resistance elements. This is particularly important in the *Enterobacteriaceae*, *Pseudomonas*, *Enterococcus* and coagulase-positive *Staphylococcus*: *S. aureus* and *S. pseudintermedius*.

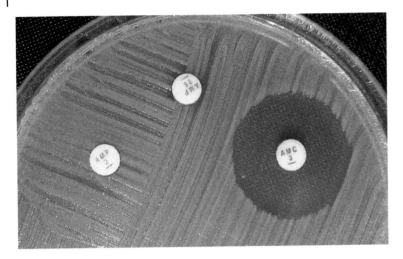

Figure 7.2 A bacterial isolate that is highly resistant to ampicillin (AMP2 and AMP25) is sensitive to the combination of amoxicillin and clavulanic acid (AMC).

Methods of Overcoming Antimicrobial Resistance

β-lactamase Stable Drugs

To combat antimicrobial resistance, drugs have been introduced which are not susceptible to the commonly encountered resistance mechanisms. These are usually semi-synthetic compounds such as cloxacillin which is not hydrolysed by the staphylococcal β-lactamases. Many cephalosporins are similarly resistant to some of these enzymes, although β-lactamases are now recognised that destroy some cephalosporins.

β-lactamase Inhibitors

An alternative approach was the introduction of β-lactamase inhibitors such as clavulanic acid. This is itself a β-lactam compound which is not inhibitory to bacteria. However, it does bind and inactivate β-lactamases in a non-competitive inhibition. When combined with amoxicillin (widely used as co-amoxiclav), the therapeutic efficacy of amoxicillin against β-lactamase-producing pathogens is often restored (Figure 7.2). More modern β-lactamase inhibitors such as tazobactam and sulbactam have been developed for combination with a penicillin.

Efflux pumps have also become the target of research to find compounds capable of inhibiting their action and so potentiate the effects of clinically relevant antibiotics. These may be useful for the treatment of infections caused by multiresistant organisms due to increased efflux and may also allow, in some cases, the utilisation of lower antibiotic doses. While some compounds have been identified, efflux pump inhibitors are still the subject of studies to show if they are safe and efficacious for clinical use. None have yet become licensed drugs for use alongside antimicrobials in humans or animals.

References

Allerton, F. and Nuttall, T. (2021). Antimicrobial use: importance of bacterial culture and susceptibility testing. *In Practice* 43: 500–510.

Ball, P.R., Shales, S.W., and Chopra, I. (1980). Plasmid-mediated tetracycline resistance in *Escherichia coli* involves increased efflux of the antibiotic. *Biochemical and Biophysical Research Communications* 93: 74–81.

Dingsdag, S.A. and Hunter, N. (2018). Metronidazole: an update on metabolism, structure–cytotoxicity and resistance mechanisms. *Journal of Antimicrobial Chemotherapy* 73: 265–279.

Fernández, L. and Hancock, R.E.W. (2012). Adaptive and mutational resistance: role of porins and efflux pumps in drug resistance. *Clinical Microbiology Reviews* 25: 661–681.

Jacoby, G.A. (2009). AmpC β-Lactamases. *Clinical Microbiology Reviews* 22: 161–182.

Komp Lindgren, P., Klockars, O., Malmberg, C., and Cars, O. (2015). Pharmacodynamic studies of nitrofurantoin against common uropathogens. *Journal of Antimicrobial Chemotherapy* 70: 1076–1082.

Partridge, S.R., Kwong, S.M., Firth, N., and Jensen, S.O. (2018). Mobile genetic elements associated with antimicrobial resistance. *Clinical Microbiology Reviews* 31: e00088–e00017.

Piddock, L.J.V. (2006). Clinically relevant chromosomally encoded multidrug resistance efflux pumps in Bacteria. *Clinical Microbiology Reviews* 19: 382–402.

Poole, K. (2005). Efflux mediated antimicrobial resistance. *Journal of Antimicrobial Chemotherapy* 56: 20–51.

8

Bacterial Typing

Distinguishing between bacterial isolates, and particularly pathogens, has seen considerable effort over the last century. Once identified as a particular species of bacteria, colonies usually look identical. Under the microscope, they have the same shape and often the same biochemical characteristics. To distinguish between different isolates, and to attempt to relate one isolate to another and perhaps show transmission of infection, special techniques have been devised to show recognisable differences. It is sometimes difficult, in the age of whole-genome sequencing, to see the depth of the problem encountered by those who first collected and examined isolates of bacteria from disease. Gradually, methods have been devised to distinguish bacterial strains that have offered greater and greater discrimination and definition until we are now at a stage where we have the ability to read and analyse the entire genome of any bacterial isolate for comparison with another.

There are many different typing schemes that have been devised for bacteria (Pitt 2007). Only the most important methods or most relevant to veterinary pathogens are noted here.

Serotyping

A common method used by early bacteriologists was to take an isolate, kill it with heat or chemicals, and inject it into an experimental animal. After several injections of the same bacteria, the animal would develop an antibody response. Blood was taken from the animal and shown to contain antibody that recognised the bacterial cells used to immunise the animal. This was often by agglutination, simple clumping of the bacteria as the antibody bound to surface antigen and bridged the bacterial cells, causing them to visibly clump together (type A). Other isolates of the same species would not all clump in the same way and so this was considered antigenically different (type B). This is an antigenic typing scheme sometimes referred to as serological typing. *Salmonella* strains were, and still are, typed in this way.

Sometimes, the surface antigens of a species were identical but soluble extracts of the bacteria would show different antigens and could be typed using a method such as precipitation to recognise the antibody–antigen reaction. β-haemolytic streptococci are typed using the Lancefield grouping system in this way.

Many typing schemes were based, in this manner and with modifications, on the antigenic differences between strains. The *Escherichia coli* serological typing scheme was based on the O antigen (lipopolysaccharide) and H antigen (flagellar protein). It was further extended to include the K antigen (polysaccharide capsule) and F antigen (fimbrial proteins). Huge efforts were made to relate O, H, K and F types to the disease caused and some relationships were recognised. Perhaps the best known is the O157:H7 serotype which causes the severe human disease haemolytic uraemic syndrome (HLS). However, more than 50% of strains of EHEC (STEC) causing HLS are not serotype O157:H7; the pathogenicity determinants are not related to the serotype determinants. There is a loose association of serotype with some disease-causing strains but ultimately serotyping has failed to inform us of pathogenicity in *E. coli*; huge research effort has been expended in refining the system and searching for relationships, and it has also failed to show the phylogenetic structure of the extraordinarily disparate group of microorganisms that we refer to as *E. coli*.

Serotyping continues to be used routinely for veterinary isolates of *Salmonella enterica*. Isolation of the pathogen from food animals in the UK is reportable as a potential zoonosis in the food chain and each isolate is serotyped using antibody to the O and H antigens (Kauffman-White scheme) to determine the serovar (Wain and Olsen 2013).

Fundamentals of Veterinary Microbiology, First Edition. Andrew N. Rycroft.
© 2024 John Wiley & Sons Ltd. Published 2024 by John Wiley & Sons Ltd.
Companion website: www.wiley.com/go/veterinarymicrobiology

Serovars are often named after the first place they were isolated and approximately 2600 serovars are currently recognised globally. These are based on the combination of an O antigen with two different H antigens. This is because many *Salmonella* strains have the capacity to produce either one or another H antigen; they are said to undergo phase change to swich between the two possibilities. Reports of positive cultures, sent to the veterinary surgeon from government-backed veterinary laboratories, will include the identity of the serovar of the *Salmonella* strain isolated. By recognising and following outbreaks of *Salmonella* infection, action can be taken to minimise transmission to human food.

Phage Typing

Many isolates of *Salmonella* from animals display the same serotype antigens and are therefore indistinguishable by typing the O and H antigens. Phage typing was introduced for the most common serovars, such as *Salmonella* serovar Typhimurium and *S.* serovar Enteritidis, to try and further discriminate between the many apparently identical strains. Phage typing uses a pattern of sensitivity to a panel of bacteriophages known to be capable of causing a lytic infection in some strains of the target bacteria, such as *S. enterica* serovar Typhimurium and serovar Enteritidis.

Phage typing gives reproducibility and a high level of discrimination. It has been critical in public health investigations and remains a valuable tool in the detection of *Salmonella* outbreaks (Kafatos et al. 2009). Nevertheless, there are difficulties with phage typing. First, the techniques require considerable training and experience to be reliable. Second, because the phage type depends on bacterial carriage of the surface receptor, this can sometimes be modified, and the phage sensitivity profile altered, by acquisition of plasmids or other genetic elements.

Multi-locus Enzyme Electrophoresis

Serotyping has too many drawbacks to be universally applicable. Furthermore, it offers only a simple binary result of reactivity with a serum, or not. Widely applicable methods were devised for typing and these have been instrumental in recognising the phylogenetic relationships between apparently related organisms.

One such method is multi-locus sequence typing (MLEE), a research technique rather than a routine discrimination method which has been used for the genetic analysis of populations. Cellular extracts of bacteria are separated by gel electrophoresis under non-denaturing conditions and enzymes are detected with specific staining methods (Boerlin 1997). Differences in mobility reflect differences in size and isoelectric point. When used with a number of enzymes, the pattern of mobility reflects the genetic make-up and phylogenetic relationship of the bacterial strains.

Multi-locus Sequence Typing

A development from and an improvement on MLEE is multi-locus sequence typing (MLST). In this, the alleles at multiple housekeeping genes are assigned directly by nucleotide sequencing, rather than indirectly from the electrophoretic mobilities of their gene products (Spratt 1999). A major advantage of this approach is that sequence data are unambiguous and amenable to electronic analysis. It has proven to be a powerful and highly reproducible tool allowing molecular typing of bacterial pathogens (Pérez-Losada et al. 2013).

Serotyping from Antigen Gene Sequence and PCR

For those microorganisms in which serotyping is important, it has sometimes become possible to replace the older, unreliable 'analogue' methods with determining the serotype by PCR of key DNA sequences, or by sequence analysis of the genes responsible for the serotype. This gives very much more certainty to identification of the serotype of a clinical isolate (Bossé et al. 2014).

Whole-genome Sequence Analysis

Over recent years, and particularly since 2005, the cost and time needed for sequencing the ~1 000 000–5 000 000 nucleotides of the bacterial genome using high-throughput sequencing technologies (referred to as 'next-generation sequencing' technologies) have decreased markedly. Comparisons between strains can now be made precisely to the nucleotide level and computing power allows rapid comparisons between strains and analysis of phylogenetic relationships (Bertelli and Greub 2013).

References

Bertelli, C. and Greub, G. (2013). Rapid bacterial genome sequencing: methods and applications in clinical microbiology. *Clinical Microbiology and Infection* 19: 803–813.

Boerlin, P. (1997). Applications of multilocus enzyme electrophoresis in medical microbiology. *Journal of Microbiological Methods* 28: 221–231.

Bossé, J.T., Li, Y., Angen, Ø. et al. (2014). Multiplex PCR assay for unequivocal differentiation of *Actinobacillus pleuropneumoniae* serovars 1 to 3, 5 to 8, 10, and 12. *Journal of Clinical Microbiology* 52: 2380–2385.

Kafatos, G., Andrews, N., Gillespie, I.A. et al. (2009). Impact of reduced numbers of isolates phage-typed on the detection of *Salmonella* outbreaks. *Epidemiology and Infection* 137: 821–827.

Pérez-Losada, M., Cabezas, P., Castro-Nallar, E., and Crandall, K.A. (2013). Pathogen typing in the genomics era: MLST and the future of molecular epidemiology. *Infection, Genetics and Evolution* 16: 38–53.

Pitt, T.L. (2007). Classification, identification and typing of micro-organisms. In: *Medical Microbiology*, 17e (ed. D. Greenwood, R. Slack, J. Peutherer, and M. Barer). Edinburgh: Churchill Livingstone.

Spratt, B.G. (1999). Multilocus sequence typing: molecular typing of bacterial pathogens in an era of rapid DNA sequencing and the internet. *Current Opinion in Microbiology* 2: 312–316.

Wain, J. and Olsen, J.E. (2013). Current and new approaches to typing of *Salmonella*. In: *Salmonella in Domestic Animals*, 2e (ed. P.A. Barrow and U. Methner). Wallingford: CABI.

9

Salmonella

Enterobacteriaceae

The term 'enterobacteria' is the name given to members of the *Enterobacteriaceae* family of Gram-negative bacilli. The term 'coliforms' is also used as a loose name for enterobacteria because they have similarities to *Escherichia coli*. This is simply a convenience word, often used in medical microbiology, to group Gram-negative bacteria which are morphologically indistinguishable, and which grow on MacConkey medium. They are facultative anaerobes that live in the intestinal tract of humans and animals. Some are primary pathogens, e.g. *Salmonella enterica*; many of the others, such as *E. coli*, may be primary or opportunistic pathogens. Others, such as *Proteus* and *Citrobacter*, only cause non-specific, incidental infections. About 28 genera of enterobacteria are now recognised, but the most important of these are *Salmonella*, *Escherichia*, *Shigella*, *Klebsiella* and *Yersinia*.

Identification of Enterobacteria

Colonies of enterobacteria all look virtually the same and they all appear as Gram-negative rods of similar shape and size under the microscope. How do we know they are enterobacteria and how are they identified?

Because enterobacteria are metabolically active and diverse, the genera (and the species within those genera) are identified by using a range of biochemical tests. This is the detection of enzyme activity, metabolic products and carbohydrate fermentations. One crucial test used to differentiate enterobacteria from some other Gram-negative bacteria is the oxidase test. Enterobacteria are always oxidase negative (they do not possess cytochrome C oxidase). They grow on MacConkey agar (grow in the presence of bile salts), are also able to reduce nitrate to nitrite and ferment glucose with the production of acid or acid and gas. The results of these tests reflect the enzyme composition of the organism and thereby its genetic structure.

Individual tests can be done but these are slow and laborious. One example of a commercially available system for multiple biochemical tests is the API 20E system by bioMérieux. It uses 20 biochemical tests to give a profile which can be used to identify the bacteria. This includes detection of enzymes such as urease and lysine decarboxylase, the fermentation of unusual sugars and sugar alcohols such as mannose and sorbitol, the utilisation of citrate as a carbon source, the formation of indole from tryptophan and the proteolytic digestion of gelatine (Figure 9.1).

Salmonella and Public Health

The members of the genus *Salmonella* are arguably the most important pathogens in the enterobacteria. They do not produce urease, they do not digest gelatine and they do not produce indole from tryptophan. They also do not ferment lactose and are therefore said to be non-lactose fermenters (NLFs). They do, however, utilise citrate as a carbon source, and they usually produce H_2S. Salmonellae are often pathogenic for animals and human beings by the oral route. The main reservoir of human and animal infection is animals – poultry, pigs, rodents, cattle, dogs and others. They cause enteritis and systemic infection (septicaemia, abortion) in animals (Barrow et al. 2022).

Fundamentals of Veterinary Microbiology, First Edition. Andrew N. Rycroft.
© 2024 John Wiley & Sons Ltd. Published 2024 by John Wiley & Sons Ltd.
Companion website: www.wiley.com/go/veterinarymicrobiology

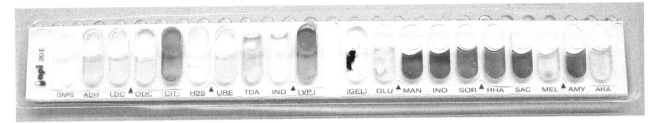

Figure 9.1 Biochemical tests to identify enterobacteria. A pure culture of the bacteria to be identified is suspended in saline and used to inoculate each of the 20 cups containing a different substrate. After incubation, the colour change indicating a positive or negative result is recorded for each cup. The tests are read in triplets. For example, if the first cup is positive, it scores 1, the second cup 2 and the third cup 4. Any that are negative score 0. The combined scoring of each triplet yields a number between 0 and 7. The eight possible combinations of + or − in three cups is recorded as a single digit for the triplet. The seven digits from the 20 cups (together with the oxidase test result) can then be used to interrogate a database and identify the organism.

Salmonella, like many bacteria, can divide every 20 minutes, at least in lab culture. They are also known to inherit new DNA by natural horizontal gene transfer (probably conjugation and transduction) from other organisms. Thus, there is the obvious opportunity for many millions of types to have evolved and diverged over the millennia that these organisms have inhabited the intestinal tracts of reptiles, amphibians, birds and mammals. It has been estimated that *E. coli* and *Salmonella* diverged from a common ancestor approximately 100–150 million years ago. This perhaps parallels the time of divergence of the placental mammals.

Classification of Salmonellae

The taxonomy of *Salmonella* has undergone changes over the last few decades and is still not firmly settled. A diverse range of different bacteria can be called *Salmonella* and the boundaries of what can be called *Salmonella* are blurred. Some of those which we call *Salmonella*, based on their biochemical characteristics and surface antigens, are probably incapable of causing enteric disease (Sanderson and Nair 2013).

The original classification scheme from 1929 was the Kauffman-White scheme. This now describes more than 2600 serovars based on their carriage of lipopolysaccharide (O) and flagellar (H) antigens (Rycroft 2013). Some serovars also carry a capsular antigen, the Vi antigen. This antigen-based system survives today but is being re-evaluated and reinvestigated by the use of DNA-based techniques which do not rely on the antigenic make-up of the bacterial surface.

Bacterial classification has been revolutionised by the advent of techniques such as multi-locus enzyme electrophoresis (MLEE) and multi-locus sequence typing (MLST). More recently, cheap, rapid, genome sequencing is being used. Ultimately, this will allow a definitive classification and comparison of strains. Yet this can also make the matter more complicated. Almost every isolate on the planet is different and possession of the right combination of functional genes to confer disease potential must be present for the organism to be capable of causing disease. Disease-causing capacity could be compromised by even a single mutation in a key gene.

In 1987, it was proposed that *Salmonella* was a genus with a single species - *Salmonella enterica*. This had six subspecies. Two years later, subspecies V was elevated to a full species and given the name *Salmonella bongori*. In 2005, this was formally accepted. The vast majority of *Salmonella* colonising and causing disease in humans and domestic animals belong to *Salmonella enterica* of subspecies I, known as subspecies *enterica*. The other subspecies (II, *salamae*; IIIa, *arizonae*; IIIb, *diarizonae*; IV, *hautenae*; and VI, *indica*) are of minor importance as pathogens of warm-blooded animals (Sanderson and Nair 2013).

Disease Caused by *Salmonella*

Salmonella serovars can be divided into three groups on the basis of their disease production. A few serovars are known to cause systemic disease in a narrow range of host species. The typhoidal salmonellae characteristically produce typhoid-like disease involving the reticuloendothelial system. These include *S.* Typhi and *S.* Paratyphi in humans and, in the case of *S.* Paratyphi B, some animals. They also include *S.* Gallinarum and *S.* Pullorum in fowl and *S.* Abortus-ovis in sheep.

Another group, which includes *S*. Dublin and *S*. Cholerae-suis, cause disease primarily in one animal species but can be pathogenic to others. The third group can cause enteritis in a wide variety of hosts, including humans. These serovars, such as *S*. Enteritidis, do not usually invade beyond the intestinal tract except where the host is unusually susceptible, such as the very young or very old or from diminished immunity for other reasons. These are also widely distributed and found in the alimentary tract of many host animals. Members of this group often pass through domestic animals with little harm to the host but they can be numerically very significant as the cause of human food-borne illness.

Transmission

The normal means of transmission of *Salmonella* is by mouth. Quite a large dose (10^5–10^8 bacteria) is required to achieve infection. This may be because of gastric acidity, normal bacterial flora and local gut immunity. The bacteria multiply in the intestine and either cause acute enteritis (enterocolitis) or invade the body to cause systemic disease. The incubation time from infection to onset of enteritis can be less than 24 hours.

Pathogenicity

Salmonella infections in animals are seen as enteritis, septicaemia or abortion, and combinations of these. It was recognised, for many years, that *Salmonella* infection led to localised enteritis and that this was associated with epithelial tissue damage. Degeneration of the microvilli can be seen when the salmonellae bacteria come into close proximity with the mucosa. Hence, considerable effort was made to identify the *Salmonella* 'enterotoxin'. This anticipated toxin proved to be elusive, and it was eventually accepted that no simple, soluble toxin was produced by *Salmonella*.

The pathogenesis of *Salmonella* infection was known to involve internalisation of the organisms by enterocytes on the mucosal surface of the alimentary tract. These findings, from mouse infection studies, tissue culture and experiments with tied-off loops of ileum in animals under anaesthesia, showed that the organisms are able to pass through the enterocytes to the underlying lamina propria. Here, the cell population includes lymphocytes, plasma cells and macrophages and the immune system is powerful. A substantial inflammatory response with neutrophils and macrophages leads to phagocytosis of the bacteria. It is also responsible for the clinical signs of diarrhoea, fever and intestinal cramping seen in *Salmonella* enteritis. The outcome of the infection is determined here. If the *Salmonella* survives and multiplies inside these professional phagocytic cells, it will lead to systemic disease. Alternatively, destruction of the pathogen at this point limits the progress of disease to enteritis (Fàbrega and Vila 2013).

Production of Enteritis by *Salmonella enterica*

Two virulence determinants were shown to be required for this key characteristic of *Salmonella* pathogenesis: (i) a type III secretion system (T3SS) encoded by *Salmonella* pathogenicity island 1 (SPI-1) and (ii) motility from active flagellae. The pathogenicity island is a contiguous length of DNA carrying genes necessary for the organism to cause disease. They are acquired by horizontal transmission and are incorporated into the genome of the pathogen either as a plasmid or by integration into the chromosome. Closely related organisms without the pathogenicity island are usually non-pathogenic.

The T3SS is a molecular syringe mechanism for injection of bacterial proteins into the epithelial cell (the injectosome). These injected effector proteins then set about causing rearrangement of the actin cytoskeleton of the host cell that induces the cell to take up the *Salmonella* bacterium (Sterzenbach et al. 2013) (Figure 9.2).

Flagellar-mediated motility is also required for efficient epithelial cell invasion. This may be because it increases the chance of contact between the bacteria and the host cells. Without their flagellae, *Salmonella* become much less able to invade and cause inflammation in the intestine.

A further property of *Salmonella* promoting gastroenteritis is now understood. During growth in the intestinal tract, enterobacteria and other organisms depend upon fermentation to generate energy and hydrogen sulfide is generated. This is toxic to the host's cells and enterocytes protect themselves by oxidation of the H_2S to thiosulfate ($S_2O_3^{2-}$). As part of the inflammation in *Salmonella* infection, neutrophils cross the mucosa into the gut lumen. Reactive oxygen intermediates produced by these neutrophils oxidise thiosulfate further to tetrathionate ($S_4O_6^{2-}$). Salmonellae possess the means to utilise tetrathionate as a terminal electron acceptor for anaerobic respiration. It confers an advantage in energy generation over other enterobacteria. This property is the basis of using tetrathionate broth for selective enrichment of *Salmonella* over other enteric bacteria in culture.

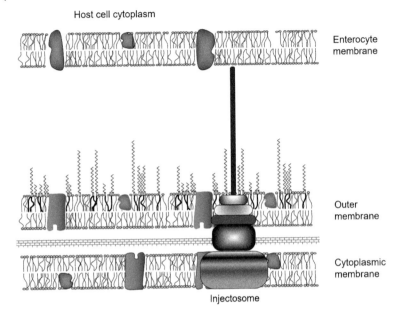

Figure 9.2 The *Salmonella* injectosome apparatus (type 3 secretion system).

The genes for this invasive process are highly conserved among salmonellae, but they are not found in closely related members of the *Enterobacteriaceae* such as *E. coli*. This is the reason why *Salmonella* serovars all have the shared property of invading epithelial cells while other, related species, do not.

Salmonella enterica Invasive Potential

On the other hand, how is it that the different serovars have such different abilities to cause disease? The ability of some serovars or strains (e.g. *Salmonella* Dublin and *S*. Typhimurium) to break out of the intestinal tract and invade the body is associated with carriage of a large plasmid. The plasmids encode genes (*spv* operon) which assist intracellular survival in macrophages and others which chelate iron *in vivo*. But the plasmid genes are themselves insufficient to allow survival in macrophages. Simply transferring the large plasmid to an *E. coli* strain would not confer the resistance to killing seen in *Salmonella*.

Another system operates. Again, this is a type 3 secretion system but encoded by SPI-2. This second T3SS delivers a number of effector proteins into the host macrophage cell, but the means by which these confer resistance to intracellular killing is not certain. Perhaps by hindering formation of the NADPH oxidase complex in the phagosome membrane, the effector proteins reduce the killing potency of the macrophage cells. Ultimately, operation of the phenotype conferred by SPI-2 allows the *Salmonella* to evade the respiratory burst in macrophages (Barrow et al. 2022).

Distant Spread

From survival and multiplication inside macrophages, such salmonellae emerge. They travel, via the lymphatics, to cause bacteraemia and set up potential foci of infection at sites distant from the intestine. In a normal animal, neutrophils control the spread of infection to other tissues. However, it is clear that some sites are less well protected and invasive *Salmonella* may localise in the reproductive tract and, in the gravid uterus, access the placenta, generate inflammation and the resulting placentitis culminates in abortion of the fetus. In this way, *Salmonella* Dublin and *S*. Typhimurium strains will cause abortion in cattle.

Diagnosis of *Salmonella* Infection

The best means to confirm *Salmonella* infection in an animal, in terms of sensitivity and specificity of the test, is culture. There are several options for culture media that can be used. There are three steps: enrichment, selective culture and identification. The methods are designed to overcome the twin problems that (i) a faecal sample may only contain very few *Salmonella* organisms per gram amongst a very large number of non-*Salmonella* bacteria and (ii) the *Salmonella* organisms appear, microscopically and in non-selective culture, to be identical to other members of the enterobacteria.

Enrichment

Enrichment is the process used for improving the chances of isolating the pathogen when only small numbers are present. It increases the proportion of the desired organism in the culture, making it more readily detected. This is especially pertinent when the animal is a carrier, shedding small numbers, perhaps intermittently.

Enrichment is carried out in liquid culture; usually selenite broth, tetrathionate broth or Rappaport-Vassiliadis (RV) broth. All of these are designed to exploit the characteristics of *Salmonella* species when compared with other enterobacteria. Selenite was first used for non-typhoid *Salmonella* isolation in 1936. A sample of faeces or tissue is incubated for 18 hours at 35 °C and it is considered reasonably effective. Tetrathionate is an alternative for *Salmonella* enrichment. Organisms which reduce tetrathionate, such as salmonellae, flourish in the medium whilst many faecal organisms are inhibited. Iodine solution is also added to the medium to improve its selective properties. Again, this is used at 35 °C for 18 hours.

Perhaps the best enrichment medium is RV broth. Originally described in 1956, it has been improved and has been found to be superior to the other *Salmonella* selective enrichment media, especially when a small inoculum of pre-enrichment broth is used. As well as being used to enrich faecal samples, it is used for food and environmental samples. The selective properties of RV were found to be further enhanced by raising the incubation temperature to 42 °C.

Selective Media

Following the enrichment step, cultures for *Salmonella* isolation are plated to selective, differential medium, sometimes more than one type of selective medium. Many of these have been devised but those most commonly in use are brilliant green agar (BG), Salmonella-Shigella agar (SS), desoxycholate citrate agar (DCA) and xylose lysine desoxycholate (XLD) medium. They are all designed to exploit characteristics of *Salmonella* species when compared with other *Enterobacteriaceae*. They all have slightly different uses, but XLD seems to give clear results with the fewest disadvantages.

XLD was described in 1965, and originally designed to detect *Shigella* in human faeces. However, it is very effective in isolation and presumptive identification of *Salmonella*. It relies on the strongly selective effect of the bile salt desoxycholate to remove most non-enterobacteria and some enterobacteria. Then, acid production from the fermentation of either lactose or sucrose, in the presence of phenol red indicator, by non-*Salmonella* organisms shows their colonies as bright yellow. Such colonies can be discarded. Most enterobacteria, except *Shigella* species, will also ferment xylose, so the inclusion of xylose is to recognise *Shigella* (usually irrelevant in animal samples). However, decarboxylation of lysine to the diamine cadaverine [$NH_2(CH_2)_5NH_2$] by *Salmonella* causes an alkaline reaction (pink colony). Added to this is the production of hydrogen sulfide. This converts the ferric ammonium citrate to ferric sulfide, which is black, acting as a clear indicator in the colony. The *Salmonella* is using sulfur, instead of oxygen, as a terminal electron acceptor in anaerobic respiration.

Identification of *Salmonella*

Once characteristic colonies have been recognised on the selective differential medium, these are called presumptive *Salmonella*: they are presumed to be but need to be confirmed. For this, a series of biochemical tests will confirm the identity of most *Salmonella*. The API system, as described above, has been in use since the early 1970s.

Once identified biochemically as *Salmonella*, an isolate is designated to a serovar on the basis of O and H agglutination with known antiserum. That is, its serovar is determined by the antigens of the LPS O-side chain and flagellae. Each new species of *Salmonella* has traditionally been named after the place where it was first isolated, e.g. *Salmonella enterica*, serovar Derby, *S.* Montevideo, *S.* London. This historically derived system has resulted in the 2600 separate serovars of the same species.

Salmonellae are grouped into nine groups (A, B, C, D, etc.) on the basis of an O antigen component unique to that group. *Salmonella* Typhimurium falls into group B because it possesses antigen 4, *S.* Dublin in group D because it has antigen 9, *S.* Cholerae-suis in group C1 with antigen 7 and so on. This is determined by slide agglutination or tube agglutination of the bacteria with specific antisera containing antibody to the individual antigen. Determining the full serovar requires specialist laboratory such as the APHA in the UK, with all the necessary anti-O and anti-H antibody reagents.

H antigen Phase Change

Most salmonellas display an H antigen and are motile. However, this antigen can switch so that the organism displays an alternative H antigen. The bacteria are said to be in 'phase 1' or 'phase 2'. Both H phase antigens need to be recognised before the organism can be fully identified to its serovar and so the identifying lab must test which H antigen is carried and then allow the bacterium to switch phase and then test for the other H antigen.

The change from one phase to another is due to a genetic switch: an invertible segment of DNA which acts as promoter for one of the H antigen genes. Either one or the other H antigen gene is transcribed. The change can be 'forced', or selected for, by a simple procedure in which the *Salmonella* is cultured on one side of a trough cut in an agar plate. Sterile, absorbent paper provides a bridge across the trough, but the paper is soaked in antiserum containing antibody to the H antigen already being expressed. Only those *Salmonella* organisms that spontaneously switch to the alternative phase can cross the bridge. Only their flagellae will not be bound by the antibody and become tangled and immobilised by the antibody. Salmonellae with the alternative phase H antigen can usually be cultured from across the other side of the trough.

The site-specific inversion of the H2 promoter region (*hin*) causes either phase 1 [H1] flagellae or phase 2 [H2] to be transcribed and expressed, never both (Figure 9.3).

Carriage

One of the important characters of *Salmonella* strains is their ability to persist in the gut or perhaps the gall bladder and continue to be excreted in the faeces after clinical recovery. This is known as active carriage. It is probably related to the ability of the bacteria to survive intracellularly where they are protected from the immune system and most antimicrobials. Carriage may also be latent so that the organism is present in the tissues and reappears in the faeces only intermittently, usually without symptoms. Long-term asymptomatic carriage is an effective means of spreading the infection to other individuals via faecal contamination of water, food and the environment.

Salmonellosis is an important zoonosis and the majority of *Salmonella* infections in humans are contracted from animals and their products – particularly poultry and cattle. Pigs also carry *Salmonella* serovars such as *S.* Derby apparently without clinical signs. Tortoises and terrapins are commonly healthy carriers of *Salmonella* that may infect humans. Snakes and other reptiles also carry *Salmonella* strains.

Stress can promote excretion of *Salmonella* in carrier animals. Stress factors include corticosteroids, antibiotics, concurrent virus infection and transport/overcrowding. This is sometimes seen in horses when under stress; they begin shedding *Salmonella* without any known contact with an infected animal or material.

Poultry Infection

There are two highly host-adapted species of *Salmonella* which infect poultry. These are *S.* Pullorum (egg-transmitted; bacillary white diarrhoea or pullorum disease) and *S.* Gallinarum (older birds; fowl typhoid). Both are now very rare as programmes for their control have largely eradicated these organisms in the UK and other developed areas (Shivaprasad et al. 2013). These include the serological detection of antibody in carrier birds. The Pullorum test is a rapid whole-blood slide agglutination test using stained Pullorum antigen which detects antibody to both *S.* Pullorum and *S.* Gallinarum (since they have the same O antigen). No anti-H because they are both non-flagellate and hence non-motile.

Far more common causes of human food poisoning from chicken meat are *S.* Typhimurium and *S.* Enteritidis (particularly phage type 4). These cause losses among young poultry, but many birds survive and go on to excrete the organism in the faeces for a long time. Infection of chicks is via the ovary to the yolk sac or from the contaminated shell immediately after hatching.

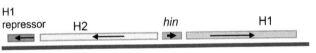

Phase 1: Transcription of H1. The H1 repressor and H2 gene **not** transcribed.

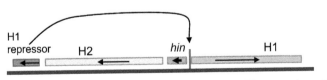

Phase 2: Invertible segment *hin* inverts: H1 repressor and H2 gene are transcribed. H1 transcription is repressed.

Figure 9.3 The genetic basis of flagellar phase change in *Salmonella*.

Other Enterobacteria

Shigella

Shigella spp. are the cause of dysentery in humans and primates. They are enteroinvasive, penetrating the intestinal mucosa and causing necrosis in patches of mucosa. They do not invade beyond the lamina propria to the bloodstream. The invasive potential is carried by a large plasmid and is related to the ability to survive inside the host cells. Some strains produce Shiga toxin which is related to the Shigatoxin of some pathogenic (STEC) strains of *Escherichia coli*.

Klebsiella

Klebsiella spp. are lactose fermenters which tend to produce large capsules which make the colonies large and mucoid. *K. pneumoniae* is the species name used for pathogenic strains. They frequently show wide-spectrum antibiotic resistance. *Klebsiella* are soil and environmental bacteria (they can non-symbiotically fix N_2), and although they are found in the gut, they are not recognised as indicators of faecal contamination of water. They are usually opportunistic pathogens in infections similar to those caused by other non-virulent enterobacteria, such as wound infections. They also cause acute mastitis in cattle and metritis leading to infertility or abortion in mares.

Proteus

Proteus species inhabit the gut and cause incidental infections such as urinary tract infection. They are highly motile and usually swarm on blood agar (but not on selective media such as MacConkey). They are NLFs and must be distinguished from *Salmonella* as they are never pathogenic in the gut. They are always urease positive within a few hours while *Salmonella* are not.

Yersinia

Yersiniae are NLFs and are facultative intracellular pathogens. Members of the genus *Yersinia* were considered enterobacteria, but they grow more slowly and at lower temperature than most other enterobacteria and in 2016 they were separated into a new family, the *Yersiniaceae*. They had been originally classified as *Pasteurella* sp. *Yersinia* species cause disease in animals but are increasingly recognised as important agents of zoonosis (Moxley 2022).

Invasive yersiniae localise inside fixed macrophages (such as Kupffer cells) where they are able to grow. They exist inside phagolysosomes and do not seem to interfere with degranulation or lysosomal fusion. They therefore seem to be resistant to the normal O_2-dependent and O_2-independent killing mechanisms. When the macrophages are destroyed by the bacteria, both in regional lymph nodes and in liver and spleen, septicaemia results. All *Yersinia* species and strains seem to be equally capable of intracellular survival, and equally virulent when injected intravenously. The differences in pathogenicity appear to be in their ability to reach the target macrophages from peripheral routes of infection. Virulence depends on carriage of plasmids.

Yersinia pseudotuberculosis var. *pestis* is the cause of bubonic plague (Black Death), a disease of rats which is transmitted by fleas – sometimes to humans – known today as sylvatic plague. It is not a cause of significant veterinary disease. It carries three plasmids, two of which are only found in this species. These encode coagulase and fibrinolytic activities on the small, 9 kb plasmid and a potent exotoxin on the 98 kb plasmid.

Y. pseudotuberculosis var. *pseudotuberculosis* resembles *Y. pestis* but is less virulent. It has only a 68 kb plasmid, loss of which results in complete avirulence. Although a number of genes on the plasmid are known, the mechanisms by which this plasmid confers virulence are not yet clear. It can produce sporadic cases of pseudotuberculosis in animals and humans, the reservoir of infection being wild birds (blackbirds and starlings) and rodents. Outbreaks of pseudotuberculosis in pigs have been traced to their eating farmyard birds infected with *Yersinia*. The organisms can penetrate epithelial cells and multiply in macrophages with granuloma formation. The main granulomatous lesions occur in the gut wall, the mesenteric lymph nodes and other organs with concurrent gastrointestinal symptoms (Moxley 2022).

Y. enterocolitica is similar but less pathogenic than *Y. pseudotuberculosis*. (It also possesses the 68 kb plasmid.) It is commonly carried in the oral cavity and gut of animals, such as pigs, from where it can contaminate the carcass and from there it can cause disease in humans. In humans, it produces enterocolitis which can last for 1–2 weeks or develop into a chronic form of the disease which lasts for many months. *Y. enterocolitica* infections are an important cause of enteric disease in farmed deer.

References

Barrow, P.A., Jones, M.A., Mellor, K.C., and Thomson, N.R. (2022). Salmonella. In: *Pathogenesis of Bacterial Infections in Animals* (ed. J. Prescott, J. MacInnes, F. Van Immerseel, et al.). Chichester: Wiley.

Fàbrega, A. and Vila, J. (2013). *Salmonella enterica* serovar Typhimurium skills to succeed in the host: virulence and regulation. *Clinical Microbiology Reviews* 26: 308–341.

Moxley, R.A. (2022). Family *Yersiniaceae*. In: *Veterinary Microbiology*, 4e (ed. D.S. McVey, M. Kennedy, M.M. Chengappa, and R. Wilkes). Chichester: Wiley.

Rycroft, A.N. (2013). Structure, function and synthesis of surface polysaccharides in *Salmonella*. In: *Salmonella in Domestic Animals*, 2e (ed. P.A. Barrow and U. Methner). Wallingford: CABI Publishing.

Sanderson, K.E. and Nair, S. (2013). Taxonomy and species concepts in the genus salmonella. In: *Salmonella in Domestic Animals*, 2e (ed. P. Barrow and U. Methner). Wallingford: CABI.

Shivaprasad, H.L., Methner, U., and Barrow, P.A. (2013). *Salmonella* infections in the domestic fowl. In: *Salmonella in Domestic Animals*, 2e (ed. P. Barrow and U. Methner). Wallingford: CABI.

Sterzenbach, T., Crawford, R.W., Winter, S.E., and Baumler, A.J. (2013). *Salmonella* virulence mechanisms and their genetic basis. In: *Salmonella in Domestic Animals*, 2e (ed. P. Barrow and U. Methner). Wallingford: CABI.

10

Escherichia coli – An Intestinal Pathogen

The fact that *Escherichia coli* is considered as a single species is curious since it is perhaps more diverse than the entire *Salmonella* genus. It is the predominant species in the aerobic Gram-negative flora of the colon of most animals and most strains in that location are harmless residents. For this reason, it is abundant in the environment where there are faeces. *E. coli* is so closely associated with faeces that it is widely used as an indicator of faecal pollution of water: rivers, beaches and drinking water. The viable *E. coli* count is used as a measure of the level of faecal pollution. While *E. coli* itself is generally harmless, the presence of faeces represents a serious hazard from other enteric pathogens: *Salmonella*, *Campylobacter*, viruses, parasites and indeed pathogenic types of *E. coli.*

Although most strains of *E. coli* are not pathogens, it is a very versatile organism capable of causing a variety of infections, both intestinal disease (enteritis and diarrhoea) and extraintestinal disease (mastitis, wound infection, urinary tract infection, septicaemia). Strains that cause disease in animals and humans do so when they are in the right location and if they possess a necessary complement of pathogenicity-related characteristics. These characteristics vary considerably and a strain pathogenic in the intestinal tract of piglets is most unlikely to possess the genetic make-up needed for it to cause urinary tract infection in a female dog.

As found in other enterobacteria, *E. coli* has an O antigen (LPS) and an H antigen (flagellae). In addition, it possesses polysaccharide K antigens and usually fimbrial (F) antigens as well. There are >150 O antigens, >55 H antigens and >70 K antigens. These antigens have been used to identify particular strains and follow patterns of disease. They were detected in labs with specialised antibody reagents using agglutination tests. Although certain combinations of these are common in nature, there are no strict rules governing the association of O, H and K antigens. These antigen combinations have therefore been used in epidemiological typing of *E. coli*: one strain being O125:K12:H42, another O122:K12:H7, and so on. Two isolates could be shown to be different or a given serotype or range of serotypes could be shown to be associated with disease.

In practice, this led to many misconceptions about the involvement of these antigens in the ability of *E. coli* to cause disease. For example, certain O types are said to be associated with enteric disease and other O types with upper UTI in humans. This reflects the clonal nature of *E. coli* strains: some clonal groups (perhaps species) carrying a limited number of O antigens are able to resist the host defences of the urinary tract while other clonal groups, also associated with a different set of O antigens, carry the pathogenicity characters to cause enteric disease. However, these are only associations and are not always reflecting the presence of the pathogenicity factors.

Serotyping with antibody was laborious and ultimately a rather fruitless exercise since the antigens were unrelated to disease production. It has been superseded by multi-locus sequence typing (MLST) and more recently by whole-genome sequencing (WGS) of strains.

E. coli as an Enteric Pathogen

Six different pathotypes of *E. coli* are currently recognised that cause disease in the intestinal tract. Much of the funding for study of these has been intended to understand human disease and much less is known about the role of *E. coli* in animal disease. The pathotypes are based on pathogenicity characteristics: enterotoxigenic (ETEC), enteropathogenic (EPEC), enterohaemorrhagic (EHEC; now better known as Shiga toxin-producing [STEC]), enteroinvasive (EIEC), diffusely

Fundamentals of Veterinary Microbiology, First Edition. Andrew N. Rycroft.
© 2024 John Wiley & Sons Ltd. Published 2024 by John Wiley & Sons Ltd.
Companion website: www.wiley.com/go/veterinarymicrobiology

adherent (DAEC) and enteroaggregative *E. coli* (EAEC). The latter three of these are not recognised pathogens of animals yet animals may, in future, be found to act as reservoirs of these pathotypes.

Adhesion Factors

Although *E. coli* is a major inhabitant of the mammalian large bowel, it is not normally found in great numbers in the small intestine. Some strains of *E. coli* possess fimbriae which attach the bacteria to the epithelium of the small intestine of particular animal species. Because these surface antigens were thought to be capsules, they were, in some cases, given K antigen numbers – in particular, K88 which is associated with adhesion to the mucosa of the ilium of the pig, and K99, for pigs and cattle. These are not polysaccharide K antigens but protein fimbriae and are now renamed with F numbers. There is now known to be a large variety of different fimbrial adhesins; at least 25 are known in human ETEC strains and there may be very many in strains affecting different animal species. The fimbriae are encoded by genes carried on plasmids.

Enterotoxigenic *E. coli* (ETEC)

Some strains of *E. coli* also carry a plasmid which encodes an enterotoxin. Two types of enterotoxin are known: a heat-labile toxin (LT) and a heat-stable toxin (ST). It was first demonstrated by a veterinary researcher, H. Williams Smith, that if plasmids carrying (i) a toxin and (ii) fimbrial genes are stably transferred to a strain of *E. coli*, that strain will become enterotoxigenic and capable of causing disease in piglets. This is now termed a diarrhoeagenic pathotype of *E. coli* (Qadri et al. 2005) (Figure 10.1).

The disease pattern in animals and humans from infection with enterotoxigenic *E. coli* (ETEC) is similar; it is a secretory diarrhoea in which fluid is actively removed from tissues to the gut lumen. In adult humans, the syndrome is sometimes termed traveller's diarrhoea; in pigs and calves it is called scours. In fact, the greatest impact is in young children and newborn animals. The fimbrial antigen or colonisation factor determines the species specificity of the disease. Strains with human CFAs (colonisation factor antigens) will not infect animals and those with K88 or 987P will not infect humans.

Heat-labile enterotoxin (LT) is an oligomeric toxin composed of an enzymatically active A subunit (30 kDa; two fragments – A1 and A2) and five identical B subunits of 12 kDa that constitute the binding portion or B oligomer. It attaches to the brush border of the epithelial cells of the small intestinal mucosa.

LT exerts its pathophysiological effects through the NAD^+-dependent ADP-ribosylation of guanine nucleotide binding proteins of the adenylate cyclase complex in eukaryotic cell membranes (Figure 10.2). ADP-ribosylation of the stimulatory subunit (G_s) by LT causes the irreversible activation of adenylate cyclase in target cells. This raises the intracellular cAMP level and causes intense hypersecretion of chloride and water into the lumen of the small intestine and inhibits reabsorption of Na^+ ions. This leads to distension of the gut with fluid and watery diarrhoea which lasts for several days. It can be fatal due to dehydration and electrolyte disturbance unless effective rehydration is enabled.

LT is antigenic. Animals develop immunity to the natural disease with local and systemic antibody to LT protein and the fimbrial antigen. Parenteral (systemic) vaccination of pigs and cattle is practised to immunise the dam in order to protect

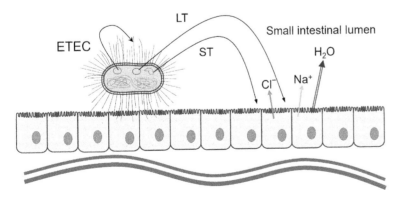

Figure 10.1 ETEC: plasmids encode adhesive fimbriae and enterotoxins LT or ST (or sometimes both). These act on enterocytes to cause water to move from the body to the intestinal lumen.

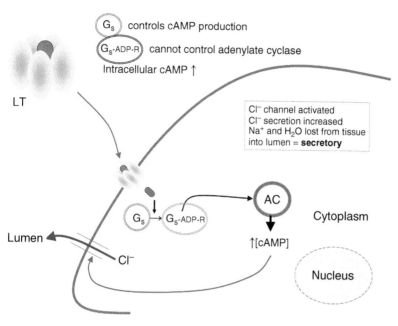

Figure 10.2 The action of LT on enterocytes causes increased cyclic AMP and reversal of the chloride pump, and leads to a secretory diarrhoea.

neonatal animals against scours via colostral antibody (passive immunity). Early vaccines used whole killed *E. coli* cells. These vaccines were not very effective and were improved by including the fimbrial antigens known to be most common in farm animal disease, such as K88, K99, 987P together with the B fragment of LT enterotoxin. In that case, the passive antibody is delivered to the mucosal surface in the young animal and can give effective protection. Unfortunately, different colonisation factors (fimbriae) together with the production of ST by many strains of ETEC mean that current vaccines are less than fully efficacious.

Heat-stable enterotoxin (ST) is a much smaller molecule. There are two forms: the STh variant, affecting humans, has 19 amino acids; the STp version, known to have action in humans and animals, has 18 amino acids. ST acts by activating microvillous guanylate cyclase in enteric epithelial cells. It does this by mimicking a natural hormone, guanylin, that is thought to ensure that the mucin layer remains moist by stimulating fluid and electrolyte secretion. ST seems to be a hyperactive form of the natural guanylin. Because it is so small, the molecule is non-antigenic and is not included in vaccines. However, efforts have been made to generate antibody by attaching ST to larger carrier molecules. These are not in commercial use at present but bioconjugation and genetic fusion methods are under investigation for the future development of improved vaccines (Zhang et al. 2010).

How do the *E. coli* strains benefit from these virulence properties? It may be that by causing diarrhoea, the bacteria are able to disseminate among the population of animals more effectively and thereby perpetuate their existence more widely than if they were to rely on colonisation through normal faecal–oral transmission.

Other mechanisms by which *E. coli* causes diarrhoea are also recognised. These mainly apply to humans but some are relevant to animals and public health.

Enteropathogenic *E. coli* (EPEC)

Enteropathogenic *E. coli* possesses an adherence factor, encoded by genes on a plasmid, known as bundle-forming pili (Bfp). The pathogen also carries genes, known as *eae* (for enterocyte attachment and effacement), that bring about close (intimate) attachment between the *E. coli* and the enterocyte. This is followed by ultrastructural changes (localised removal in the microvilli of the enterocyte, known as effacement) and actin pedestal formation. One of these genes, *eaeA*, encodes a protein known as intimin. Another (*tir*) encodes the translocated intimin receptor (Tir). *E. coli* uses a type 3 secretion system, resembling a molecular syringe, to inject Tir from the pathogen into the host cell. Tir inserts itself into the host cell membrane; intimin, on the *E. coli* outer membrane, is then bound to Tir. This anchors the EPEC to the enterocyte and causes the close association. Further steps lead to actin polymerisation which causes pedestal formation. This is associated with an intense inflammatory response. While the actin is polymerised inside enterocytes, the same pathogen is able to block actin polymerisation in phagocytic cells: an antiphagocytic mechanism to evade uptake of the EPEC by neutrophils and macrophages.

Attaching and effacing lesions in the lining of the gut were first recognised in 1983. EPEC is known to be a serious cause of disease in young children in the developing world and also in previously unexposed susceptible adults. It is known to be a relatively rare, but serious, cause of severe enteritis in the dog. By implication, the dog may therefore be a source of EPEC infection for humans although there is little evidence to suggest it is regularly transmitted from dog to owner.

Enterohaemorrhagic *E. coli* (EHEC)

Enterohaemorrhagic *E. coli* was first recognised in the early 1990s in the USA as a cause of an outbreak of haemorrhagic colitis in children followed, in many cases, by acute renal failure. Similar disease outbreaks of haemolytic uraemic syndrome (HUS) were seen and all were found to be associated with an *E. coli* of serotype O157:H7. It was traced to ground beef used to make burgers, and cooking practice had been inadequate to kill the offending bacteria in the centre of the burger.

The pathogenic organism was named enterohaemorrhagic *E. coli*. It was often found to be of serovar O157:H7 but EHEC strains were gradually discovered that were of different serovars and in fact, approximately 50% of strains causing HUS are non-O157 yet carry the necessary genes to cause the pathological effects. EHEC strains are essentially the same as EPEC strains (see above) but they produce an additional toxin, known as Shiga-like toxin (SLT) because of its similarity to the toxin of *Shigella dysenteriae*. For this reason, pathogenic *E. coli* strains previously known as EHEC are now correctly referred to as STEC (Croxen et al. 2013).

Two SLTs are now recognised: Stx-1 and Stx-2. These are encoded on a temperate phage genome and only by infection of the strain with the phage and expression of those phage genes does that strain acquire the ability to produce one of the toxins. It is Stx-2 that is most associated with strains of STEC that cause HUS in humans. Of course, since the phage is a carrier of these toxin genes, that same phage can enter lytic phase and infect related, pathogenic strains, causing them also to become capable of producing the Stx.

Confusingly, the Stx previously went by the name vero toxin (VT). A vero toxin is a toxin whose activity damages vero (African green monkey kidney) cells. This cell line is particularly susceptible, and production of cytopathic effects has been used to detect new and different toxin activities. Other, quite unrelated toxins have therefore been described as vero toxins in microbial pathogenicity.

STEC remains an important pathogen. While animals suffer little disease from this pathotype, outbreaks of serious, life-changing disease in humans continue to be seen throughout the developed world. The disease is usually transmitted from uncooked meat, primarily beef. This is because STEC can be carried in young beef cattle without clinical signs. In some cases, the meat may become surface contaminated with intestinal contents at slaughter. Remarkably, the infective dose for a human is approximately 10 viable bacteria. This is 0.0001% of the infective dose (10^7 CFU) of *Salmonella* required to cause disease in a human subject. Previously cooked foods contaminated with uncooked meat juices or incompletely cooked burgers in which STEC is protected from lethal heating continue to be sources of the infection.

Enteroaggregative *E. coli* (EAEC)

Enteroaggregative *E. coli* are responsible for a persistent form of diarrhoea in children. They adhere to the small intestinal mucosa in clumps, or aggregates, rather than evenly across the tissue surface. They produce a fibrillar adhesin and an enterotoxin similar to ST known as enteroaggregative ST and a pore-forming RTX-like toxin.

Enteroinvasive *E. coli* (EIEC)

Enteroinvasive *E. coli* causes a dysentery-like illness (bloody, mucoid diarrhoea) and the strains invade epithelial cells by inducing endocytosis and pass across the gut wall to the lamina propria. This is very similar to the pathogenesis of dysentery caused by *Shigella* species. It is restricted to humans and non-human primates (Croxen et al. 2013).

Diffusely Adherent *E. coli* (DAEC)

Diffusely adherent *E. coli* strains have been associated with urinary tract infections and diarrhoea in children aged 18 months to 5 years. They are not, to date, associated with enteric disease in animals.

References

Croxen, M.A., Law, R.J., Scholz, R. et al. (2013). Recent advances in understanding enteric pathogenic *Escherichia coli*. *Clinical Microbiology Reviews* 26: 822–880.

Qadri, F., Svennerholm, A.-M., Faruque, A.S.G., and Sack, R.B. (2005). Enterotoxigenic *Escherichia coli* in developing countries: epidemiology, microbiology, clinical features, treatment, and prevention. *Clinical Microbiology Reviews* 18: 465–483.

Zhang, W., Zhang, C., Francis, D.H. et al. (2010). Genetic fusions of heat-labile (LT) and heat-stable (ST) toxoids of porcine enterotoxigenic *Escherichia coli* elicit neutralizing anti-LT and anti-STa antibodies. *Infection and Immunity* 78: 316–325.

11

Escherichia coli as an Extraintestinal Pathogen

Escherichia coli causes many soft tissue infections in adult animals. Other enterobacteria such as *Klebsiella* and *Proteus* produce clinical signs that are not distinguishable from those of *E. coli*, although the epidemiology varies between species. *E. coli* is the most common organism infecting the urinary tract (anatomical proximity), causing pyometra in the dog and cat, and is a common cause of acute mastitis in lactating animals. It is also a common cause of wound infections of many types (Manges et al. 2019).

  E. coli (and all other enterobacteria) are Gram-negative, facultative anaerobes. They will voraciously consume oxygen when it is available but can grow in low oxygen and anaerobically when the need arises. They are motile by peritrichous flagellae and oxidase negative. They have a formidable synthetic capability and will grow using no more than ammonium sulfate solution, inorganic phosphate and glucose (with a few trace elements) although adaptation to such a medium takes several hours of lag phase.

  In clinical practice, *E. coli* is readily cultured for identification on rich medium such as blood agar and MacConkey's medium. It produces lactose-fermenting colonies on MacConkey that are easily recognised. Nevertheless, for more accurate identification, biochemical tests are used. These include production of indole from tryptophan; inability to utilise citrate as a carbon source or to split urea into NH_3 and CO_2 (urease test). It is also negative in the Voges Proskauer (VP) test for production of acetoin but positive in the methyl red test which detects the production of stable acids such as lactic acid and acetic acid from the fermentation of glucose. Although pre-prepared tests such as API 20E can be used for this, biochemical tests take 1–2 days to obtain the result and are not usually necessary. Furthermore, PCR-based testing for *E. coli*-specific genes, if needed, are now much quicker and unequivocal. Serotyping the O, H and K antigens, that was once common as investigators used serotypes as epidemiological markers and sought links between carriage of serotype antigens of *E. coli* and pathogenicity (Ørskov et al. 1977), is now rarely conducted, yet serotypes are still quoted as a way of describing strains, for example in the constituents of animal vaccines.

  Analysis of thousands of natural and clinical isolates of *E. coli* from humans and other sources by multilocus enzyme electrophoresis (MLEE) indicated that the species could be subdivided into four groups, designated A, B1, B2 and D, plus a minor group E that has largely been ignored because it clustered inconsistently in subsequent analyses (Wirth et al. 2006). This has been superseded by multilocus sequence typing (MLST) which offers genetically based typing and perhaps better reflects relationships between strains and associations with pathogenicity. The current classification, based on seven housekeeping genes, again divides the species into five phylogroups: A, B1, B2, D and E, but with many further subgroupings (Kaas et al. 2012). There remains only a loose relationship between phylogroup and pathogenicity class.

  Whole-genome sequencing is now so advanced that it is further revolutionising the taxonomic tree of organisms like *E. coli* and allowing deeper insight into their evolution and genetic exchange.

Pathogenicity

Pathogenic characters that enable *E. coli* to invade are those that allow survival and growth in the tissues. These include α-haemolysin which may be cytotoxic; high-affinity iron acquisition systems such as the siderophores enterochelin and aerobactin; K antigens (polysaccharide capsules) which prevent phagocytosis or mimic the antigens of the host body and increase resistance to complement; and fimbriae that allow specific attachment to mucosal surfaces and tissue surfaces.

Fundamentals of Veterinary Microbiology, First Edition. Andrew N. Rycroft.
© 2024 John Wiley & Sons Ltd. Published 2024 by John Wiley & Sons Ltd.
Companion website: www.wiley.com/go/veterinarymicrobiology

In some cases, *E. coli* may reach the bloodstream to cause bacteraemia and sepsis. Other members of the enterobacteria cause similar infections, but their relative importance reflects their lower numbers in the normal gut flora and the relatively virulent nature of some *E. coli* strains.

Pathogenesis

Specific syndromes caused by relatively virulent *E. coli* are recognised. In newly hatched chickens, *E. coli* may cause a septicaemia: avian colibacillosis. The organism gains access to the bird either by contamination of the egg surface with faeces or via infection of the ovary of the hen. Infection is via the respiratory tract; bacteraemia appears to be an essential element of the clinical disease. Colibacillosis is seen clinically as acute colisepticaemia, subacute fibrinopurulent serositis and a chronic granulomatous disease of the viscera. Strains causing the disease are termed avian pathogenic *E. coli* (APEC). They are predominantly of serovars O1, O2 and O78 and carry a variety of colonisation factors, invasive and antiphagocytic mechanisms and iron chelating systems (Dziva and Stevens 2008). Colibacillosis in older birds may due to inhalation of *E. coli* in dust. The respiratory infection then spreads to the bloodstream, causing acute colisepticaemia. The acute, invasive phase is characterised by airsacculitis, pericarditis and perihepatitis. It is often secondary to virus or mycoplasma infection and environmental stress.

In neonatal calves, piglets, foals and lambs, virulent *E. coli* strains can penetrate the intestinal mucosa or gain access via the umbilicus, to cause joint-ill, peritonitis or systemic disease: colisepticaemia. It is probable that *E. coli* bacteria often gain access to the bloodstream in small numbers but that adequate colostrum intake prevents establishment of infection. It is the 'invasive' strains of *E. coli* that survive the host defences while most strains do not. These are not to be confused with the enteroinvasive strains (EIEC, see above). Virulence of strains is dependent upon those adhesive properties, complement resistance and Fe uptake ability but also influenced by husbandry including hygiene, ammonia, excessive dust, viral infections and changes in temperature.

Once established in the blood of a young animal, the infection will progress rapidly to death from endotoxin, the release of inflammatory effectors, vascular damage, hypotensive shock and circulatory collapse. One of the confusing aspects of colisepticaemia, promulgated for many years, was the association with diarrhoea in terminally sick animals. Enteric disturbance in this case arises from the effects of the systemic disease rather than a direct effect of *E. coli* or toxins in the gut.

Urinary Tract Infection

Escherichia coli is the most common causative agent of urinary tract infection (UTI) in cats and dogs. Much of the understanding of pathogenesis and the attributes of strains causing UTI has come from research into human disease but this can probably be extrapolated to animal disease, particularly since much of the evidence has come from animal models of infection, particularly the mouse.

Urinary infections are most commonly caused by uropathogenic (UPEC) strains of *E. coli* that ascend the urethra to the bladder (Lloyd et al. 2009). These differ from other (commensal) *E. coli* strains by possessing additional genetic material, often carried on pathogenicity islands, that encode components contributing to pathogenicity. These include haemolysin, secreted proteins, specific LPS O-antigen and capsule types, iron acquisition systems and fimbrial adhesins. They are most common among females because the bacterial strains are carried in the colon and the route from rectum to urethral opening is much shorter in female than male animals. The female urethra is also much shorter.

Most bacteria that gain access to the urethra are removed by the flushing action of urine. Hence, in animals with impaired micturition or urine retention, there is a greater chance of UTI. Nevertheless, UPEC strains adhere, very effectively, to the epithelium of the urethra and bladder. Type 1 fimbriae (those responsible for mannose-sensitive haemagglutination) are now known to contribute to adhesion in humans and almost certainly the development of urinary infection of animals. Most *E. coli* strains produce type 1 fimbriae. They can bind mannose residues in the glycoproteins on bladder epithelium via their tip protein, FimH. Another adhesin is the P-fimbriae (aptly named, but originating from their association with pyelonephritis) which are regularly found in UPEC strains but not on benign *E. coli*. These bind to a disaccharide (D-galactose-D-galactose) which is found on a ceramide lipid in the membrane of host bladder cells.

Other adhesins probably play a role and there may be those that specifically recognise receptors on cells of the dog or the cat.

A more recently recognised property of UPEC is their ability to invade, and hide, in bladder epithelial cells (the uroepithelium). It appears, from research in human UTI, that type 1 fimbriae stimulate the uroepithelium to internalise the bacteria. When infected with *E. coli*, the uroepithelium is more readily shed from the bladder than uninfected cells. This removal of infected uroepithelium may constitute a defence mechanism. However, some cells infected with bacteria are not shed and the UPEC are protected from removal by the normal urinary flushing and, indeed, from some antimicrobial treatments such as β-lactams which cannot penetrate the epithelial cells. These infected cells may also serve as a reservoir for recurrence of UTI in the future. Recurrence of UTI is a recognised problem in humans and certainly, we have seen evidence of multiple, sequential *E. coli* infections in the cat.

Evidence suggests that the profound inflammatory response from UPEC infection in the bladder is attributable to the combined, even synergistic, effects of endotoxin and P-fimbriae. As part of the response, neutrophils cross the bladder mucosa into the lumen of the bladder. These are considered essential for eventually clearing the infection. However, there is also some evidence that toxins from UPEC play a role in the pathogenesis. Urinary strains of *E. coli* have long been recognised as haemolytic. This is due to secretion of α-haemolysin (HlyA), an RTX group cytolysin closely related to those crucial to virulence in many other Gram-negative pathogens. HlyA is encoded on a plasmid in some strains and the chromosome in others. It is known to be a potent neutrophil and macrophage toxin but may also have important action in stimulating cytokine release and subtle damage to other cell types – even at very low concentration. UPEC strains unable to produce P-fimbriae or HlyA through mutation are unable to cause UTI in a mouse model, while their isogenic parental strains (same genetic background) colonise the bladder and kidney and kill a proportion of the mice. Notably, a very similar cytolytic toxin is produced by *Proteus* species isolated from UTI.

Another toxin, known as cytotoxic necrotising factor (CNF-1), may also be involved in the pathogenicity of UPEC strains. In addition, UPEC strains carry effective iron acquisition mechanisms and those infecting the kidney are almost always resistant to the bactericidal action of complement.

Treatment of UTI is with antibiotics. However, because of the common recurrence of these infections, multiple treatments may be needed and many strains express resistance to the common antimicrobial drugs used, such as amoxicillin and trimethoprim/sulfonamide.

Vaccination Against UTI

A vaccine to prevent *E. coli* UTI in humans and animals would be a great achievement (Brumbaugh and Mobley 2012). One approach has been to use the FimH protein on the tip of type 1 fimbriae as a vaccine antigen to induce antibody that would prevent adhesion of the *E. coli* to the uroepithelium. This is a highly conserved antigen, and is carried by more than 90% of UPEC strains, so FimH was an appropriate candidate. Although early studies (1997) of vaccination in mice reported a 99% reduction in bladder colonisation, later research (2011) showed a different result. Immunisation with FimH induced antibodies that recognised FimH. However, they did not inhibit the adhesive function. On the contrary, the antibodies enhanced FimH-mediated binding to mannosylated glycoprotein receptor and substantially increased bacterial adhesion to uroepithelial cells.

Watery Mouth of Lambs

Watery mouth is a disease caused primarily by *E. coli*. It is named from the excessive salivation in neonatal lambs that accompanies the depression as the animal becomes sick. This is due to colostrum deprivation, rapid overgrowth of *E. coli* in the small intestine (perhaps associated with gastrointestinal hypomobility), translocation of *E. coli* to the circulation, release of endotoxin and death (Collins and Carson 2022). No special toxins or bacterial pathogenicity factors are required. It is the endotoxaemia that is responsible for the clinical signs and organ failure (King and Hodgson 1991). Host susceptibility, through inadequate passive immunity, is predisposing for the disease.

Control by using early and adequate colostrum intake is therefore most important. Treatment is usually with oral or parenteral antibiotic and can be successful if given early enough. However, a high proportion of strains of *E. coli* are resistant to antimicrobials such as oxytetracycline and streptomycin that are normally used in the sheep.

Oedema Disease in Pigs

Oedema disease is a worldwide fatal disease of piglets, typically seen after weaning. Piglets show swollen eyelids due to oedema, sometimes accompanied by diarrhoea. They also show ataxia, nervous signs from acute necrotising panencephalopathy, recumbence and sudden death. This is due to colonisation with *E. coli* producing the Stx2e toxin, which is closely related to the shiga-like toxin of EHEC (STEC) (see Chapter 10). The STEC *E. coli* strains attach to the glycosphingolipids located on the enterocytes of weaned piglets using the F18 fimbriae or occasionally F6. When the toxin is absorbed from the gut (an enterotoxaemia), it causes damage to the vascular endothelium which results in oedema, haemorrhage and microthrombus formation.

Control of oedema disease was based on use of prophylactic antibiotics. However, antimicrobial therapy of the disease is not effective because once clinical signs are seen, the toxin has already been absorbed and spread throughout the body. The global pressure to reduce the preventive use of antibiotics such as colistin in agriculture has given increasing priority to vaccine development (Fricke et al. 2015). Vaccination using the F18 antigen has not been successful in preventing oedema disease. However, immunisation using inactivated toxin has shown good protection and more recently, recombinant, genetically altered Stx2e toxoid has been shown to be effective in protecting pigs (Oanh et al. 2012).

The question of whether Stx2e-producing strains of *E. coli* are pathogenic for humans arises. Those EHEC strains that produce the closely related toxins Stx2, Stx2c, etc. cause severe human disease (haemorrhagic colitis and haemolytic uraemic syndrome). Humans must have regular contact with Stx2e-producing STEC. However, epidemiological studies show no association between Stx2e *E. coli* and human diarrhoea. It is suggested that these STEC bacteria cannot colonise or may infect but do not cause disease in humans (Beutin et al. 2008).

Wound and Soft Tissue Infections

Escherichia coli is a very common contributor to many different infections that might be considered secondary or opportunistic. Wound infections are often contaminated with faeces and the infections that arise are sometimes mixed. Here, an *E. coli* strain carrying the most efficient package of virulence determinants may quickly dominate the site. Sometimes, the *E. coli* will act in concert with a strict anaerobe, also derived from faeces, by mopping up any oxygen and so create an anaerobic niche for the anaerobe to thrive. Strict anaerobes (*Prevotella*, *Bacteroides* or *Clostridium*, for example) often produce very potent enzymes and toxins that quickly kill tissue cells, create a necrotic milieu and spread the infection.

Bovine Mastitis

In the UK, *E. coli* is responsible for approximately 25% of clinically apparent lactating mastitis in cows (Bradley et al. 2007). Acute *E. coli* intramammary infection is usually transient, lasting 2–3 days, but a proportion (between 5% and 20%) are persistent and this appears to be strain related. Persistent strains have been shown to invade cultured mammary epithelial cells more effectively and were found to have greater motility *in vitro*. More recently it has been shown that persistent strains produce colanic acid: a slime polysaccharide produced by *E. coli* under suboptimal conditions, such as osmotic and oxidative stress. Colanic acid has been largely ignored but is now associated with bacterial resistance to serum complement.

Vaccines are used to protect against *E. coli* mastitis. The severity of clinical signs of coliform mastitis has been shown to be reduced by immunisation with the *E. coli* J5 vaccine. This is a mutant strain, lacking the O-antigen in the lipopolysaccharide (known as a rough strain) so that the LPS core antigen (R-antigen) is exposed on the surface. Although this would make it relatively non-pathogenic, it is in any case delivered as a killed vaccine. The mechanism by which it confers protection may not be simply generation of anti-*E. coli* antibody in the milk; in any case, the R-antigen is not exposed on the surface of pathogenic *E. coli* causing mastitis because it is masked by the O-antigen. Instead, there is evidence to suggest this may be a complex immunological process in which T-lymphocytes enhance the neutrophil effector response needed for bacterial clearance.

Antimicrobial Resistance

Escherichia coli, along with some of the other enterobacteria, is one of those infection-causing bacteria that has become very unpredictable in its susceptibility to antimicrobial drugs. Once rare, strains causing disease are now regularly found to be resistant to multiple antimicrobials (Figure 11.1).

While they might appear unconnected, there is a connection between disease-causing ability and antimicrobial resistance. Particularly among strains circulating in human and veterinary hospitals, recombination (effectively the sexual mixing of genes) has led to the improved fitness of strains that can colonise sick individuals, resist antimicrobial treatment and transmit to another individual. The genetic elements for invasion and survival in the host are being co-inherited with genetic elements for resistance. At the same time, there is evolution of elements such as those

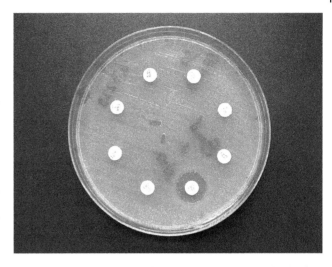

Figure 11.1 Multi-resistant *E. coli* from urinary tract infection in a six-year-old female dog.

encoding β-lactamase to be active against a wider spectrum of drugs and β-lactamase inhibitors such as clavulanic acid. Screening measures (e.g. for carbapenemase-producing *Enterobacteriaceae*) and thoughtful stewardship of important drugs will help to alleviate the trend towards highly resistant, aggressive strains of *E. coli* in bacterial disease.

References

Beutin, L., Krüger, U., Krause, G. et al. (2008). Evaluation of major types of Shiga toxin 2e-producing *Escherichia coli* bacteria present in food, pigs, and the environment as potential pathogens for humans. *Applied & Environmental Microbiology* 74: 4806–4816.

Bradley, A.J., Leach, K.A., Breen, J.E. et al. (2007). Survey of the incidence and aetiology of mastitis on dairy farms in England and Wales. *Veterinary Record* 160: 253–258.

Brumbaugh, A.R. and Mobley, H.L.T. (2012). Preventing urinary tract infection: progress toward an effective *Escherichia coli* vaccine. *Expert Review of Vaccines* 11: 663–676.

Collins, R. and Carson, A. (2022). Watery mouth disease in lambs. *Veterinary Record* 190: 28–29.

Dziva, F. and Stevens, M.P. (2008). Colibacillosis in poultry: unravelling the molecular basis of virulence of avian pathogenic *Escherichia coli* in their natural hosts. *Avian Pathology* 37: 355–366.

Fricke, R., Bastert, O., Gotter, V. et al. (2015). Implementation of a vaccine against Shigatoxin 2e in a piglet producing farm with problems of oedema disease: case study. *Porcine Health Management* 1: 6.

Kaas, R.S., Friis, C., Ussery, D.W., and Aarestrup, F.M. (2012). Estimating variation within the genes and inferring the phylogeny of 186 sequenced diverse *Escherichia coli* genomes. *BMC Genomics* 13: 577.

King, T. and Hodgson, C. (1991). Watery mouth in lambs. *In Practice* 13: 23–24.

Lloyd, A.L., Henderson, T.A., Vigil, P.D., and Mobley, H.L.T. (2009). Genomic islands of uropathogenic *Escherichia coli* contribute to virulence. *Journal of Bacteriology* 191: 3469–3481.

Manges, A.R., Geum, H.M., Guo, A. et al. (2019). Global extraintestinal pathogenic *Escherichia coli* (ExPEC) lineages. *Clinical Microbiology Reviews* 32: e00135–e00118.

Oanh, T.K., Nguyen, V.K., de Greve, H., and Goddeeris, B.M. (2012). Protection of piglets against edema disease by maternal immunization with Stx2e toxoid. *Infection and Immunity* 80: 469–473.

Ørskov, I., Ørskov, F., Jann, B., and Jann, K. (1977). Serology, chemistry, and genetics of O and K antigens of *Escherichia coli*. *Bacteriological Reviews* 41: 667–710.

Wirth, T., Falush, D., Lan, R. et al. (2006). Sex and virulence in *Escherichia coli*: an evolutionary perspective. *Molecular Microbiology* 60: 1136–1151.

12

Campylobacter – Hyperendemic on the Farm

Campylobacter spp. are curved Gram-negative bacteria. They are microaerophilic and extremely sensitive to drying. The thermophilic campylobacters, which include *C. jejuni*, *C. upsaliensis* and *C. coli*, are enteric organisms. They are zoonotic, the leading cause of human bacterial food-borne enteric disease. The non-thermophilic members of the genus, *C. fetus,* cause infertility and abortion in cattle and sheep.

Campylobacters were first associated with disease by John McFadyean and Stewart Stockman from cases of ovine abortion in 1913 (McFadyean and Stockman 1913). They were largely ignored as rather insignificant, rare animal pathogens until the 1970s when it was realised that they were a cause of human enteric disease. Since then, it has become clear how widespread *Campylobacter* is and the disease burden it confers on both animals and the human population (Butzler 2004).

At least part of the reason for this was the difficulty of selective culture of *Campylobacter* from faeces. Only once the techniques for selective isolation were worked out, and microaerophilic culture was routinely used, was *Campylobacter* sought in clinical diagnostic laboratories (Dekeyser et al. 1972; Skirrow 1977).

Campylobacter fetus subsp. *fetus*

Campylobacter fetus subspecies *fetus* is associated with sporadic abortion in cattle and sheep. It is responsible for about 10% of all ovine abortions investigated in the UK. It can be naturally carried in the intestinal tract without causing harm. When material contaminated with *C. fetus* is ingested during the last trimester of pregnancy, the organisms invade, reach the blood and bacteraemia ensues. The organisms localise in the placenta, causing inflammation and necrosis, and abortion can occur.

Campylobacter fetus subsp. *venerealis* is associated with infertility in female cattle. The organism is harboured on the prepuce of the mature bull without clinical signs or inflammation. When transmitted to the female genital tract, the bacteria cause an inflammatory reaction. This persistent inflammatory stimulation prevents implantation until the bacteria are cleared from the uterus. The bacteria are cleared from the upper genital tract but may persist in the vagina: IgA may block opsonising antibody required for clearance. They may then be transmitted to other bulls at later service. It is therefore a venereal infection of cattle: infectious infertility.

Campylobacter jejuni

Campylobacter jejuni is an important enteropathogen of humans and some animal species (Moore et al. 2005) (Figure 12.1). This species causes 90% of *Campylobacter* infections in humans. It grows over a wide range of temperatures (30–47 °C), with optimal growth at 42 °C (Stintzi 2003). It is the largest source of food poisoning in the UK, causing five times the number of cases attributed to *Salmonella enterica*.

Campylobacter jejuni is very widely distributed in the farm environment; cattle, sheep, dogs and, most importantly, farmed poultry and wild birds carry the bacteria in the intestinal tract. The components enabling successful colonisation of the chicken intestinal tract are many and complex (Ruddell et al. 2021). Its widespread distribution on the farm means that it is hyperendemic: all the animals are regularly exposed to it by the faecal–oral route and passive (colostral) protection

Fundamentals of Veterinary Microbiology, First Edition. Andrew N. Rycroft.
© 2024 John Wiley & Sons Ltd. Published 2024 by John Wiley & Sons Ltd.
Companion website: www.wiley.com/go/veterinarymicrobiology

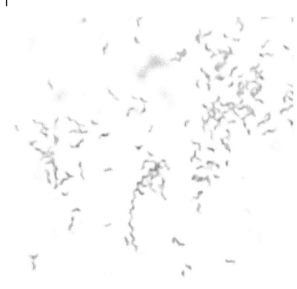

Figure 12.1 Microscopic appearance of *Campylobacter jejuni* stained by Gram stain.

is helpful while active immunity develops. However, in the hygienic environment of the human or pet dog, there is no regular exposure and such animals are highly susceptible to infection.

At slaughter, the intestinal contents of the broiler chicken may contaminate the abdominal cavity, and this further contaminates the skin when the carcass passes through the wash tank. Therefore, a high proportion of birds can be moderately or heavily contaminated with *Campylobacter*. Handling the meat can then allow access. Much chicken meat is frozen and the bacteria remain viable in the abdominal cavity, especially when the organisms are bathed in protein-rich meat juices. When thawing of frozen chicken is inadequate, so that cooking is incomplete, bacteria may remain viable or grow during cooking and then be ingested by humans.

Campylobacteriosis, the infection caused by *C. jejuni*, is an acute gastroenteritis with symptoms ranging from watery to bloody diarrhoea and inflammation of the ileum and jejunum. Human infection with *C. jejuni* may sometimes lead to other complications, such as the peripheral neuropathies Guillain–Barré syndrome and Miller Fisher syndrome (Allos 2001).

The mechanism by which *C. jejuni* causes gastroenteritis involves colonisation, attachment, invasion and toxin production. Following intake by a susceptible host in a relatively low infectious dose, *C. jejuni* resists stomach acid by upregulation of stress responses inside the bacteria. The organism penetrates the mucus layer of the small intestine and proximal colon to reach the apical surface of the intestinal epithelial cells. Mucus is crucial in the colonisation of *C. jejuni*, as mucin is a chemoattractant for *C. jejuni* and facilitates the increased flagellar gene expression and motility required to reach the underlying epithelium (Callahan et al. 2021). Once *C. jejuni* has transited through the mucus layer, the bacterium is able to adhere to and invade into the epithelium. Colon damage is characterised by necrosis of absorptive epithelial cells, erosion of the mucosa, crypt abscesses and infiltration of inflammatory cells, primarily neutrophils, into the mucosa. Functional flagella are important as virulence factors. Non-flagellate bacteria do not colonise *in vivo* and are less invasive *in vitro*.

Pathogenicity

Despite analysis of the genome sequence of many strains, the components responsible for pathogenicity of *C. jejuni* are still not well understood. Disease depends on functions such as chemotaxis, motility, adhesion and invasion of host epithelial cells and cytotoxin production. A highly variable polysaccharide capsule is produced. These are complex heteropolysaccharides that are modified with unusual and exotic sugars. This extensive variation in structure probably has a key role in the evasion of the host immune response. In addition, there is biofilm formation, and lipo-oligosaccharide production, secretion systems and various colonisation factors contribute to survival in the host, transmission and infection. The pathogen is able to proliferate following attachment to host cells and this is followed by internalisation into intestinal epithelial cells and secretion of the cytolethal distending toxin (CDT), causing host cell apoptosis (Figure 12.2).

Disease in Animals

The importance of *C. jejuni* is as a food-borne zoonosis of public health concern. In poultry, it so easily colonises the intestinal tract (cecum) and is so difficult to eradicate, without causing any disease, that it is considered a commensal (part of the normal gut flora) of gallinaceous birds (Young et al. 2007). Similarly, *C. coli* is most commonly present in pigs, where it seems to cause little disease, and *C. upsaliensis*, *C. lari* and *C. helveticus* can be found in dogs and cats showing no clinical signs. Many farm animals regularly carry *Campylobacter* organisms in the gut but, either through immunity acquired in early life or from lack of susceptibility to the pathogen, they do not become diseased. Simultaneous colonisation with different species is sometimes present (Thépault et al. 2020). This reinforces the notion that simple infection with a *Campylobacter* sp. is not itself to be equated with disease causation.

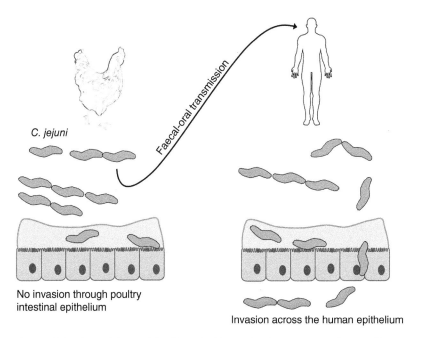

C. jejuni

Faecal-oral transmission

No invasion through poultry
intestinal epithelium

Invasion across the human epithelium

Figure 12.2 *Campylobacter jejuni* is carried in poultry but causes no disease. The organisms colonises the mucus layer of the intestinal epithelium but penetrates no further. In humans, the organism, which is usually acquired by ingestion of faecal-contaminated poultry, attaches to the intestinal epithelial cells and invades across the epithelium, causing inflammation and diarrhoea.

Nevertheless, *Campylobacter* does cause disease in animals. Farm animals suffer outbreaks of disease that has been attributed to *Campylobacter*, but these are mild and self-limiting. Winter dysentery in calves was associated with *Campylobacter* but this is now recognised as being due to a coronavirus. In dogs, particularly kept in households under hygienic conditions, *Campylobacter* infection may cause acute diarrhoea, similar to human disease, with abdominal pain, mucus and blood (Skirrow 1981). This can inevitably spread to human owners. The infection may also be transferred from human owner to animal. Cats seem to suffer little with *Campylobacter* disease but do carry the organism and in particular circumstances this may be causing enteritis.

Control

Since most *Campylobacter* infections are acquired by consuming or handling poultry, the obvious way to control the number of human infections would be to limit contamination of poultry flocks. However, the near-universal contamination of poultry with *Campylobacter* and the heavy bacterial burden in the flocks make elimination of *Campylobacter* in chickens impractical, if not impossible. Vaccination of poultry to encourage the immune system to remove what is effectively a commensal organism is fraught with problems (antigenic variety, lack of effect, cost–benefit) and is not likely to be used unless there is a major change to our understanding of the host–pathogen relationship.

Methods that have been effective for controlling *Salmonella* infection in poultry are generally ineffective against campylobacters. Biosecurity measures on poultry farms are of limited value when wild birds or even insects may carry the organism into a flock. The most effective barrier to *Campylobacter* infection of humans is the hygienic handling and preparation of foods of animal origin to reduce cross-contamination. Cooks are prone to licking their fingers. Simple hand washing immediately after handling meat is adequate. Utensils, such as chopping boards in contact with raw meat, should be cleaned before use for any food that is not going to be further cooked. Washing utensils with soapy water dilutes out and effectively disinfects any contamination. Also, meat must be adequately cooked to kill the pathogen.

Industrialised production, processing and distribution of chicken may increase the level of carriage and assist in distribution to the population. Alternative strategies for control might involve decontamination of poultry carcasses by radiation or chlorination, but these are currently not acceptable to the public as feasible methods of control of the bacterial contamination of foods (Allos 2001).

Controversy over Antibiotic Treatment

When animals do become unwell with enteritis, and there is reason to believe *Campylobacter* is involved, there is pressure (often from the owner) for the vet to treat with antimicrobials. Cases in which *Campylobacter* enteritis has been diagnosed in dogs, and then spread to the human owners, are not without precedent. However, most cases of campylobacteriosis are self-limiting and seldom require antimicrobial therapy (Butzler 2004). In humans, while the disease is most unpleasant, maintenance of hydration and electrolyte balance, rather than antibiotic treatment, is the basis of treatment for *Campylobacter* enteritis. Most patients with *Campylobacter* infection do not require antibiotics at all. There is every reason to follow this guidance in companion animals.

Nevertheless, there are specific clinical circumstances in which antibiotics should be used. These include high fever, bloody stools, prolonged illness (more than seven days), pregnancy, concurrent infection and an immunocompromised state (Allos 2001). If therapy is indicated, erythromycin is considered the drug of choice based on efficacy, low toxicity and low cost. When erythromycin is used in genuine *Campylobacter* enteritis, and the strain is sensitive to the drug *in vitro*, it is reported to cause the clinical signs to disappear rapidly (Butzler 2004).

Other Curved Gram-negative Bacteria

Helicobacter

These curved or spiral-shaped, microaerophilic, Gram-negative rods were discovered in the stomach of humans in 1987. In humans, the most common and best known gastric *Helicobacter* species is *Helicobacter pylori*. This is highly adapted for human colonisation of the human stomach and is present in half of the world's population. The organism colonises as a commensal, yet it is implicated in the development of peptic ulcers, gastritis and gastric cancer (adenocarcinoma and lymphoma) in people (Joosten et al. 2016). Dogs, cats and pigs are reservoir hosts for other *Helicobacter* species, such as *H. heilmannii*, now considered to be zoonotic for humans.

In animals, several *Helicobacter* species have been detected in the stomach (Haesebrouck et al. 2009). Gastric *Helicobacter*-like organisms in dogs (sometimes called *Gastrospirillum*) have been known for more than a century but were never cultivated. *H. felis* and non-*H. pylori Helicobacter* species (NHPH) such as *H. heilmannii* are found in both the dog and cat. There is some evidence that infection causes clinical gastritis and histological evidence confirms a clear association between *Helicobacter* and stomach lesions. The pathogenic significance of *Helicobacter* in these animals remains unclear and is probably strain dependent or related to host differences (Joosten et al. 2016).

The pig regularly carries *H. suis*. As many as 60–80% of pigs are colonised in the stomach by *H. suis* at slaughter weight. *H. suis* causes gastritis in experimentally and naturally infected pigs and is associated with ulcers of the non-glandular part of the stomach (near the oesophagus).

There is epidemiological evidence that *Helicobacter* species such as *H. suis* are associated with neurological disorders in humans, particularly Parkinson's disease, and the zoonotic significance of this pathogen may change as further investigations progress.

Lawsonia

The single species *Lawsonia intracellularis* is the causative agent of porcine intestinal adenopathy: PIA. This chronic disease of growing pigs is now known as porcine proliferative enteropathy (PE) and is characterised by proliferation of intestinal mucosa enterocytes leading to gross thickening of the ileal wall. The lesions may progress to an acute form known as proliferative haemorrhagic enteritis. Proliferative enteropathy is commercially important in the intensive pig industry. Large numbers of pigs may be affected, causing significant losses in weight gain (Lawson and Gebhart 2000).

Lawsonia intracellularis underwent a number of name changes. The organism is a curved Gram-negative rod but unlike *Campylobacter* or *Helicobacter*, it is an obligate intracellular pathogen. From the shape, and the lack of other features normally seen in culture, the organism was referred to as a '*Campylobacter*-like organism'. Unlike *Campylobacter*, it is weakly acid fast (like *Brucella* and *Chlamydia*). It was later named *ileal symbiont intracellularis* and then, following comparison of the 16S rRNA, it was reclassified as *Desulfovibrio desulfuricans*, an environmental organism that uses sulfate as an electron acceptor in anaerobic mud. Eventually, it was settled as a single species in the new genus *Lawsonia* (McOrist et al. 1995). *Lawsonia* is propagated in cell culture, and it cannot be grown in laboratory media (Lawson et al. 1993).

The effects of the disease were described, and the disease reproduced in pigs by oral inoculation of intestinal mucosa from diseased pigs, as early as 1931. The organism was first seen and described as a curved rod inside porcine intestinal epithelial cells from pigs with adenomatous changes and thickening of tissues of the intestinal tract (especially the ileum) during the 1970s in Edinburgh.

Pathogenesis

Lawsonia intracellularis is documented as present in 94% of pig herds. It is transmitted by the faecal–oral route and colonises the epithelial tissue of the small intestine. This causes adenomatous changes (proliferation and thickening) of the mucosa and gradually the lesion progresses to the large intestine. The mechanism is not fully established but it is thought that the bacteria infect dividing cells of the crypts between villi. This is reminiscent of canine parvovirus infection. It appears to be dependent upon actively dividing cells for its own growth and the dividing *Lawsonia* cause hyperplasia and proliferation of the crypt cells. This leads to an excess of immature epithelial cells that have not differentiated to produce the normal microvilli. These cells replace the normal epithelial cells of the villi and because they lack the normal surface microvilli, absorption is impaired and a malabsorptive diarrhoea ensues. There is an associated hypoproteinaemia, perhaps again like canine parvovirus, from leakage of tissue fluid proteins from the damaged villous surface.

The pathogenicity factors contributing to survival and invasion are not known. Some clues have been found from analysis of the genome sequence. These include genes for an adhesin, a type 3 secretion system, a putative haemolysin and an autotransporter, but these are not conclusive and have not been related to the pathogenesis of the disease. It appears that the bacteria cause signalling effects and disruption of normal pathways in the enterocyte. Cells infected with *Lawsonia* upregulate genes associated with the G_1 phase of the cell cycle to cause transcription and translation and proliferation of immature crypt cells. Failure of the crypt cells to differentiate into goblet and absorptive cells results in inadequate function and diarrhoea.

Diagnosis

Clinical signs of proliferative enteropathy are considered to be non-specific. Demonstration of the causative organism in live animals is based on PCR of faecal samples. At postmortem, characteristic appearance of the gut and histopathology are used to recognise the disease. Immunohistochemistry allows specific recognition of the pathogen in tissue sections.

Control

Traditionally, antimicrobials have been used regularly in the feed of commercial pigs to control enteric and respiratory disease. This has been effective in controlling and preventing disease due to *Lawsonia*. However, with the drive to reduce the quantity of antimicrobials used in pork production, alternative means of prevention or control are needed.

Fortunately, natural infection with *L. intracellularis* confers considerable immunological protection against the disease. Both a live, attenuated, oral vaccine and a killed, injectable vaccine are available for use in the pig (Jacobs et al. 2019). Both are considered to be effective in reducing lesions of proliferative enteropathy and shedding of *L. intracellularis*.

Equine Proliferative Enteropathy

Lawsonia intracellularis is now accepted as the causative agent of equine proliferative enteropathy (Page et al. 2014). This mostly affects foals around six months of age but varies from two to 12 months with fever, oedema, weight loss, diarrhoea and colic (Pusterla and Gebhart 2009). Older horses can also suffer from proliferative enteropathy. Antemortem diagnosis using faecal PCR has become widely available. Strains that are host-adapted to the pig are not able to cause disease in the horse and conversely, *Lawsonia* from equine lesions is not able to cause disease in pigs.

References

Allos, B.M. (2001). *Campylobacter jejuni* infections: update on emerging issues and trends. *Clinical Infectious Diseases* 32: 1201–1206.

Butzler, J.-P. (2004). *Campylobacter*, from obscurity to celebrity. *Clinical Microbiology and Infection* 10: 868–876.

Callahan, S.M., Dolislager, C.G., and Johnson, J.G. (2021). The host cellular immune response to infection by *Campylobacter* spp. and its role in disease. *Infection and Immunity* 89: e00116–e00121.

Dekeyser, P., Gossuin-Detrain, M., Butzler, J.P., and Sternon, J. (1972). Acute enteritis due to a related vibrio: first positive stool cultures. *Journal of Infectious Diseases* 125: 390–392.

Haesebrouck, F., Pasmans, F., Flahou, B. et al. (2009). Gastric helicobacters in domestic animals and nonhuman primates and their significance for human health. *Clinical Microbiology Reviews* 22: 202–223.

Jacobs, A.A.C., Harks, F., Hazenberg, L. et al. (2019). Efficacy of a novel inactivated *Lawsonia intracellularis* vaccine in pigs against experimental infection and under field conditions. *Vaccine* 37: 2149–2157.

Joosten, M., Lindén, S., Rossi, M. et al. (2016). Divergence between the highly virulent zoonotic pathogen *Helicobacter heilmannii* and its closest relative, the low-virulence "*Helicobacter ailurogastricus*" sp. nov. *Infection and Immunity* 84: 293–306.

Lawson, G.H.K. and Gebhart, C.J. (2000). Proliferative enteropathy. *Journal of Comparative Pathology* 122: 77–100.

Lawson, G.H.K., McOrist, S., Jasni, S., and Mackie, R.A. (1993). Intracellular bacteria of porcine proliferative enteropathy: cultivation and maintenance in vitro. *Journal of Clinical Microbiology* 31: 1136–1142.

McFadyean, J. and Stockman, S. (1913). *Report of the Departmental Committee appointed by the Board of Agriculture and Fisheries to inquire into Epizootic Abortion. III. Abortion in Sheep.* London: HMSO.

McOrist, S., Gebhart, C.J., Boid, R., and Barns, S.M. (1995). Characterization of *Lawsonia intracellularis* gen. nov., sp. nov., the obligately intracellular bacterium of porcine proliferative enteropathy. *International Journal of Systematic Bacteriology* 45: 820–825.

Moore, J.E., Corcoran, D., Dooley, J.S.G. et al. (2005). Campylobacter. *Veterinary Research* 36: 351–382.

Page, A.E., Slovis, N.M., and Horohov, D.W. (2014). *Lawsonia intracellularis* and equine proliferative enteropathy. *Veterinary Clinics of North America. Equine Practice* 30: 641–658.

Pusterla, N. and Gebhart, C. (2009). Equine proliferative enteropathy caused by *Lawsonia intracellularis*. *Equine Veterinary Education* 21: 415–418.

Ruddell, B., Hassall, A., Sahin, O. et al. (2021). Role of *metAB* in methionine metabolism and optimal chicken colonization in *Campylobacter jejuni*. *Infection and Immunity* 89: e00542–e00520.

Skirrow, M.B. (1977). Campylobacter enteritis: a "new" disease. *British Medical Journal* 2: 9–11.

Skirrow, M.B. (1981). Campylobacter enteritis in dogs and cats: a 'new' zoonosis. *Veterinary Research Communications* 5: 13–19.

Stintzi, A. (2003). Gene expression profile of *Campylobacter jejuni* in response to growth temperature variation. *Journal of Bacteriology* 185: 2009–2016.

Thépault, A., Rose, V., Queguiner, M. et al. (2020). Dogs and cats: reservoirs for highly diverse *Campylobacter jejuni* and a potential source of human exposure. *Animals* 10: 838.

Young, K.T., Davis, L.M., and DiRita, V.J. (2007). *Campylobacter jejuni*: molecular biology and pathogenesis. *Nature Reviews Microbiology* 5: 665–679.

13

Leptospira – Using Urine to Spread

Leptospirosis is an infectious disease of animals throughout the world. It is also a zoonotic disease, transmitted from animals to humans, that has been described by WHO as the most widespread zoonosis in the world. Different animals carry specific *Leptospira* serovars as a chronic infection in the renal tubules as a maintenance host. Other animals, including humans, then become infected as accidental (incidental) hosts.

Leptospira are tightly coiled, very thin spirochaetes. They are Gram-negative rods with an outer membrane and lipopolysaccharide (LPS). This LPS dominates the surface antigenicity and the O-antigen can be modified when under selective pressure to evade an immune response (Haake and Zückert 2015). They cannot be visualised by bright-field microscopy with normal staining because they are no more than 0.1 μm in width. Silver staining can be used to make the organisms appear thicker. Alternatively, dark-field microscopy can be used to see the live bacteria (Figure 13.1). When set up correctly, the light passes through the bacteria but not directly into the objective lens. Only light refracted by objects passes into the lens and is focused. The person viewing them sees a black background (like the night sky) and the spirochaetes appear (like the stars) as bright, moving bacteria. This shows the organisms as very highly motile and surprisingly long: between 6 and 20 μm (Adler and de la Peña Moctezuma 2010).

Leptospira organisms are obligate aerobes. They utilise long-chain fatty acids as a carbon and energy source. They are not able to grow on conventional bacteriological media. Instead, they can be cultured in special broth medium such as EMJH which is supplemented with oleic acid and serum albumin. They also require vitamins B2 (riboflavin), B12 (cobalamin) and ammonium salts. Incubation temperature is usually 28–30 °C and primary isolation may take several weeks. Once adapted to the artificial medium, they may grow well in 7–10 days. Colonies can be grown on a solid medium but successful culture requires some experience and careful handling.

Pathogenic leptospires were originally named *L. interrogans*. The name was given because observation of the organism in 1907 found they had hooked ends – rather like a question mark. The non-pathogenic species were called *L. biflexa* (Levett 2001).

Leptospira, as for other spirochaetes, are motile by flagellae which are located not externally but in the periplasmic space, between the cytoplasmic and outer membranes. For historical reasons, these are known as axial filaments but they are internalised polar flagellae, attached to the ends of the organism. They rotate within the periplasm and cause opposite rotation of the bacteria because of the equal and opposite reaction of the body of the organism in response to the rotation of the flagellum (Newton's third law of motion). This rotation of the bacterial cell is then translated into motility because of the spiral (corkscrew) shape of the organism. Rotation causes it to move through liquid like a drill pulls into wood.

Analysis of the genome shows there are two circular chromosomes of around 3000 and 4000 kb. The majority of the genes do not have counterparts (orthologues) in other spirochaetes. This shows the great divergence of *Leptospira* from other members of the Spirochaete group. Furthermore, spirochaetes are now placed in their own phylum, reflecting their distinction from other bacteria and a very long history of independent evolution.

Classification of *Leptospira*

The organisms are impossible to differentiate on morphology and biochemically they are rather inactive. It is the antigenic differences between the bacteria that have been used to recognise differences between strains. The antigenic heterogeneity is in the carbohydrate component of the LPS and antiserum was applied to the live bacteria in the microscopic

Fundamentals of Veterinary Microbiology, First Edition. Andrew N. Rycroft.
© 2024 John Wiley & Sons Ltd. Published 2024 by John Wiley & Sons Ltd.
Companion website: www.wiley.com/go/veterinarymicrobiology

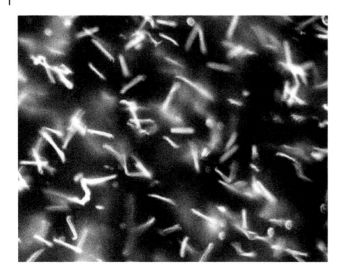

Figure 13.1 Under dark-field microscopy, the unstained *Leptospira* bacteria appear as bright, highly motile, refractile bodies against a dark background.

agglutination test. Using this, *L. interrogans* was subdivided into several serogroups and within each of these are numerous serotypes which are known as serovars. In total, 24 serogroups containing more than 200 serovars of pathogenic leptospires were recognised and serotyping remains important for epidemiological investigations since serovars and serogroups are related to the host reservoirs involved in pathogen transmission. Unfortunately, serotyping is conducted by only a few reference laboratories in the world and so is not generally available.

More recent classification has used genotyping and molecular-based methods such as multilocus enzyme electrophoresis (MLEE) data. This has determined 16 different 'genomospecies'. A genomospecies is a term used to suggest that we can recognise sufficient difference between strains that they could be considered a different species. Yet, the designation of a species in the bacterial world is far from settled or clear. Ultimately, genome sequence analysis, of which hundreds currently exist, is now being used to discriminate and classify *Leptospira* organisms.

Based on genomic analyses, the saprophytic species now comprise *Leptospira biflexa* and six other species. There are eight pathogenic species currently recognised: *Leptospira interrogans*, *L. kirschneri*, *L. borgpetersenii*, *L. santarosai*, *L. noguchii*, *L. weilii*, *L. alexanderi* and *L. alstoni*. A third group, the intermediate *Leptospira* species, is now recognised. These are of uncertain pathogenicity and the group comprises a further five species. Studies have now demonstrated that there is no clear relationship between serogroups/serovars and the groups based on genomic analysis. Hence, a classification system based on genetic relationships is used in conjunction with antigenic classification.

The Maintenance Host and the Accidental Host

Leptospira serovars are host-adapted to live in many different animal species. These are the reservoir or maintenance hosts. In such a host, they cause long-term, carrier infection without engendering a strong inflammatory or immune response. The organisms colonise the kidney tubules, causing a chronic infection, from where they are excreted in the urine. In a reservoir host, the infection is endemic within the population of that species and the organism is readily transferred between animals through direct contact or contact with urine.

Successful infection of a host for which the *Leptospira* is not host-adapted (an accidental host) often results in acute disease in that animal, but there is then no carrier state and no onward transmission.

Transmission

Many *Leptospira* serovars are maintained by circulating in small mammals and are considered as parasites of rodents. *Leptospira* serovars have specific host preferences. Rats are asymptomatic maintenance hosts for several pathogenic leptospires, including the Icterohaemorrhagiae serogroup. Similarly, house mice are the reservoir for the Ballum serogroup (Figure 13.2).

Figure 13.2 The transmission of *Leptospira* among animals and humans.

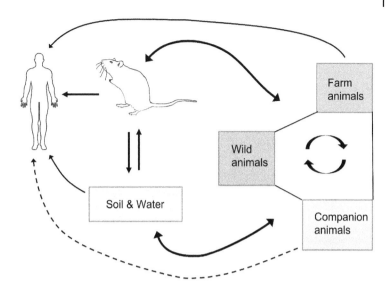

In the accidental host, the organisms cause a more severe disease in which the organisms multiply in the liver, cause liver damage and haemorrhage, migrate via the blood to other organs and may cause death. Humans are an accidental host for *Leptospira*. The degree of disease in humans depends on the infecting serovar. It will include one or more of severe headache, fever, renal dysfunction, hepatic disease, myocarditis and meningoencephalitis. Severe human leptospirosis, usually due to *L. interrogans* serovar Icterohaemorrhagiae, is known as Weil's disease. This has typical presentation of jaundice, acute renal failure and bleeding. A more recently described pulmonary haemorrhage syndrome is also sometimes seen.

Pathogenesis

Leptospira organisms are able to survive in an aquatic environment. From urine deposited in the environment, they may gain access to other maintenance host animals or into accidental hosts via breaks in the skin or by contact with mucous membrane (oral, nasal, genital, conjunctival). They are not normally able to cross the intact skin barrier.

Once they have penetrated to the tissues, leptospires establish a systemic infection by crossing tissue barriers and by haematogenous spread. Leptospires are known to enter host cells transiently during invasion but they are not considered facultative intracellular pathogens. The organisms circulate in blood, reaching 10^7 organisms per ml, and are not destroyed by the innate immune system such as the alternative complement system. This is probably using a complement factor H binding protein on the *Leptospira* surface. Factor H prevents complement activation and C3b deposition and the amplification loop on cell surfaces and so inhibits opsonophagocytosis and complement-mediated bactericidal action. A similar factor H binding function is seen on the M-protein of β-haemolytic streptococci. An acquired immune response is indeed needed to eliminate the pathogen from blood.

Damage to vascular endothelium is a recognised feature in acute leptospirosis. This causes haemorrhage, capillary leakage and vasculitis. Infection also activates the coagulation system such that intravascular coagulation occurs in some cases. The pathogenesis also includes the production of proinflammatory cytokines that mediate inflammation and damage to organ tissues.

In the maintenance host, the *Leptospira* organisms become localised to the renal tubules. From here, they are excreted for many months at high concentration.

Pathogenicity Factors of *Leptospira*

There are few components of *Leptospira* that are actually known to be involved in causing disease and host tissue damage (Adler 2014; Ko et al. 2009). There are proteins on the surface that may be involved in adhesion and entry into host cells, and in binding factor H to inhibit opsonisation by complement. Iron uptake systems are present and a haem-oxygenase that is able to release ferrous iron from haem. Motility is considered an essential property for disease and there are genes for a pore-forming haemolysin, a collagenase and a sphingomyelinase that are not present in saprophytic leptospires. There is evidence that the profile of gene expression is altered by temperature and osmolality. If so, and functions needed for disease are only expressed in conditions found inside the animal, it may be difficult to recognise factors needed for pathogenicity while the pathogen is growing *in vitro*.

Leptospirosis in Dogs

Only a very few serovars are of real significance in animal disease in the UK and Western Europe. *L. interrogans* serovar Canicola is considered to be host-adapted to the dog yet it can cause severe, sometimes fatal, renal disease in young pups. Speculatively, *L. canicola* may not be so host-adapted for the domesticated dog and perhaps the true reservoir host of this serovar is the fox or the wolf from which domestic dogs have been derived relatively recently.

Another serovar, *L. interrogans* serovar Icterohaemorrhagiae, is also seen in the dog. Rats act as a reservoir host for this serovar. It is associated with more severe disease in the dog and is the cause of Weil's disease in humans.

Since vaccination of the dog against leptospirosis using these two serovars has been widely practised for several decades, different serovars have emerged as causing disease in parts of Europe. These are serovars Australis, Sejroe, Bratislava, Pomona and Grippotyphosa and commercial vaccines are now including additional serovars to control these infections.

Leptospirosis in Cats

Serological evidence suggests cats are sometimes infected with *Leptospira* serovars but since there appears to be relatively little disease, cats may be acquiring the infection but this is generally subclinical. When disease is seen, it usually manifests as pyrexia, jaundice and reduced appetite but there may also be a role for infection in the aetiology of chronic kidney disease (Murphy 2018).

Leptospirosis in Cattle

The disease is common in cattle in which the important serovar is Hardjo. Confusingly, serovar Hardjo antigens can be found in two unrelated genomospecies: *L. interrogans* and *L. borgpetersenii*. It is the latter, *L. borgpetersenii serovar* Hardjo, that is responsible for most cattle infection. It appears that cattle are a maintenance host for this serovar and may also harbour Pomona and Grippotyphosa. However, *Leptospira* infection is responsible for sudden loss of milk yield (sometimes referred to as milk-drop or 'flabby bag'), infertility and abortion, usually in the third trimester of pregnancy. Leptospirosis was the cause of substantial numbers (>30%) of investigated bovine abortions and probably continues to be so, although testing for the disease is not widespread at present.

Outbreaks of leptospirosis in cattle tend to be associated with co-grazing with sheep, suggesting sheep also carry the organism as a maintenance host. It is also transmitted at service by shared bulls and where there is a shared source of water.

Vaccination of cattle is available. Again, this includes only the most common serovars as killed vaccine and is mainly used to control and prevent abortions.

Leptospirosis in Pigs

Pigs are a maintenance host for serovar Pomona. They also carry serovars Tarassovi and Bratislava. These are known to cause reproductive tract disease. Acute disease can happen in pigs when infected as accidental host with serovars such as Icterohaemorrhagiae.

Zoonotic Disease

Leptospirosis is zoonotic. Disease is transmitted to farmers and farm workers via urine splash and the aerosol this generates, from cattle in milking areas. If small quantities of infected urine gain access to the mouth, nose or eyes, or to an open wound, the bacteria can invade, enter the bloodstream and lead to leptospirosis. This usually takes the form of an influenza-like illness with severe frontal headache in humans. There are also innumerable accounts of transmission to humans through water in which rats and other rodents have urinated. Activities such as swimming in ponds and rivers, canoeing and windsurfing in fresh water are associated with outbreaks of the disease. Approximately 50 cases per year are reported in the UK but more undiagnosed cases will occur and be considered as flu-like illness.

Other Risk Factors

The incidence of leptospirosis is higher in warmer climates and it is seasonal. Warm, humid climates with high rainfall favour survival of *Leptospira* in the environment. Combined with the effect of climate is the greater contact, direct or indirect, between humans and infected livestock and wild animals. Conversely, dry conditions are very unsuitable for survival of *Leptospira*: it rapidly dies in a desiccating environment.

I have heard it stated that leptospirosis occurs in places where there are microbiologists interested in *Leptospira*. The disease seems to follow certain individuals as they move in their work. These individuals are the specialists working in this particular field. Infection and disease will be occurring and yet be missed unless the means for laboratory diagnosis is available. Once cases are identified, there is an improved awareness among health professionals. It seems the influence of individuals capable of seeking and recognising the organism, or the antibody, is crucial.

References

Adler, B. (2014). Pathogenesis of leptospirosis: cellular and molecular aspects. *Veterinary Microbiology* 172: 353–358.

Adler, B. and de la Peña Moctezuma. A. (2010). *Leptospira* and leptospirosis. *Veterinary Microbiology* 140: 287–296.

Haake, D.A. and Zückert, W.R. (2015). The leptospiral outer membrane. *Current Topics in Microbiology and Immunology* 387: 187–221.

Ko, A.I., Goarant, C., and Picardeau, M. (2009). *Leptospira*: the dawn of the molecular genetics era for an emerging zoonotic pathogen. *Nature Reviews Microbiology* 7: 736–747.

Levett, P.N. (2001). Leptospirosis. *Clinical Microbiology Reviews* 14: 296–326.

Murphy, K. (2018). Leptospirosis in dogs and cats: new challenges from an old bacteria. *In Practice* 40: 218–229.

14

Lyme Disease – Ticks and Dogs

Borrelia burgdorferi

Lyme disease (also known as Lyme borreliosis) was first recognised in 1975 in children showing signs of arthritis in Old Lyme, a small town near the estuary of the Connecticut River in the USA. It was not until 1983 that the organism was identified, and the first animal case was described in 1984. It is now an increasingly diagnosed cause of disease in horses, cattle and dogs (Chang et al. 2000). The disease agent is a spirochaete, *Borrelia burgdorferi*, which is transmitted by ticks. In fact, the agent of Lyme disease is more than one species and these are referred to as *B. burgdorferi sensu lato* (in the broad sense). Other related species capable of causing Lyme disease include *B. garinii* and *B. afzelii*. These are being grouped under a new genus named *Borreliella* (Adeolu and Gupta 2014). Here we refer to *B. burgdorferi* in that broad sense as the agent(s) of Lyme disease.

This is a Gram-negative organism with a very thin body and a loosely spiralled morphology. It can be cultured using BSK II liquid medium as described by Alan Barbour in 1984 with an optimum temperature between 34 and 37 °C but is not cultured for routine diagnosis. At temperatures above 39 °C, no growth occurs and the organism becomes non-viable.

The organism is unusual in three ways. First, it has a segmented genome comprising a linear chromosome of about 910 kb together with at least 17 plasmids, some of which are circular and some linear. The plasmids vary in size from 5 to 55 kb and carry genes of (as yet) unknown function although loss of certain linear plasmids has been associated with loss of infectivity of the organism, indicating that these plasmids carry functions essential for maintenance of *B. burgdorferi in vivo*. Second, although it is Gram-negative, it has no recognisable lipopolysaccharide. Finally, it uses manganese instead of iron; iron is not required and is not used by the pathogen. *B. burgdorferi* was found to contain none of the usual iron-containing proteins or the genes for such proteins in the genome sequence. The intracellular iron concentration was estimated by Posey and Gherardini (2000) to be less than 10 atoms per cell, far fewer than would be required if iron was a required element.

Epidemiology

The ticks acting as reservoir are *Ixodes scapularis* and *I. pacificus* in the USA, and *I. ricinus* in the UK (Kurokawa et al. 2020). When an infected tick bites into the skin, it allows the *Borrelia* to enter the epidermis. Blood from the host animal pools in the skin and bacteria enter this pool. From there, they are able to enter the dermis and spread into the skin. In humans, the associated inflammation leads to a red rash (erythema) with a characteristic 'target' appearance. This inflammation is not visible in animals with a hair coat. After a period of a few days, during which the pathogen adapts and multiplies, it enters the subcutaneous tissues and the blood. At this stage, the body of the animal responds with fever and lethargy while the pathogen migrates to localise in two relatively protected sites, the nervous system and the joints of the animal, which results in neurological damage and arthritis respectively.

The reservoir of Lyme disease is in wildlife, particularly rodents and deer. This is where it persists; there is no vertical transmission in the tick vector. Infection of the tick happens when a larval-stage tick bites an infected animal, usually a rodent. The next season, the tick spreads infection as a nymph by again mostly feeding from rodents. In the season when the ticks are adult, they will also feed from deer; the blood is needed for the reproductive cycle of the tick and this again infects the deer. Dogs, horses and humans are inadvertent hosts (Figure 14.1).

Fundamentals of Veterinary Microbiology, First Edition. Andrew N. Rycroft.
© 2024 John Wiley & Sons Ltd. Published 2024 by John Wiley & Sons Ltd.
Companion website: www.wiley.com/go/veterinarymicrobiology

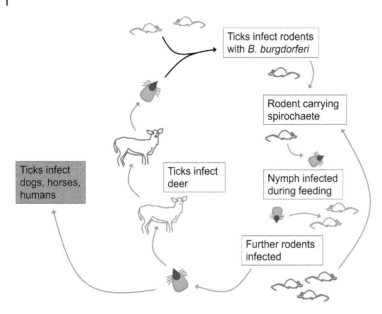

Figure 14.1 Transmission of *Borrelia burgdorferi*.

Pathogenesis

The virulence determinants are unclear. *B. burgdorferi* apparently uses a large and diverse set of adhesins, several of which have been experimentally shown to contribute to the ability of the bacterium to cause infection and disease in mice (Coburn et al. 2013).

No obvious toxins are produced but clearly the organism has the means to evade immune recognition or at least avoid destruction by the innate immune system. The inflammation observed in persistently infected animals is due to the host response at the site of infection, which can be induced by spirochaete antigens, including lipoproteins (Kurokawa et al. 2020).

One feature that is essential is motility. This is considered necessary for evasion of clearance by the host. However, it is also likely to be essential for invasion across the skin into the tissues. Spirochaetes are normally highly motile but *flaB* mutants of *B. burgdorferi* have no periplasmic flagellae and are non-motile and rod-shaped. These mutants are unable to establish infection in mice and do not survive well in the tick vector (Figure 14.2).

Diagnosis

Diagnosis of Lyme disease mainly relies on detection of antibody in infected individuals but the serological test, using ELISA, generally has low specificity (false positives can occur). This is because subclinical infection is common and cross-reactive antibody may also be present. Furthermore, antibody levels can be slow to rise in genuine cases so that false negatives may also occur. PCR is now successfully used on blood for direct detection of the pathogen (Branda and Steere 2021).

Treatment and Control

Treatment is with antimicrobials and there are now established protocols of prolonged, combined antimicrobial therapy in order to penetrate the sites where the infection is secreted (Wormser and Schwartz 2009). Prevention by vaccination is a worthwhile goal. The vaccine in use (LYMErix™ OspA) is based on the outer surface protein OspA. This protein is abundant on the surface of the spirochaete grown in lab culture. Unfortunately, it is now known that OspA is not expressed when *B. burgdorferi* is growing in the body of the animal (or human). OspA is expressed in the tick mid-gut but is not expressed during tick feeding (on contact with animal tissues and blood). The protective immunity from vaccination with OspA is thought to operate by the effects of the antibody on the bacteria while inside the tick.

A second outer membrane lipoprotein, OspC, expressed by the spirochaete during feeding, and also while in the animal body, is a candidate for inclusion in next-generation vaccines under development (Marconi et al. 2020). Unfortunately, in the US alone there are approximately 25 different OspC types. While an immune response can confer protection against the

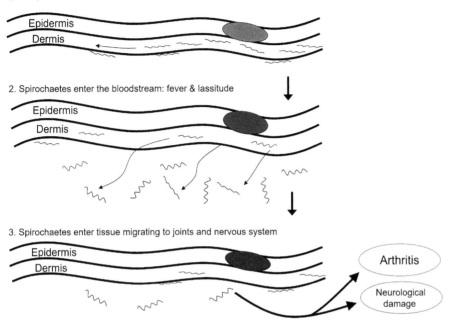

1. Tick bites, blood pools at the lesion, bacteria enter the pool, spread into skin. Inflammation leads to red rash

Epidermis
Dermis

2. Spirochaetes enter the bloodstream: fever & lassitude

Epidermis
Dermis

3. Spirochaetes enter tissue migrating to joints and nervous system

Epidermis
Dermis

Arthritis

Neurological damage

Figure 14.2 Pathogenesis of Lyme disease following the tick bite.

same type, this is relatively ineffective against infection with other types. *B. burgdorferi* strains are now defined by their OspC genotype which is associated with their ability to invade in the body and determines the pattern and severity of disease in animals and in experimental models of infection.

Recent evidence has shown that *B. burgdorferi* can shield itself from immunogenic proteins with the highly variable VlsE surface protein. The VlsE antigen is essential for persistence in the mammalian host and undergoes antigenic switching through recombination events in the *vlsE* locus and 15 silent *vls* cassettes (Kurokawa et al. 2020). This high degree of heterogeneity, as well as the shielding and antigenic switching, complicates the development of an effective vaccine.

References

Adeolu, M. and Gupta, R.S. (2014). A phylogenomic and molecular marker-based proposal for the division of the genus *Borrelia* into two genera: the emended genus *Borrelia* containing only the members of the relapsing fever *Borrelia*, and the genus *Borreliella* gen. nov. containing the members of the Lyme disease Borrelia (*Borrelia burgdorferi* sensu lato complex). *Antonie Van Leeuwenhoek* 105: 1049–1072.

Branda, J.A. and Steere, A.C. (2021). Laboratory diagnosis of Lyme borreliosis. *Clinical Microbiology Reviews* 34: e00018–e00019.

Chang, Y.-F., Novosol, V., McDonough, S.P. et al. (2000). Experimental infection of ponies with *Borrelia burgdorferi* by exposure to Ixodid ticks. *Veterinary Pathology* 37: 68–76.

Coburn, J., Leong, J., and Chaconas, G. (2013). Illuminating the roles of the *Borrelia burgdorferi* adhesins. *Trends in Microbiology* 21: 372–379.

Kurokawa, C., Lynn, G.E., Pedra, J.H.F. et al. (2020). Interactions between *Borrelia burgdorferi* and ticks. *Nature Reviews Microbiology* 18: 587–600.

Marconi, R.T., Honsberger, N., Winkler, M.T. et al. (2020). Field safety study of VANGUARD® crLyme: a vaccine for the prevention of Lyme disease in dogs. *Vaccine* X 6: 100080.

Posey, J.E. and Gherardini, F.C. (2000). Lack of a role for iron in the Lyme disease pathogen. *Science* 288: 1651–1653.

Wormser, G.P. and Schwartz, I. (2009). Antibiotic treatment of animals infected with *Borrelia burgdorferi*. *Clinical Microbiology Reviews* 22: 387–395.

15

Brachyspira

Brachyspira species, originally *Treponema* spp. and then *Serpulina* spp., are Gram-negative spirochaetes with an open spiral shape (very few turns to the organism). They were originally found associated with porcine intestinal disease but there are now nine species recognised, some of which are pathogenic and others not, infecting different animal species and humans (Hampson 2018).

Brachyspira hyodysenteriae

Brachyspira hyodysenteriae is an anaerobic spirochaete. The organism can be cultured on blood agar using the antimicrobial spectinomycin as a selective agent. It then forms an almost invisible film of growth rather than individual colonies. *B. hyodysenteriae* can be differentiated from the morphologically similar non-pathogenic spirochaete *B. innocens* by the production of a complete zone of β-haemolysis on blood agar. This is now known to be more than coincidental association; the haemolysin gene has been isolated and shown to be an important factor in the virulence of *B. hyodysenteriae*. The related species *B. hampsonii* and *B. suanatina* are also recognised causes of severe porcine enteric disease and are similarly strongly haemolytic (Costa et al. 2014; Rohde et al. 2014) (Figure 15.1).

Pathogenesis

Brachyspira hyodysenteriae causes swine dysentery, a mucohaemorrhagic colitis with diarrhoea in pigs. Gross lesions are restricted to the large intestine. There is variable thickening of the mucosal tissues with haemorrhage, fibrinonecrotic exudate and often abundant mucus production (Wilberts et al. 2014). The disease causes severe dehydration, loss of condition and 30% mortality in weaned pigs (7–20 weeks of age) (Quintana-Hayashi et al. 2019). This association was first demonstrated by Taylor and Alexander in Cambridge in 1971. However, it also became apparent that other members of the lower intestinal flora are necessary for the full effects of the spirochaete to be seen. It has now been suggested that normal enteric bacteria such as *Bacteroides* and *Prevotella* species, that are able to degrade sulfated mucins, may induce the decreased expression of these mucins. This may enable *Brachyspira* to breach the protective mucus layers and access the underlying epithelial cells (Wilberts et al. 2014).

Brachyspira pilosicoli

In addition, a syndrome associated with similar bacteria and known as spirochaetal diarrhoea or porcine intestinal spirochaetosis has been recognised for some time. It is milder than swine dysentery with moderate diarrhoea and reduced growth rate. Many of the organisms isolated from field cases are a recently recognised species known as *B. pilosicoli*. This is a weakly haemolytic spirochaete which can be characterised by specific biochemical tests and is of increasing importance as a cause of porcine intestinal spirochaetosis (PIS) in the field but also avian intestinal spirochaetosis (AIS) and human intestinal spirochaetosis (HIS) (Hampson 2018).

Fundamentals of Veterinary Microbiology, First Edition. Andrew N. Rycroft.
© 2024 John Wiley & Sons Ltd. Published 2024 by John Wiley & Sons Ltd.
Companion website: www.wiley.com/go/veterinarymicrobiology

Figure 15.1 The morphology of *Brachyspira hyodysenteriae* alongside other Gram-negative bacteria visible in a smear of porcine faeces after Gram staining.

References

Costa, M.O., Hill, J.E., Fernando, C. et al. (2014). Confirmation that "*Brachyspira hampsonii*" clade I (Canadian strain 30599) causes mucohemorrhagic diarrhea and colitis in experimentally infected pigs. *BMC Veterinary Research* 10: 129.

Hampson, D.J. (2018). The spirochete *Brachyspira pilosicoli*, enteric pathogen of animals and humans. *Clinical Microbiology Reviews* 31: e00087–e00017.

Quintana-Hayashi, M.P., Venkatakrishnan, V., Haesebrouck, F., and Landen, S. (2019). Role of sialic acid in *Brachyspira hyodysenteriae* adhesion to pig colonic mucins. *Infection and Immunity* 87: e00889–e00818.

Rohde, J., Habighorst-Blome, K., and Seehusen, F. (2014). "*Brachyspira hampsonii*" clade I isolated from Belgian pigs imported to Germany. *Veterinary Microbiology* 168: 432–435.

Wilberts, B.L., Arruda, P.H., Kinyon, J.M. et al. (2014). Comparison of lesion severity, distribution, and colonic mucin expression in pigs with acute swine dysentery following oral inoculation with "*Brachyspira hampsonii*" or *Brachyspira hyodysenteriae*. *Veterinary Pathology* 51: 1096–1108.

16

Pasteurella

The genus *Pasteurella* is a member of the *Pasteurellaceae* family. This is a group of delicate, Gram-negative bacteria with genera and species that are commensals, opportunistic pathogens and primary pathogens. Rather unfortunately, the relationships of the different groups of the family *Pasteurellaceae* were usually based on cultural and disease-related criteria, and analysis based on genomic and phylogenetic criteria has revealed that many species were incorrectly classified. A substantial number of these organisms (such as *Yersinia*, *Bibersteinia* and *Mannheimia* species) have therefore been renamed.

Pasteurella species are usually small, short rods, sometimes coccobacilli. All are facultative anaerobes. They are oxidase-positive and have a characteristic catarrhal odour in culture. They may show bipolar staining, but this property is inconsistent and difficult to see in such small bacteria. They are common inhabitants of the oral cavity, nasopharyngeal and upper respiratory mucosa of many domestic and wild animals. Many *Pasteurella* species are opportunistic pathogens that can cause endemic disease and are associated increasingly with epizootic outbreaks (Wilson and Ho 2013).

Pasteurella multocida

Pasteurella multocida has quite large, grey colonies on blood agar. The colonies are often very glossy and one colony runs into another because of the large quantity of capsular polysaccharide produced (Figure 16.1). As a simple guide to recognising colonies in culture, it does not grow on MacConkey agar. There are three subspecies of *P. multocida* but the significance of these is limited. These are subsp. *multocida*, subsp. *galicida* and subsp. *septica*.

Pasteurella multocida is an important primary and secondary pathogen. It causes fowl cholera (a septicaemia) in chickens and turkeys, and epizootic haemorrhagic septicaemia, a fatal septicaemic disease of cattle and buffalo in Africa and Asia. It is also involved in atrophic rhinitis of pigs and 'snuffles' (enzootic pasteurellosis) in rabbits.

Pasteurella multocida also causes disease as a secondary pathogen (an opportunistic infection following primary viral, mycoplasmal or other infection), particularly in the respiratory tract. For example, it is often isolated from pig enzootic pneumonia lesions where it probably causes much more damage than the initial mild infection with a mycoplasma or virus.

Five capsular serotypes (A, B, D, E, F) are recognised. The original typing system was tedious to perform and rather inaccurate but PCR-based typing, using detection of key capsule genes, is now used with much greater clarity. Types A and D are found as normal flora in the upper respiratory tract of animals. Type A capsular polysaccharide is composed of hyaluronic acid and, because this is also found in connective tissue, it is very poorly immunogenic. These are responsible for the majority of secondary infections due to *Pasteurella*. Type B is the cause of haemorrhagic septicaemia of cattle in Asia and southern Europe; type E causes haemorrhagic septicaemia in Africa. The strain designated as type C, if it ever truly existed, was lost. There are also 16 serovars of lipopolysaccharide produced, designated 1–16 and an adhesin, filamentous haemagglutinin (Mégroz et al. 2016). Apart from the basis of the typing scheme, capsular polysaccharide and lipopolysaccharide form the bacterial surface and are key to evasion of the innate host defences by resisting phagocytosis and both antimicrobial peptide and complement-mediated bactericidal activity.

Fundamentals of Veterinary Microbiology, First Edition. Andrew N. Rycroft.
© 2024 John Wiley & Sons Ltd. Published 2024 by John Wiley & Sons Ltd.
Companion website: www.wiley.com/go/veterinarymicrobiology

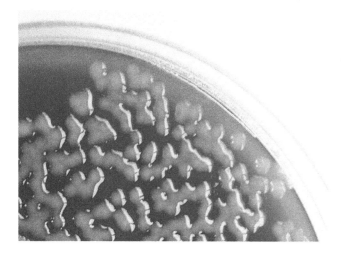

Figure 16.1 *Pasteurella multocida* colonies showing mucoid colonies coalescing because of the large quantity of hyaluronic acid capsule.

Fowl Cholera

Pasteurellosis in poultry is often asymptomatic or seen as mild disease such as conjunctivitis and chronic sinusitis. It can also develop into pneumonia but then suddenly progress into fatal disseminated fowl cholera. Fowl cholera is a septicaemia of all kinds of poultry caused by *P. multocida* types A or D. Infection is via the respiratory tract. It then gains access to the circulation and evades phagocytic clearance in birds. The organism grows in the bloodstream and the organ failure and circulatory collapse from endotoxin and cytokine response lead to severe illness and often death. Infection probably spreads from infected bird to susceptible bird via respiratory secretions into the nose or eyes and on feed and water. Fowl cholera can be a devastating disease with high mortality (Christensen and Bisgaard 2000).

Despite extensive investigation, no bacterial virulence trait or obvious mechanism has been found to correlate with the severity of disease or its incidence. Previously commensal *P. multocida* appear to be capable of causing full-blown fowl cholera. It is as though a bacterial factor necessary for disease is switched on, or upregulated, but the environmental or host factors that contribute to this switching, or influence the severity of invasion, remain unknown.

Considerable effort has been made over decades to use vaccines and antimicrobials in the control and treatment of fowl cholera. These have been partially successful, but outbreaks still occur and early detection and intervention are crucial to the outcome of an outbreak (Chung et al. 2005).

Haemorrhagic Septicaemia

Haemorrhagic septicaemia (HS) is a serious, acute, highly fatal and highly prevalent disease in livestock. It is seen particularly in cattle and buffalo in tropical regions of the world: Asia, India, Africa, southern Europe and the Middle East. HS is caused primarily by *P. multocida* serotypes B:2 and E:2 and is thought to occur at the later stages of pasteurellosis disease. HS is also seen in pigs, sheep, goats and deer, mostly associated with serotype B:2 strains. HS may be asymptomatic or unnoticed until the acute stage, which is characterised by rapid onset and progression. Clinical signs of upper respiratory disease and fever are followed by respiratory distress, sepsis and widespread haemorrhaging. This is usually fatal in 24–72 hours. As with fowl cholera, despite efforts over three decades, very little is known about the virulence mechanisms involved in the transition from mild pasteurellosis to acute severe disseminated disease (Moustafa et al. 2015).

Vaccination against HS has not been easy because of the sporadic nature of the disease and the very wide distribution of working buffalo and cattle in the regions where the disease occurs. Killed bacterial vaccines have been used and a live avirulent *aroA*-deficient mutant was produced and shown to be effective in preventing disease (Dagleish et al. 2007). However, development and licensing of vaccines such as this for small numbers in economically poorer, developing regions is not a financial priority for veterinary biologicals.

Mass die-offs among herds of Asian Saiga antelope in Kazakhstan have been recorded on a regular but apparently unpredictable basis. Hundreds of thousands of these ancient antelope have been recorded as dying almost simultaneously in the Asian Steppe in the spring time, coinciding with parturition. This has now been attributed to HS caused by *P. multocida* type B (Fereidouni et al. 2019). The disease affects the adults and calves then die from starvation. Various trigger factors, including high temperatures coupled with high atmospheric humidity, have been proposed as environmental factors promoting bacterial invasion and lethal disease.

Atrophic Rhinitis

Atrophic rhinitis is a disease seen only in pigs but is found in most pig-rearing countries of the world. It is unusual because two infections happen in sequence for the disease to occur. Piglets become infected in the nasopharynx with *Bordetella bronchiseptica* before the age of about three weeks. Most strains of *B. bronchiseptica* produce an ADP ribosylation toxin known as dermonecrotic toxin. This can lead to poor development of the bone in the turbinate scrolls of the porcine snout, known as turbinate atrophy. On top of this, pigs may become further infected with a strain of *P. multocida* producing the osteolytic toxin (known as PMT). This is a 143 kDa protein toxin encoded by the *toxA* gene in approximately 10% of type A and D strains of *P. multocida* (Peng et al. 2019). It is an extremely potent mitogen for eukaryotic cells through activation of a spectrum of G proteins. Overgrowth of the toxigenic *Pasteurella* leads to full-blown atrophic rhinitis in which the turbinate scrolls are destroyed along with considerable inflammation in the snout tissues and general poor growth and development of the animal (Figure 16.2).

While the *Bordetella* toxin is thought to interfere with the growth of osteoblasts, the osteolytic toxin from *Pasteurella* is thought to have complex signalling effects on both osteoblasts and osteoclasts, stimulating the latter to resorb bone. This is also a systemic mitogenic and other signalling effect at the cellular level in pigs. The effect of this is seen most clearly in the turbinate scrolls of piglets from about five weeks old such that the snout becomes deformed: shortened and twisted. The disease also has effects elsewhere in the animal, causing poor growth and hence reduced production.

Atrophic rhinitis is of economic significance but also a welfare concern. Disease can be treated or prevented with antimicrobials. It is also prevented by vaccination using products containing killed *B. bronchiseptica* and toxoid of the PMT.

Rabbit Snuffles (Enzootic Pasteurellosis)

Pasteurella multocida is a well-recognised cause of disease and mortality in rabbits. This is an upper respiratory infection, known as 'snuffles', that may spread to visceral organs. It is often enzootic in rabbit colonies and infection is transmitted early in life to young rabbits from the nasal secretions of infected adult animals. Once established, the *Pasteurella* may then spread to the middle ear, sinuses, lower respiratory tract and the genitals (Mancinelli 2019).

Different LPS of capsular types A and D are involved. Whether PMT production plays a role in rabbit disease has not been established but an atrophic rhinitis-like syndrome has been described in rabbits. Prior infection with *B. bronchiseptica* does appear to facilitate colonisation by *P. multocida*.

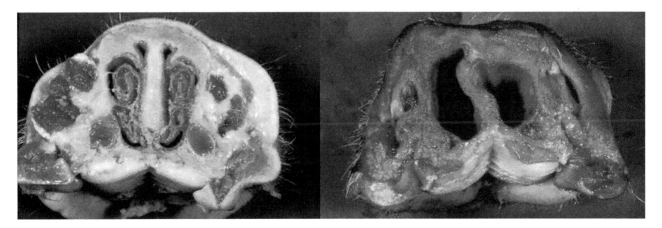

Figure 16.2 Porcine atrophic rhinitis. (Left) A section through the snout showing normal nasal turbinates. (Right) The inflammatory and destructive effect of atrophic rhinitis.

Attempts to prevent disease by vaccination have not so far been successful. However, some unvaccinated, untreated rabbits exposed to *P. multocida* resist infection altogether and of those with infection, a significant number resist disease. Treatment with antibiotics (such as fluoroquinolones) over a prolonged period is needed to control chronic infection.

Secondary Infection

Pasteurella multocida is also a secondary invader in different species following initial infection with virus or mycoplasma, or other predisposing events that facilitate bacterial invasion of the lungs. For instance, it is isolated from pulmonary lesions of porcine and bovine respiratory disease complex (PRDC and BRDC).

It is also seen in 50% of dog bite wounds and 75% of cat bite wounds. It is the most aggressive organism commonly causing infection following dog bites in humans (Wilson and Ho 2013).

References

Christensen, J.P. and Bisgaard, M. (2000). Fowl cholera. *Revue Scientifique et Technique* 19: 626–637.

Chung, J.-Y., Wilkie, I., Boyce, J.D., and Adler, B. (2005). Vaccination against fowl cholera with acapsular *Pasteurella multocida* A:1. *Vaccine* 23: 2751–2755.

Dagleish, M.P., Hodgson, J.C., Ataei, S. et al. (2007). Safety and protective efficacy of intramuscular vaccination with a live *aroA* derivative of *Pasteurella multocida* B:2 against experimental hemorrhagic septicemia in calves. *Infection and Immunity* 75: 5837–5844.

Fereidouni, S., Freimanis, G.L., Orynbayev, M. et al. (2019). Mass die-off of Saiga antelopes, Kazakhstan, 2015. *Emerging Infectious Diseases* 25: 1169–1176.

Mancinelli, E. (2019). Respiratory disease in rabbits. *In Practice* 41: 121–129.

Mégroz, M., Kleifeld, O., Wright, A. et al. (2016). The RNA-binding chaperone Hfq is an important global regulator of gene expression in *Pasteurella multocida* and plays a crucial role in production of a number of virulence factors, including hyaluronic acid capsule. *Infection and Immunity* 84: 1361–1370.

Moustafa, A.M., Seemann, T., Gladman, S. et al. (2015). Comparative genomic analysis of Asian haemorrhagic septicaemia-associated strains of *Pasteurella multocida* identifies more than 90 haemorrhagic septicaemia-specific genes. *PLoS One* 10: e0130296.

Peng, Z., Wang, X., Zhou, R. et al. (2019). *Pasteurella multocida*: genotypes and genomics. *Microbiology and Molecular Biology Reviews* 83: e00014–e00019.

Wilson, B.A. and Ho, M. (2013). *Pasteurella multocida*: from zoonosis to cellular microbiology. *Clinical Microbiology Reviews* 26: 631–655.

17

Pseudomonas and *Burkholderia*

Pseudomonas

Members of the genus *Pseudomonas* may appear to be rather similar to the enterobacteria in microscopic morphology, colony size and appearance. However, metabolically, they are entirely distinct from enterobacteria and these microorganisms are in a different taxonomic family. Pseudomonads are motile, aerobic, Gram-negative rods. They produce cytochrome C oxidase in their cytoplasmic membrane (so they are strongly oxidase positive in the oxidase test, while all enterobacteria are oxidase negative). Although other species of *Pseudomonas* are known, only *P. aeruginosa* is of any consequence in animal disease. Others, such as *P. syringae*, are plant pathogens or environmental microorganisms.

Pseudomonas aeruginosa does not ferment carbohydrates but instead only uses respiratory metabolism to generate energy and the organism will not grow under anaerobic conditions. *P. aeruginosa* often secretes pyocyanin, a distinctive greenish/blue pigment which diffuses into the medium. Some strains instead secrete pyoverdin (green) or pyorubin (pink). In addition, they have a characteristic smell and a metallic sheen to the surface of their colonies that help in their quick identification.

Habitat

Pseudomonas aeruginosa is free-living and widely distributed in the environment. It is present in soil and water and can be isolated from various living sources, including plants and animals where they cause no harm. It is also found in antiseptics, soap, sinks, mops, medicines, and physiotherapy and hydrotherapy pools. *P. aeruginosa* is seldom a member of the normal microbial flora in animals but it more readily colonises animals when the normal flora is altered or when there is tissue damage or trauma.

Pathogenicity

Pseudomonas aeruginosa is relatively non-pathogenic but nevertheless is a common cause of a variety of genuinely opportunistic infections which are difficult to treat. It is particularly able to cause infection in hospitals where sick animals, damaged tissue and widespread use of antibiotics favour colonisation and invasion of tissue by *Pseudomonas*. Arising from the large genome, encoding substantial metabolic flexibility, it can grow on very little nutrient and may survive in solutions of some disinfectants such as dilute cetrimide (a quaternary ammonium compound).

The pathogenicity factors of *P. aeruginosa* include the LPS which assists it in surviving phagocytosis; fimbriae for adhesion; exotoxin A, an ADP-ribosylating toxin that inhibits host protein synthesis; quorum sensing; biofilm formation; elastase, which destroys elastin in lung parenchyma and blood vessel walls; and other proteases and hydrolytic enzymes.

Pseudomonas aeruginosa is sometimes mistakenly referred to as an encapsulated pathogen. It produces an alginate slime, a hydrophilic polysaccharide that is a major component of the biofilm generated, but no true capsule is produced. This biofilm, in which the organism effectively hides from immune defences and antimicrobials, is an effective means of long-term survival of *Pseudomonas* in host tissues.

Fundamentals of Veterinary Microbiology, First Edition. Andrew N. Rycroft.
© 2024 John Wiley & Sons Ltd. Published 2024 by John Wiley & Sons Ltd.
Companion website: www.wiley.com/go/veterinarymicrobiology

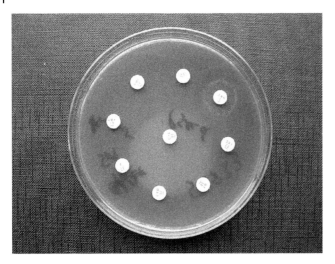

Figure 17.1 *Pseudomonas aeruginosa* in culture displaying the characteristic green pigment (pyocyanin) and no susceptibility to a variety of antimicrobials in the paper discs.

Antimicrobial Resistance

One of the major characteristics of *P. aeruginosa* is multiple antibiotic resistance (Figure 17.1). This is seen as resistance *in vitro* and borne out by failure of clinical response to treatment. Indeed, treatment of other infections with broad-spectrum antibiotics can be a factor that encourages *P. aeruginosa* infection: a microbiological vacuum is created which is filled by overgrowth of *P. aeruginosa*. For example, chronic canine otitis externa that has failed to resolve with treatment often yields a pure culture of *P. aeruginosa* (Barnard and Foster 2017).

Some antimicrobial resistance is intrinsic due to the very effective barrier of the pseudomonal outer membrane. The outer membrane protein OprD normally functions as a porin channel for basic amino acids and small peptides. This forms a narrower channel than the OmpF porin of *E. coli*, causing a lower permeability in *P. aeruginosa* than *E. coli* (Losito et al. 2022). This is exacerbated when there is a deficiency of OprD, or mutational changes in the protein, causing further restriction of the channel and resistance to carbapenems, particularly imipenem (Li et al. 2012; Moradali et al. 2017).

Resistance is also mediated by carriage of large plasmids (R-factors) carrying many resistance genes. These encode enzymes such as extended spectrum β-lactamases (ESBL) and carbapenemases, including metallo-β-lactamase (MBL). These are acquired through the accumulation and evolution of resistance genes on mobile genetic elements. Chromosomal genes are also involved in resistance through mutational changes that cause overexpression and altered function of existing multidrug efflux pumps. An example is the MexAB-OprM efflux pump that actively expels antimicrobial molecules such as fluoroquinolones, tetracyclines, macrolides, novobiocin, sulfonamides, trimethoprim, chloramphenicol, β-lactams (including carboxypenicillins, aztreonam, third-generation cephalosporins such as ceftazidime and cefotaxime, penems such as faropenem, and the carbapenems meropenem and panipenem, but not imipenem and biapenem) and β-lactamase inhibitors (Lister et al. 2009).

Pathogenesis

In animals, *P. aeruginosa* causes canine otitis following previous infection and *Otodectes cynotis* infestation. Such psoroptic ear mite infestations are often treated with preparations that include a parasiticide but also antibiotics, antifungals and a steroid. The external ear canal is inflamed but the normal bacterial and fungal yeast micro-organisms are destroyed. Sometimes, this damaged tissue, without competing bacterial flora and antibiotic, creates an excellent opportunity for *P. aeruginosa* to thrive – if it is present. Similar opportunities arise in other animals in other body sites and are frequently associated with the removal of competing microflora with antibiotic treatments.

Human infections follow a similar pattern and have greatly informed our understanding of *Pseudomonas*. Infections are common in burn wounds where severely damaged skin tissue and antimicrobial treatment combine to facilitate infection with *P. aeruginosa*. The lungs of individuals with the chronic, inherited disease cystic fibrosis are also susceptible because infections persist from the failure to remove secretions from the respiratory tract. Persistent infection causes chronic fibrosis and requires long-term antimicrobial treatment. *P. aeruginosa* colonises these sites and is then very difficult to clear. Moreover, exposure to antimicrobials encourages the overproduction of efflux mechanisms both through mutation in the control of this expression and from the changes in gene expression in response to the drugs.

Antibiotics for Treating *Pseudomonas* Infection

To combat this, special antibiotics with activity against *Pseudomonas* have been developed. Early examples of drugs used for *Pseudomonas* infection were gentamicin, tobramycin, carbenicillin and polymyxin B. Third-generation cephalosporins such as ceftazidime were developed in the 1980s to address the need for long-term therapy of *Pseudomonas* infections in humans with cystic fibrosis. Fluorinated 4-quinolones such as ciprofloxacin were also effective, and enrofloxacin was introduced about 1992 for animal treatment. However, the efficacy of this drug has gradually been eroded for treatment of infections due to *P. aeruginosa* (and some other Gram-negatives). The proportion of *Pseudomonas* from animal infections showing resistance to this drug, and the MIC, has gradually risen over the three decades since its first use.

Resistance to all these drugs is recognised in *P. aeruginosa* and this resistance continues to evolve as bacterial populations are exposed to the selection pressure of these agents. As an example, strains of *P. aeruginosa* naturally carry an inducible AmpC cephalosporinase. Wild-type strains produce only low basal levels of AmpC and are susceptible to the antipseudomonal penicillins, penicillin-β-lactamase inhibitor combinations, cephalosporins and carbapenems. However, when AmpC is overproduced by mutation of the control mechanism, the strain develops resistance to all β-lactams, with the exception of the carbapenems (Lister et al. 2009).

Newer antibacterial combinations of β-lactam/β-lactamase inhibitors have been introduced such as imipenem-relebactam, ceftazidime-avibactam and ceftolozane-tazobactam. Drugs with novel mechanisms of entry are also being developed such as the siderophore cephalosporin cefiderocol that penetrates by linking to ferric iron, allowing it to use iron carriers to permeate the bacterial outer membrane (Losito et al. 2022). Overall, however, there is a progressive increase in multidrug resistance with time among strains prevailing in hospital settings, and options for therapy of *Pseudomonas* infections can sometimes be very limited.

Burkholderia

Burkholderia mallei, a non-motile Gram-negative rod, was once called *Pseudomonas mallei*. It is a facultative intracellular pathogen that causes glanders (particularly in horses) in parts of the Middle East, Asia, Eastern Europe and Africa. *B. mallei* is an obligate animal pathogen, normally found only in infected horses. It is not found in the environment and animals other than equidae are accidental hosts. The organism gains access to the lymphatics via the nasopharyngeal mucosa and spreads to other parts of the body. Lesions in the lymphatics may ulcerate to the surface (known as farcy). The organism gains access to the bloodstream and thence to the lungs. The lung lesions are tuberculosis-like granulomas. When lesions are present in the upper respiratory tract, they rupture to release pus which is highly infectious and released from the nostrils. Glanders may be diagnosed serologically.

Burkholderia pseudomallei

Burkholderia pseudomallei causes mellioidosis, primarily in South-east Asia and northern Australia where the organism is present in the environment, particularly soil and water. The disease is similar to glanders but affects primarily rodents, although it has been seen in a variety of species and also affects humans. The lesions are caseous nodules which may be present in a variety of tissues of the reticuloendothelial system (fixed and wandering phagocytic macrophages of liver, spleen and lymphatic system), the joints, lungs and upper respiratory tract.

References

Barnard, N. and Foster, A. (2017). *Pseudomonas* otitis in dogs: a general practitioner's guide to treatment. *In Practice* 39: 386–398.

Li, H., Luo, Y.-F., Williams, B.J. et al. (2012). Structure and function of OprD protein in *Pseudomonas aeruginosa*: from antibiotic resistance to novel therapies. *International Journal of Medical Microbiology* 302: 63–68.

Lister, P.D., Wolter, D.J., and Hanson, N.D. (2009). Antibacterial-resistant *Pseudomonas aeruginosa*: clinical impact and complex regulation of chromosomally encoded resistance mechanisms. *Clinical Microbiology Reviews* 22: 582–610.

Losito, A.R., Raffaelli, F., del Giacomo, P., and Tumbarello, M. (2022). New drugs for the treatment of *Pseudomonas aeruginosa* infections with limited treatment options: a narrative review. *Antibiotics* 11: 579.

Moradali, M.F., Ghods, S., and Rehm, B.H. (2017). *Pseudomonas aeruginosa* lifestyle: a paradigm for adaptation, survival, and persistence. *Frontiers in Cellular and Infection Microbiology* 7: 39.

18

Bordetella

Bordetellae are small Gram-negative coccobacilli which have a respiratory metabolism. They do not ferment carbohydrates such as glucose, are therefore strictly aerobic, and are oxidase positive. There are nine species of *Bordetella* although only four are considered to be of consequence in disease. *B. bronchiseptica* appears to be the evolutionary progenitor of *B. pertussis* and *B. parapertussis*. *B. bronchiseptica* is the pathogen of animals (Gerlach et al. 2001). This species can be motile and will grow on MacConkey agar.

Bordetella bronchiseptica

Bordetella bronchiseptica is a respiratory pathogen of world-wide distribution that infects many animal species (dogs, cats, pigs, rabbits) but not ruminants. It is closely related to *B. pertussis* and *B. parapertussis*, the causative agents of whooping cough in humans. Colonisation of a host by *B. bronchiseptica* can result in asymptomatic carriage or lead to a range of diseases, including fatal pneumonia.

A general term for the disease is bordetellosis which includes rhinitis, tracheitis, bronchitis and bronchiolitis. The organism is able to colonise the ciliated respiratory epithelium of young animals, particularly following primary virus infection. Many infections are inapparent and clinical disease is associated with mildly exudative inflammation of the ciliated airway to give nasal discharge, cough and low-grade fever. In the dog, this is termed canine infectious tracheobronchitis (kennel cough). Where canine distemper is the virus infection, colonisation with *B. bronchiseptica* leads to a lethal bronchopneumonia. This was the case following phocine (seal) distemper in the late 1980s in which many of the seals were killed by the secondary *B. bronchiseptica* infection.

Pathogenicity

Colonisation requires adhesive factors, of which fimbriae, filamentous haemagglutinin and the outer membrane protein pertactin have been characterised (Mattoo and Cherry 2005). An adenylate cyclase enzyme is also produced by *B. bronchiseptica*. This is actually an RTX group cytotoxin fused to adenylate cyclase (Cya). The pore-forming toxin part of the molecule damages cells and the adenylate cyclase activity is functionally active against neutrophils and macrophages at the site of bacterial activity (Gueirard et al. 1998). The effect of the toxin is to inhibit removal of the organism from the airway.

A heat-labile (or dermonecrotic toxin) is also secreted and this is required for turbinate atrophy in the pig. In piglets, it causes mild atrophic rhinitis (turbinate hypoplasia). While this is self-healing, it favours colonisation by *P. multocida* which produces osteolytic toxin and leads to severe atrophic rhinitis (Rutter 1989). For this, colonisation with *B. bronchiseptica* must take place in the first few weeks of life.

Regulation of Virulence in *Bordetella*

Virulence genes of *B. bronchiseptica* are regulated in a co-ordinated fashion depending on the environment in which the bacteria find themselves. This was known as 'phenotypic modulation' and is regulated by the two-component signal transduction system Bvg, for *Bordetella* virulence gene. It was originally discovered in *B. pertussis* (Weiss and Falkow 1984) and

Fundamentals of Veterinary Microbiology, First Edition. Andrew N. Rycroft.
© 2024 John Wiley & Sons Ltd. Published 2024 by John Wiley & Sons Ltd.
Companion website: www.wiley.com/go/veterinarymicrobiology

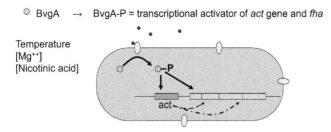

Figure 18.1 Co-ordinated transcriptional activation of virulence factors via Bvg in *Bordetella*.

was later found to apply in *B. bronchiseptica*. In the absence of chemical modulators, at 37 °C, the BvgAS system activates the expression of a large set of virulence factors together (Gestal et al. 2019) (Figure 18.1).

The bacteria are then virulent, known as Bvg$^+$. In the presence of 40 mM $MgSO_4$ or 10 mM nicotinic acid or low temperature (25 °C), the genes for expression of virulence factors are switched off: the bacteria are non-virulent, known as Bvg$^-$. In the Bvg$^-$ form, *B. bronchiseptica* expresses flagellae and becomes motile. The switch is mediated by the products of a two-component regulatory locus (*bvgAS*), (Figure 18.2).

In Bvg$^+$, adhesins and toxins associated with virulence are synthesised. These include filamentous haemagglutinin, fimbriae, pertactin, adenylate cyclase toxin and dermonecrotic toxin. In addition, a type 3 secretion system is induced. This is used to translocate effector proteins using a needle-like injection apparatus directly into eukaryotic cells and disrupt host cell signalling, and induces necrotic-like cell death (Mattoo and Cherry 2005).

Bvg$^+$ may be important for colonisation of the respiratory tract. Bvg$^-$ may be considered as 'starvation mode' in which the bacteria avoid wastage and survival in the environment. It may also be better for fitness in the later stages of infection, including persistence in the host. An intermediate phase is also hypothesised in which a subset of Bvg$^+$ phase-specific factors is expressed which may facilitate respiratory transmission.

In addition to phenotypic modulation, the expression of virulence genes is also regulated by a genetic event known as phase variation. This is thought to be the result of a reversible frameshift mutation in the *bvg* locus that is inherited.

Pathogenesis

Bordetella bronchiseptica infection is a cause of tracheobronchitis (kennel cough) in dogs. This is characterised by congestion of the mucosal lining of the trachea and bronchi and a mucoid or mucopurulent exudate. Kennel cough is usually a complex infection initiated by virus or mycoplasma with subsequent bacterial infection and so is usually ascribed the term canine respiratory disease complex in which *B. bronchiseptica* may or may not be a major component. Disease is also seen in pigs as described elsewhere. Upper respiratory infection in young piglets is a prerequisite to turbinate atrophy and, alongside toxigenic *Pasteurella multocida*, leads to atrophic rhinitis with hypoplasia and destruction of the turbinate scrolls (see Chapter 16).

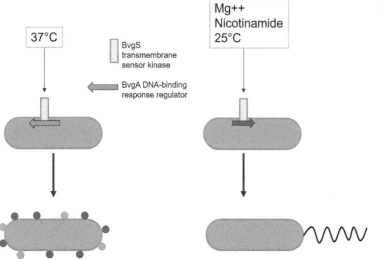

Figure 18.2 BvgAS two-component signal transduction system.

Feline respiratory infection with *B. bronchiseptica* is also seen. Serological evidence suggests infection takes place at an early age in kittens. Infection of older cats is detected in approximately 10% overall, but the majority of this is in catteries and not household pets.

Vaccination using a live, attenuated strain of *B. bronchiseptica* administered into the nostrils has been employed since the 1970s in the UK. Elsewhere, in Europe and the USA, vaccines are killed, whole cells given by subcutaneous injection.

The original strain used in the commercial UK vaccine was a pig strain, held for many years in storage. When retrieved and recultured, it was developed into the commercial vaccine. No reason for the strain to be avirulent was known and no effort seems to have been made to demonstrate that it lacked the ability to cause bordetellosis. It was perhaps optimistically assumed that since it was derived from a pig, it was unlikely to cause disease in a dog. Protection derived from this vaccine in the field seems to have been weak. Attempts to improve vaccination were made in the 1990s when rationally defined *aroA* mutants of *B. bronchiseptica*, shown to have reduced pathogenicity, were developed and these have been marketed as live, intranasal vaccines for both the dog and the cat.

Other *Bordetella* Species

Bordetella avium causes rhinotracheitis in turkey poults. Again, the organism colonises ciliated tracheal epithelium, leading to inflammation. *B. parapertussis* is known in two groups: human-adapted *B. parapertussis* (*B. parapertussis$_{hu}$*) that causes a milder form of pertussis-like disease in humans and also an ovine-adapted *B. parapertussis* (*B. parapertussis$_{ov}$*) that causes chronic respiratory infection of sheep. As with *B. pertussis*, it has no environmental reservoir. Human and ovine strains of *B. parapertussis* represent distinct clonal lineages that diverged independently from *B. bronchiseptica*. Evidence suggests that there is little or no transmission between the sheep and human reservoirs.

References

Gerlach, G., von Wintzingerode, F., Middendorf, B., and Gross, R. (2001). Evolutionary trends in the genus *Bordetella*. *Microbes and Infection* 3: 61–72.

Gestal, M.C., Whitesides, L.T., and Harvill, E.T. (2019). Integrated signaling pathways mediate *Bordetella* immunomodulation, persistence and transmission. *Trends in Microbiology* 27: 118–130.

Gueirard, P., Druilhe, A., Pretolani, M., and Guiso, N. (1998). Role of adenylate cyclase-hemolysin in alveolar macrophage apoptosis during *Bordetella pertussis* infection *in vivo*. *Infection and Immunity* 66: 1718–1725.

Mattoo, S. and Cherry, J.D. (2005). Molecular pathogenesis, epidemiology, and clinical manifestations of respiratory infections due to *Bordetella pertussis* and other *Bordetella* subspecies. *Clinical Microbiology Reviews* 18: 326–382.

Rutter, M. (1989). Atrophic rhinitis. *In Practice* 11: 74–80.

Weiss, A.A. and Falkow, S. (1984). Genetic analysis of phase change in *Bordetella pertussis*. *Infection and Immunity* 43: 263–269.

19

Delicate Gram-negative Bacteria

Of the bacterial pathogens causing specific animal diseases, some are rather fastidious and easily killed once outside the body. These have been referred to as delicate Gram-negatives and include *Brucella*, *Moraxella* and *Taylorella* species.

Brucella

The *Brucella* species are small, Gram-negative, non-motile coccobacilli. They are unusual in having two circular chromosomes, known as chromosomes I and II. The genome sequences of the different *Brucella* species are very similar and it has been suggested that they are really a single species with biovars that are adapted to a particular host animal. However, the current view is that they should be considered as individual species.

Because these species have been considered very similar, it was a specialist task to differentiate between them using metabolic and serological characteristics. In addition, they are delicate to culture and must be handled with care in containment level 3 facilities to avoid exposure of personnel and escape into the environment. Six species were recognised based originally on the animal from which they were isolated. These are host-adapted to their respective animals: *B. abortus* in cattle, *B. melitensis* in goats and sheep, *B. suis* in pigs, *B. ovis* in sheep, *B. canis* in dogs and *B. neotomae* in desert woodrats (Whatmore 2009).

With whole-genome sequencing, it became clear that brucellae have probably evolved from saprophytic soil bacteria and it is also now recognised that there is considerable genetic diversity within the genus and several new species have been distinguished from many different animals including marine mammals, reptiles, fish and amphibians (Whatmore and Foster 2021).

Pathogenesis

The *Brucella* genus causes a substantial burden of disease in livestock and zoonotic infection of global importance. In animals, *Brucella* causes generalised infections, with a bacteraemic phase followed by localisation in the reproductive organs and reticuloendothelial system. *Brucella* species are facultative intracellular pathogens which survive and multiply in host cells by inhibiting lysosome-phagosome fusion. Intracellular bacteria generally produce chronic diseases characterised by granulomatous inflammatory reactions.

When ingested, brucellae can penetrate nasal, oral or pharyngeal mucosa. These are phagocytosed and progress to the regional lymph nodes. These enlarge (lymphatic and reticuloendothelial hyperplasia) and inflammation is induced. If the organisms are not killed at this stage, they will spread to other organs (liver, spleen, placenta, mammary gland, epididymis) where they cause a chronic granulomatous immune reaction.

The four-carbon sugar alcohol erythritol is found in the uterine tissues of cattle. It acts as a growth stimulant for *Brucella* and causes tissue tropism for this region (Smith et al. 1962). The organisms then cause infection of the fetus and placenta with massive proliferation of the bacteria in these tissues, leading to abortion (Jain et al. 2012) (Figure 19.1). Evidence has also been presented to suggest that erythritol may encourage the brucellae to leave the intracellular niche of the trophoblasts in the placental region and replicate extracellularly. It is also known to upregulate virulence-associated genes so that those organisms expelled with a placenta are actively expressing the virulence factors required to establish further

Fundamentals of Veterinary Microbiology, First Edition. Andrew N. Rycroft.
© 2024 John Wiley & Sons Ltd. Published 2024 by John Wiley & Sons Ltd.
Companion website: www.wiley.com/go/veterinarymicrobiology

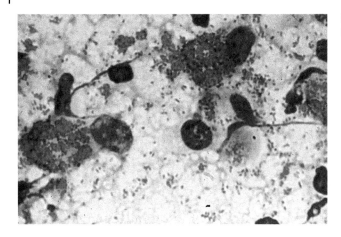

Figure 19.1 *Brucella abortus* (red coccobacilli) in placental tissue, stained by modified Ziehl-Neelsen stain.

infection. When ingested by another animal host, these primed bacteria may be more able to efficiently generate a successful infection (Petersen et al. 2013).

Zoonotic Disease

Human infection with *B. abortus* was once common. Among the general population, infection was acquired mainly through ingestion of unpasteurised dairy products. There are now very few reports of indigenously acquired human cases of brucellosis in the developed world because almost all milk is pasteurised and because the programme to eradicate bovine brucellosis has been largely successful.

Most zoonotic disease is due to infection with the three species *B. abortus*, *B. melitensis* or *B. suis*. *Brucella*, particularly *B. melitensis*, is considered to infect more than 500 000 people annually (Seleem et al. 2010) and *B. melitensis* is considered to be the *Brucella* sp. most virulent for humans. Human infection from other species has been only rarely reported.

The incubation period in humans is normally 2–3 weeks but may be several months. The onset is insidious with malaise, headache, night sweats and weakness and is known as undulant fever. Chronic brucellosis is associated with fatigue, myalgia, fever and depression. It can persist for months.

In the wider world where brucellosis is still present, the disease still occurs in farmers, farm workers and veterinary surgeons who have close contact with animals (placenta and abortions) and in those consuming infected animal products (unpasteurised milk).

A few human cases of undulant fever (or Malta fever from *B. melitensis*) continue to be reported in the UK and northern Europe; these are often associated with consumption of raw milk or unpasteurised cheese consumed in regions of the world where the infection persists. Brucellosis due to *B. melitensis* has never been reported in animals in the UK. Control of human brucellosis remains dependent on control of animal disease and the effective implementation of appropriate food safety regulations.

Anecdotally, an older colleague (Professor John E. Smith) once told me how he, as a veterinary microbiologist in the 1950s, used to diagnose brucellosis by sniffing the placentas of aborted calves. Those positive for brucellosis apparently had a distinctive aroma. By his account, it was a useful method although whether it was ever evaluated for sensitivity and specificity against an accepted reliable method was never mentioned. Unsurprisingly, John caught undulant fever from this traditional veterinary practice for which, in his typically stoical way, he then refused treatment in order to ensure that he gained a good solid immunity. It took 10 months for the disease to resolve, illustrating (apart from the predictable outcome of a rather *laissez-faire* attitude to disease transmission) the persistent nature of the pathogen and the time needed to develop an effective immune response.

Pathogenicity

Brucella species are unusual among pathogens in apparently not producing any of the normally recognised bacterial virulence determinants such as adhesive fimbriae and toxins (Seleem et al. 2008). The key to pathogenicity is intracellular survival and there must be components that are used to enable this. One virulence determinant that has now been recognised is VirB, a type IV secretion system.

Brucella abortus gaining access to a host animal is taken up by professional phagocytic cells. It cannot grow in neutrophils but is also not destroyed by them and so viable organisms are ultimately carried to preferred host cells: macrophages, monocytes, dendritic cells and epithelial cells. Once inside these cells, *Brucella* is contained in a *Brucella*-containing vacuole (BCV) and this avoids fusion with the lysosomes. A two-component regulatory system in the bacterial membrane, BvrR/BvrS, detects the acidic conditions in the BCV and activates transcription of genes for the VirB system in the *Brucella*. These are effector proteins that modulate host secretory functions to remodel BCVs into replication-permissive organelles (Altamirano-Silva et al. 2021). The organisms grow in this vacuole, spread to adjacent cells and are released from the cell by unknown mechanisms.

Control

In the UK, as in much of northern Europe, North America and Australasia, brucellosis has been successfully controlled in farm livestock and is now considered largely eradicated. This has been through testing and culling, and by a successful vaccination programme. However, in most other parts of the world, it remains a major animal health and zoonotic problem.

Testing for Brucellosis

Major tools for the control of brucellosis are serological tests. Screening of bulk milk using the milk ring test and serological testing of beef cattle using the rose Bengal plate test, ELISA tests and the complement fixation test have been very effective. These tests mainly detect antibody to the surface lipopolysaccharide. This dominant antigen (a linear homopolymer of β-1,2-linked 4,6-dideoxy-4-formamido-β-D-mannopyranosyl subunits) is common to virulent and some vaccine strains (below), so the distinction between infection and immune response from vaccination is problematical.

Vaccination Against Brucellosis

Vaccine strain S19 was the widely used live vaccine in the control of brucellosis. It is a spontaneously attenuated strain discovered in 1923 and has been used worldwide since the early 1930s to prevent brucellosis in cattle. Young animals were vaccinated (90–180 days); vaccination in older animals caused the antibody titre to be more persistent which would interfere with serological testing. It was replaced in some regions during the 1990s by strain RB51. This is a lipopolysaccharide O-antigen-deficient mutant of a virulent strain of *B. abortus* which carries an insertion sequence in the wboA glycosyl transferase gene. Unlike S19, it therefore cannot induce antibodies to the *Brucella* LPS O-antigens that are detected by the serodiagnostic tests for brucellosis (Schurig et al. 1991).

Being live vaccines, both S19 and RB51 are effective in generating the cell-mediated immune response needed for protection. Vaccination with killed *B. abortus* strain 45/20 is safer, causing fewer side-effects (abortions in cattle and accidental cases of operator infection) and like RB51 is O-antigen deficient, but it does not induce the strong cell-mediated response needed to protect animals. Another vaccine strain is used widely in Europe. The live, attenuated *B. melitensis* strain Rev-1 is used for vaccinating sheep and goats against *B. melitensis* disease. Rev-1 vaccination is protective but still interferes in the classic serodiagnostic tests for *B. melitensis* and can both induce abortions and be excreted in milk when used in adult animals (Barrio et al. 2009).

Moraxella bovis

Moraxella bovis is the cause of infectious bovine keratoconjunctivitis (IBK; sometimes known as pink eye or New Forest eye). It is a Gram-negative coccobacillus that is a commensal of the upper respiratory tract in cattle and probably spread between animals by flies (Postma et al. 2008). *M. bovis* is classified in a separate family of bacteria, the *Moraxellaceae*. The species was subdivided into seven distinct serogroups (A–G) based on fimbrial antigens (Moore and Lepper 1991).

Pathogenicity

Moraxella bovis is considered an opportunistic pathogen and concurrent viral or mycoplasma infection can help to initiate the infection. The organism adheres specifically to the conjunctival surface by means of fimbriae (Ruehl et al. 1993).

Antibody to the pili generated by vaccination can be protective (Lepper et al. 1992). However, mucosal surface immunity tends to be short-lived and so protection declines rapidly. A cytolysin is also produced: this is MbxA, an RTX group toxin (Billson et al. 2000). This is essential for the pathogen to cause conjunctivitis (Beard and Moore 1994). Like many other Gram-negatives, *M. bovis* acquires iron for growth using specific proteins (Fenwick et al. 1996).

Taylorella equigenitalis

The single species *Taylorella equigenitalis* is the cause of contagious equine metritis (CEM). This is a sexually transmitted (venereal) infection of all types of horses. *Taylorella* is a delicate, non-motile, microaerophilic, Gram-negative coccobacillus.

The organism appears to have originated in continental Europe and was first imported into the UK in carrier mares from Ireland. It was recognised and reported in Newmarket as a previously unrecognised pathogen, initially called *Haemophilus equigenitalis*, in 1977.

Pathogenesis

Taylorella equigenitalis resides on the mucosal surface of the penis of stallions where it is considered a commensal, causing no recognisable clinical signs. Stallions are the primary source of infection, from where the pathogen is passed to the genital tract of the mare at breeding, causing an endometritis with a mucopurulent discharge from the vagina in approximately 30–40% of cases of exposure. This inflammation in the uterus hinders implantation of the conceptus, causing infertility. Most animals recover from this infection and become free of the organism while a small proportion become carriers where the pathogen will persist, long term, in the external genitalia of the infected mare.

The bacterial components involved in colonisation, survival in the host, specificity for equids, persistence on the mucous membrane and endometritis are not known.

Control of Transmission

The infection has been seen in North and South America, Japan, southern Africa and Australia; it has been detected in at least 30 countries in Europe. Currently, it is assumed that the main reservoir of *T. equigenitalis* is continental Europe where the pathogen is enzootic within the resident non-thoroughbred population, particularly wild ponies (Schulman et al. 2013).

Detection of the organisms in carrier animals is crucial to prevent them from infecting other horses, particularly in the stud farm breeding of thoroughbred horses. Detection is by careful sampling, transport of samples and culture. PCR has been used for many years as an adjunct to the relatively difficult culture, with PCR found to be marginally more sensitive than culture (Mawhinney 2020). In the UK, only bacteriology laboratories accredited by, and thence registered with, the Horse Race Betting Levy Board can provide a report stating whether a horse is infected or free of the organism. Apart from occasional outbreaks, the UK has remained free of CEM for a number of years.

Artificial Breeding

While infection of thoroughbreds by natural breeding has become very rare due to the careful testing of breeding horses and implementation of disease surveillance, more recently transmission through artificial breeding (using chilled semen) has re-emerged among breeding of non-thoroughbred horses. It is therefore vital that testing of breeding animals and the semen used to inseminate mares is also used as a means of control (Schulman et al. 2013).

References

Altamirano-Silva, P., Cordero-Serrano, M., Méndez-Montoya, J. et al. (2021). Intracellular passage triggers a molecular response in *Brucella abortus* that increases its infectiousness. *Infection and Immunity* 89: e00004–e00021.

Barrio, M.B., Grilló, M.J., Muñoz, P.M. et al. (2009). Rough mutants defective in core and O-polysaccharide synthesis and export induce antibodies reacting in an indirect ELISA with smooth lipopolysaccharide and are less effective than Rev 1 vaccine against *Brucella melitensis* infection of sheep. *Vaccine* 27: 1741–1749.

Beard, M.K. and Moore, L.J. (1994). Reproduction of bovine keratoconjunctivitis with a purified haemolytic and cytotoxic fraction of *Moraxella bovis*. *Veterinary Microbiology* 42: 15–33.

Billson, F.M., Harbour, C., Michalski, W.P. et al. (2000). Characterization of hemolysin of *Moraxella bovis* using a hemolysis-neutralizing monoclonal antibody. *Infection and Immunity* 68: 3469–3474.

Fenwick, B., Rider, M., Liang, J., and Brightman, A. (1996). Iron repressible outer membrane proteins of *Moraxella bovis* and demonstration of siderophore-like activity. *Veterinary Microbiology* 48: 315–324.

Jain, N., Boyle, S.M., and Sriranganathan, N. (2012). Effect of exogenous erythritol on growth and survival of *Brucella*. *Veterinary Microbiology* 160: 513–516.

Lepper, A.W.D., Moore, L.J., Atwell, J.L., and Tennent, J.M. (1992). The protective efficacy of pili from different strains of *Moraxella bovis* within the same serogroup against infectious bovine keratoconjunctivitis. *Veterinary Microbiology* 32: 177–187.

Mawhinney, I. (2020). Ten years of *Taylorella equigenitalis* ring trial results comparing culture and polymerase chain reaction. *Revue Scientifique et Technique* 39: 717–724.

Moore, L.J. and Lepper, A.W. (1991). A unified serotyping scheme for *Moraxella bovis*. *Veterinary Microbiology* 29: 75–83.

Petersen, E., Rajashekara, G., Sanakkayala, N. et al. (2013). Erythritol triggers expression of virulence traits in *Brucella melitensis*. *Microbes and Infection* 15: 440–449.

Postma, G.C., Carfagnini, J.C., and Minatel, L. (2008). *Moraxella bovis* pathogenicity: an update. *Comparative Immunology, Microbiology and Infectious Diseases* 31: 449–458.

Ruehl, W.W., Marrs, C., George, L. et al. (1993). Infection rates, disease frequency, pilin gene rearrangement, and pilin expression in calves inoculated with *Moraxella bovis* pilin-specific isogenic variants. *American Journal of Veterinary Research* 54: 248–253.

Schulman, M.L., Maya, C.E., Keys, B., and Guthrie, A.J. (2013). Contagious equine metritis: artificial reproduction changes the epidemiologic paradigm. *Veterinary Microbiology* 167: 2–8.

Schurig, G.G., Roop, R.M., Bagchi, T. et al. (1991). Biological properties of RB51: a stable rough strain of *Brucella abortus*. *Veterinary Microbiology* 28: 171–188.

Seleem, M.N., Boyle, S.M., and Sriranganathan, N. (2008). *Brucella*: a pathogen without classic virulence genes. *Veterinary Microbiology* 129: 1–14.

Seleem, M.N., Boyle, S.M., and Sriranganathan, N. (2010). Brucellosis: a re-emerging zoonosis. *Veterinary Microbiology* 140: 392–398.

Smith, H., Williams, A.E., Pearce, J.H. et al. (1962). Foetal erythritol: a cause of the localization of *Brucella abortus* in bovine contagious abortion. *Nature* 193: 47–49.

Whatmore, A.M. (2009). Current understanding of the genetic diversity of Brucella, an expanding genus of zoonotic pathogens. *Infection, Genetics and Evolution* 9: 1168–1184.

Whatmore, A.M. and Foster, J.T. (2021). Emerging diversity and ongoing expansion of the genus *Brucella*. *Infection, Genetics and Evolution* 92: 104865.

20

Mannheimia, Actinobacillus and Other Pasteurellaceae

Mannheimia

Mannheimia haemolytica was previously named *Pasteurella haemolytica*. Normally, it lives in the oropharynx of healthy cattle and other ruminants, but it is also an opportunistic pathogen. It is the cause of epizootic (epidemic) pneumonia in cattle (shipping or transit fever; bovine pneumonic pasteurellosis) and in sheep (pasteurellosis).

These organisms were previously subdivided into two biovars: those that fermented the disaccharide sugar trehalose and those that fermented the 5-carbon monosaccharide arabinose, known as the T and A biovars respectively. The arabinose fermenters (A-biovar; 12 capsule types) became five different species of which the important pathogen is *M. haemolytica*. The trehalose fermenters (T-biovar; four capsule types) became known as *Pasteurella trehalosi* but in 2007 were renamed *Bibersteinia trehalosi* (Blackall et al. 2007).

Mannheimia haemolytica

Strains of *M. haemolytica* are usually β-haemolytic on blood agar and, unlike *P. multocida*, grow on MacConkey agar. They produce a pore-forming leucotoxin (Lkt) which kills leucocytes of ruminants. It is this leucotoxin that is causing the weak haemolysis observed on blood agar. Lkt is a member of the RTX group of toxins, closely related to the α-haemolysin of *E. coli* and the Apx toxins of the pig respiratory pathogen *A. pleuropneumoniae*. This toxin is crucial for the pathogenicity of the bacteria to cause pneumonia (Petras et al. 1995). Like *P. multocida*, *M. haemolytica* strains carry different capsular and LPS types. The types most commonly seen in pneumonic pasteurellosis are capsular types 1 and 2 (previously A1 and A2).

Bovine Pneumonic Pasteurellosis

Mannheimia haemolytica is a normal commensal in the upper respiratory tract of cattle, goats, sheep and some non-ruminant animals. Disease occurs when animals, particularly young animals, are stressed through transport, adverse weather or when mild virus infections such as PI-3, IBR, BVD or BRSV damage the mucosal epithelium of the upper airway. Bacterial pathogens, particularly *Mycoplasma bovis*, can also initiate respiratory disease. The *Mannheimia* are then capable of invading into the lower respiratory tract. This is known as bovine respiratory disease complex (BRDC) because it is a mixed set of circumstances and pathogens. Once the disease becomes established in the lungs in one animal, it can spread via respiratory secretions (aerosol) through coughing. Other animals inhale the droplets and so the pathogen gains direct access to the lower airway in large numbers. This overcomes the clearance mechanisms that normally prevent small numbers of the pathogen from invading.

Mannheimia haemolytica causes a more rapid and more severe disease course than *P. multocida*. This is due to the effect of the leucotoxin in actively killing and lysing macrophages and neutrophils. Bacterial pneumonia develops very rapidly, particularly in calves (Figure 20.1). If initial signs of disease, such as depression and reduced appetite, are not recognised and treatment is delayed, the outcome of the disease is often poor. Delayed detection and treatment are closely related to the duration and severity of bovine pneumonia. Calves that recover from bacterial pneumonia often have irreversible lung damage. This results in calves that are chronically unhealthy; they never grow as well as if they had not become diseased (Figure 20.2).

Fundamentals of Veterinary Microbiology, First Edition. Andrew N. Rycroft.
© 2024 John Wiley & Sons Ltd. Published 2024 by John Wiley & Sons Ltd.
Companion website: www.wiley.com/go/veterinarymicrobiology

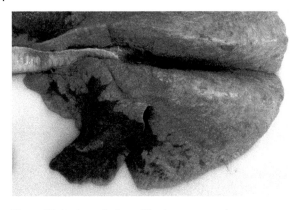

Figure 20.1 Lung lesion of bovine pneumonic pasteurellosis (uncomplicated *M. haemolytica* infection).

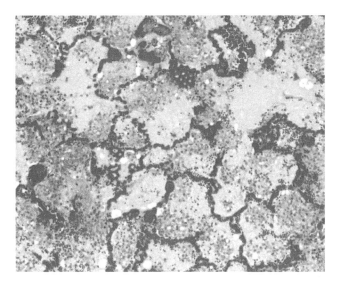

Figure 20.2 Acute pasteurellosis. Alveolar spaces are filled with pink fibrinous fluid; large numbers of inflammatory cells (mostly degenerating neutrophils) and erythrocytes have infiltrated the tissue.

Mannheimia haemolytica is a component of calf pneumonia in at least 75% of cases of BRDC. While virus infection is self-limiting and usually mild, bacterial pneumonia can be fatal. It is therefore the bacterial component that must be addressed in any outbreak. Treatment with antibiotics such as florfenicol or tulathromycin is usually highly effective but some resistance is found among strains of *P. multocida* and *M. haemolytica* to the older drugs such as amoxicillin and tetracycline. Antimicrobial resistance among *Pasteurellaceae* is not particularly common although it is reported to be high in fattening yards in the USA. It is increased because animals and herds may be simultaneously infected with *M. haemolytica* strains carrying different resistance profiles.

Resistance is usually plasmid mediated and is most often found in establishments where a high level of antibiotic use through guesswork has been common. The habit of trying an antibiotic and then changing the drug if it is ineffective, until one is found that causes a clinical improvement, is poor practice. Alongside empirical treatment, taking a representative sample to detect and identify the pathogen by culture, and recognising the drugs it is likely to be resistant to by doing a sensitivity test, avoids the unnecessary exposure of the entire microbial flora of the herd to antimicrobial selection pressure.

Vaccination has been used effectively to control the virus infections initiating damage. However, vaccination against the bacterial disease has not always been effective and straightforward. While vaccines are widely marketed with strong claims of efficacy, killed whole organisms (bacterins) often failed to prevent disease on the farm. Supplementing the vaccines with Lkt toxin was found, in some cases, to make the disease outbreak more severe. A vaccine containing *M. haemolytica* organisms grown under conditions of iron limitation was shown to be most effective. Iron starvation of the bacteria in culture causes them to produce the surface proteins (transferrin-binding proteins) that would be displayed by bacteria growing in the body; they need these in the iron-poor environment of body tissues. These are important protective antigens. The combination of Lkt and *M. haemolytica* type A1 and A2 grown under iron-restricted conditions is probably considered the most effective type of product available for vaccination so far.

Mannheimia haemolytica is also a pathogen of sheep, causing pneumonia in adult sheep and in lambs less than three months old, as septicaemia, severe pleuritis and pericarditis. It is also a cause of mastitis in lactating ewes and goats.

Bibersteinia trehalosi

Bibersteinia trehalosi (previously the T-biovar of *M. haemolytica*) is a cause of acute or peracute septicaemia in older lambs (5–12 months) that have been moved from a relatively poor grassland to a lush grass diet. It is also associated with pneumonia in sheep.

The pathogen produces a leucotoxin that is very closely related to the Lkt of *M. haemolytica* and which is essential for virulence (Murugananthan et al. 2018).

Histophilus somni

Histophilus somni (previously *Haemophilus somnus*) is normally commensal in the genital tract and transiently found in the upper respiratory tract. As an opportunist, it is a component of BRDC alongside *P. multocida* and *M. haemolytica*. It is also a rare cause of septicaemia leading to infectious thromboembolic meningoencephalitis and myocarditis with necrosis in cattle 6–20 months old, particularly in the USA but also parts of Europe including the UK. Fever, staggering and dyspnoea, followed by somnolence, paralysis and death is the usual disease progression.

Actinobacillus

Another member of the *Pasteurellaceae* family, *Actinobacillus* is again a small, Gram-negative, non-motile coccobacillus.

Actinobacillus lignieresi

Actinobacillus lignieresi is the cause of wooden tongue in cattle. It is a commensal of the mouth of cattle and sheep. If the oral mucosa is damaged (as often happens in mild trauma), the organism penetrates and causes a granuloma, termed actinobacillosis. The infection is therefore endogenous, sporadic and chronic in its course. Lesions may be in the tongue, cheeks or lips, but also sometimes in the lower gut and the lungs through aspiration. There is often spread of the organism from the local lesion to the lymphatics. There is formation of fibrous tissue in the lesions which leads to the characteristic hardening of the tissues and the name 'wooden tongue' in cattle. In sheep, the lesions are thick-walled abscesses. Feeding is impaired and animals lose condition. Spontaneous recovery is unlikely but antibiotic therapy is effective.

Actinobacillus equuli

Actinobacillus equuli is a normal inhabitant of the oral cavity and intestinal tract of equids. New-born foals may pick up the organism and develop acute septicaemia within 24 hours of birth. This is known as 'sleepy foal disease'. Although it is associated with failure to suckle, this sign may be a result of the developing infection rather than the reason for development of the infection. The pathogenicity is not understood, but an RTX group cytotoxin is present in some strains of the organism and this is likely to influence the failure of the innate defences to clear the infection.

There are two subspecies: *A. equuli* subsp. *equuli* and *A. equuli* subsp. *haemolyticus*. Both subspecies carry the *aqxCABD* operon for RTX cytolysin but only *A. equuli* subsp. *haemolyticus* produces an active RTX toxin (Huang et al. 2015). Since both have been independently isolated from different sites in the same foal at postmortem, this implies that infection is due to an immunological deficit of the very young foal rather than the chance invasion of a virulent strain (Rycroft et al. 1998).

Joint infections and purulent nephritis are also seen in cases in which animals survive the initial blood-borne infection. The reason why foals older than a few days do not suffer the infection is not clear. The development of an innate immunity or protection from the intake of passive antibody from the mare are both possibilities.

Poor performance in thoroughbreds is associated with mild respiratory disease. Epidemiological investigations using culture of transtracheal wash have suggested a link between inflammatory airway disease and the presence of *Actinobacillus* species. These are variously classified as *A. equuli*, *A. suis* or haemolytic *A. lignieresi* (Wood et al. 2005).

Actinobacillus pleuropneumoniae

Actinobacillus pleuropneumoniae is a major respiratory pathogen of the pig. It is unusual in that most strains fail to grow on blood agar because they require an exogenous source of β-nicotinamide adenine dinucleotide (NAD) as a co-factor for metabolic activity. Most bacteria synthesise their own NAD so this pathogen is often cultured on heated blood agar (chocolate agar) in which the NAD naturally present in blood plasma is preserved. This is because an NADase enzyme in the erythrocytes is destroyed by the heating. For this reason, the pathogen was originally classified as a *Haemophilus* species, alongside others that required NAD for growth, but was moved to *Actinobacillus* in the 1980s.

The organism is also identified with another cultural test: the CAMP effect. This is the production of a co-haemolytic effect on sheep blood agar in close proximity to a *Staphylococcus* growing on the same culture plate. The *Staphylococcus* produces excessive NAD and so the *Actinobacillus* is then able to grow on the blood agar. The *Staphylococcus* must be one also producing the β-toxin sphingomyelinase. This sensitises the erythrocytes so the Apx toxins are then able to fully lyse them and this is seen as a strong haemolytic effect.

Pathogenicity

There are currently 18 different serovars of *A. pleuropneumoniae* based on polysaccharide capsular antigen. In practice, serotyping is now done by detection of capsule synthesis genes by PCR. Of far greater significance is the production of RTX group, pore-forming toxins: the Apx toxins (Frey 2019). These rapidly destroy macrophages and neutrophils and probably have potent effects on other cell types in the body. There are three Apx toxins and the combination of toxins secreted follows the serotype: many produce ApxI and ApxII while others produce ApxII and ApxIII. Some serovars produce only one Apx toxin.

The Apx toxins are known to be essential for pathogenicity and the combination of toxins that a strain secretes influences the virulence of the strain. It also seems to be related to the cross-protectivity derived from prior infection. The action of the Apx toxins in lysing neutrophils, as they are increasingly attracted to a developing focus of infection, leads to a mass of highly inflamed tissue and necrotic debris (Bossé et al. 2002).

Other bacterial factors known to be required for bacterial pathogenicity are the capsular polysaccharide and the iron acquisition system. Mutants lacking capsule are unable to cause disease and have been used as live vaccines. Mutants lacking either of the transferrin binding proteins, TbpA or TbpB, are also much less virulent. These proteins are part of a system that enables the bacteria to obtain iron from porcine transferrin carrying iron. It does not enable the bacteria to glean iron from other species of animal and perhaps that is one reason why *A. pleuropneumoniae* causes pulmonary disease known to be specific for the pig and no other species.

Pathogenesis

Contagious porcine pleuropneumonia (CPP) is a highly contagious disease which can spread rapidly in pig herds and kill animals in a day. Lesions develop quickly as a region of inflammation which attracts neutrophils. The neutrophils are lysed by toxin releasing further inflammatory mediators. The lesion causes oedema, haemorrhage and fibrinous deposits around the necrotic centre. Lesions can engulf almost the entire diaphragmatic or other lung lobes and animals die from pulmonary oedema, haemorrhage and respiratory failure. If the animal recovers, the lesions wall off the focus of infection as an abscess. Most commonly, it is seen as a chronic problem in which there is a level of herd immunity and while many animals can be affected, only sporadic deaths occur. While it is most often seen in animals of 7–15 weeks of age, fatalities due to CPP in piglets as young as three weeks are sometimes seen (Figure 20.3).

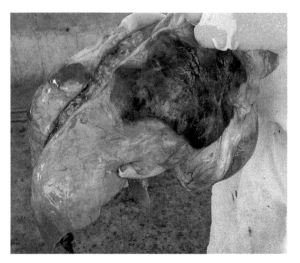

Figure 20.3 Acute pleuropneumonia lesions in the lungs of a pig.

Control

Control of the disease with antibiotics has usually been empirical and sometimes chaotic. As with treatment of calf pneumonia, it is under these circumstances that antimicrobial resistance is most often seen but pigs are often medicated with antimicrobials *en masse* through the water or feed, making the problem worse. (I have seen examples of prescription antimicrobials being used on a weekly rotation: changing the drug each week and starting the whole cycle again after four weeks, on an open-ended basis, in an attempt to control disease.)

Vaccination is practised but protection and control are hard to achieve. Whole killed bacteria, originally derived from the causative organism, adjuvanted with Al(OH)$_3$ (on-farm vaccines), have been used but not with great success. They have been found to exacerbate the disease situation in some cases. The vaccines containing Apx toxin have proven most effective but are far from perfect, with incomplete protection and some significant side-effects from endotoxin contamination of the material. Inclusion of Apx toxin in the vaccine is not itself toxic to the animal because the activity of the Apx toxins is short-lived. Despite efforts over a long period, control of bacterial pneumonia in animals at an affordable cost has been a hard nut to crack.

Actinobacillus suis

Actinobacillus suis is closely related to *A. pleuropneumoniae* but produces a milder form of respiratory disease. It is usually seen in high health status pigs that are free of *A. pleuropneumoniae*. It can, however, also be involved in septicaemia, enteritis, meningitis, arthritis, skin lesions and abortion. *A. suis* produces variants of the ApxI and ApxII cytolysins normally found in strains of *A. pleuropneumoniae*. The organism also carries transferrin-binding activity, adhesins, O and K polysaccharide antigens and fibronectin-binding protein (MacInnes et al. 2012).

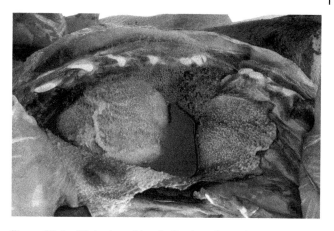

Figure 20.4 Fibrin deposition (yellow) on the surface of the heart, lungs and other organs of a pig with acute *G. parasuis* infection. Copious serous fluid is present in the thoracic cavity.

Glaesserella parasuis

Another delicate Gram-negative member of the *Pasteurellaceae* family is *Glaesserella parasuis*. Like some of the others, this organism requires NAD for growth and was originally classified as *Haemophilus* but renamed in 2019 (Dickerman et al. 2019). There are 15 serovars, based on capsular polysaccharide, although many strains are as yet untypable (Howell et al. 2015). Strains are harboured in the healthy nasal cavity of pigs.

Glaesserella parasuis is the causative agent of Glässer's disease in pigs. This occurs as sporadic outbreaks of a fibrinous polyserositis that includes pericarditis, peritonitis and pleuritis with high morbidity and mortality in pigs of 3–10 weeks old (Figure 20.4). Arthritis is common and meningitis is also sometimes seen.

The organism can also contribute to respiratory disease following enzootic pneumonia or virus infection and may result in major losses for the pig-rearing industry. Animals that survive may have chronic arthritis or intestinal obstruction due to adhesions.

Pathogenicity of *G. parasuis* is not well understood. Some serovars are widespread and appear more pathogenic than others and the capsule is recognised as essential for virulence. However, there is no direct correlation between capsular type and virulence of the isolate. Other factors must therefore contribute to disease (Zhang et al. 2014). No RTX cytolytic toxin is known and while the presence of a cytolethal distending toxin has been suggested as necessary for pathogenicity, the evidence to support this is limited to *in vitro* studies.

Treatment of outbreaks with antibiotics is effective and vaccination with commercial products, or on-farm vaccines prepared from the strain isolated from disease, is also used with positive effect.

Gallibacterium anatis

Gallibacterium anatis, formerly *Pasteurella anatis*, is found in the upper respiratory tract and lower genital tract of healthy birds. It is also an opportunistic invader causing salpingitis (inflammation of the oviduct) and peritonitis. The most probable route to the reproductive organs is via ascending infection from the cloaca. This leads to decreased egg production, lowered animal welfare and increased mortality and is considered a serious economic and welfare problem in poultry production.

Like many other pathogenic members of the *Pasteurellaceae* family, it produces an RTX-toxin. GtxA is responsible for cytotoxic activity against avian macrophages. Loss of the toxin attenuates the pathogen (Persson and Bojesen 2015). There are fimbriae that may be needed for progressive attachment in the avian reproductive tract. The role of other components such as polysaccharide capsule and metalloproteases remains to be understood.

Avibacterium paragallinarum

This is one of the more recent genera of organisms that now includes organisms previously classified as *Haemophilus* species and *Pasteurella* (Blackall et al. 2005).

The agent of infectious coryza (infectious upper respiratory inflammation) of poultry is *A. paragallinarum* (Blackall and Soriano-Vargas 2020). Several components are now recognised as contributing to pathogenicity. These include an RTX cytolysin, AvxA, that is toxic for avian macrophage cells, the polysaccharide capsule, transferrin binding proteins specific for acquiring iron from ovotransferrin and fimbriae (FlfA) that are necessary for colonisation.

References

Blackall, P.J. and Soriano-Vargas, E. (2020). Infectious coryza and related bacterial infections, Ch 20. In: *Diseases of Poultry*, 14e (ed. Swayne, D.E. (ed.)). Oxford: Wiley.

Blackall, P.J., Christensen, H., Tim Beckenham, T. et al. (2005). Reclassification of *Pasteurella gallinarum*, [*Haemophilus*] *paragallinarum*, *Pasteurella avium* and *Pasteurella volantium* as *Avibacterium gallinarum* gen. nov., comb. nov., *Avibacterium paragallinarum* comb. nov., *Avibacterium avium* comb. nov. and *Avibacterium volantium* comb. nov. *International Journal of Systematic and Evolutionary Microbiology* 55: 353–362.

Blackall, P.J., Bojesen, A.M., Christensen, H., and Bisgaard, M. (2007). Reclassification of [*Pasteurella*] *trehalosi* as *Bibersteinia trehalosi* gen. nov., comb. nov. *International Journal of Systematic and Evolutionary Microbiology* 57: 666–674.

Bossé, J.T., Janson, H., Sheehan, B.J. et al. (2002). *Actinobacillus pleuropneumoniae*: pathobiology and pathogenesis of infection. *Microbes and Infection* 4: 225–235.

Dickerman, A., Bandara, A.B., and Inzana, T.J. (2019). Phylogenomic analysis of *Haemophilus parasuis* and proposed reclassification to *Glaesserella parasuis*, gen. nov., comb. nov. *International Journal of Systematic and Evolutionary Microbiology* 70: 180–186.

Frey, J. (2019). RTX toxins of animal pathogens and their role as antigens in vaccines and diagnostics. *Toxins* 11: 719.

Howell, K.J., Peters, S.E., Wang, J. et al. (2015). Development of a multiplex PCR assay for rapid molecular serotyping of *Haemophilus parasuis*. *Journal of Clinical Microbiology* 53: 3812–3821.

Huang, B.F., Kropinski, A.M., Bujold, A.R., and MacInnes, J.I. (2015). Complete genome sequence of *Actinobacillus equuli* subspecies *equuli* ATCC 19392[T]. *Standards in Genomic Sciences* 10: 32.

MacInnes, J.I., Mackinnon, J., Bujold, A.R. et al. (2012). Complete genome sequence of *Actinobacillus suis* H91-0380, a virulent serotype O2 strain. *Journal of Bacteriology* 194: 6686–6687.

Murugananthan, A., Shanthalingam, S., Batra, S.A. et al. (2018). Leukotoxin of *Bibersteinia trehalosi* contains a unique neutralizing epitope, and a non-neutralizing epitope shared with *Mannheimia haemolytica* leukotoxin. *Toxins* 10: 220.

Persson, G. and Bojesen, A.M. (2015). Bacterial determinants of importance in the virulence of *Gallibacterium anatis* in poultry. *Veterinary Research* 46: 57.

Petras, S.F., Chidambaram, M., Illyes, E.F. et al. (1995). Antigenic and virulence properties of *Pasteurella haemolytica* leukotoxin mutants. *Infection and Immunity* 63: 1033–1039.

Rycroft, A.N., Woldeselassie, A., Gordon, P.J., and Bjornson, A. (1998). Serum antibody in equine neonatal septicaemia due to *Actinobacillus equuli*. *Veterinary Record* 143: 254–255.

Wood, J.L.N., Newton, J.R., Chanter, N., and Mumford, J.A. (2005). Association between respiratory disease and bacterial and viral infections in British racehorses. *Journal of Clinical Microbiology* 43: 120–126.

Zhang, B., Tang, C., Liao, M., and Yue, H. (2014). Update on the pathogenesis of *Haemophilus parasuis* infection and virulence factors. *Veterinary Microbiology* 168: 1–7.

21

Chlamydia – A Stealthy Pathogen

Chlamydiae are obligate intracellular parasites; they will not grow on artificial media but require living eukaryotic cells in which to grow. Because of their intracellular development and growth cycle, they were (until 1954) thought to be viruses. However, they have characteristics that clearly show them to be Gram-negative bacteria, with an outer membrane, lipopolysaccharide, ribosomes and both DNA and RNA.

Members of the family *Chamydiaceae* have a biphasic development cycle. The infective form of the organism is known as an elementary body (EB). These are extracellular and they stimulate invasion of host cells using a type three secretion system to transfer effector proteins into the host cell (Wilkat et al. 2014). They then subvert the host cell defences in a complex series of steps (Elwell et al. 2016). The elementary body is transformed to the intracellular, reproductive form known as the reticulate body (RB) which multiplies by binary fission. These form large intracellular colonies inside the host cell vacuole and then go through a maturation process to become elementary bodies. The progeny are then released from the host cell as the vacuole bursts out so that these elementary bodies can go on to infect many more host cells (Figure 21.1).

There has been controversy over whether *Chlamydia* contain peptidoglycan as a bacterial wall component. Some evidence, such as the effective use of β-lactams (amoxicillin) in treatment of *Chlamydia* infection, suggests that they contain cross-linked peptidoglycan. They also activate the host cell system for detecting peptidoglycan: the nucleotide-binding oligomerisation domain-containing 1 (NOD1). However, peptidoglycan has not been detected using the usual methods and there is no homologue of FtsZ, a protein normally used by bacteria for directing cell division in conjunction with peptidoglycan. It appears that there is a peptidoglycan-like material and biosynthesis of this is required for the localisation of two recently described septal proteins – RodZ and NlpD (Jacquier et al. 2015). As has been suspected for 40 years, *Chlamydia* makes a different form of peptidoglycan to that recognised in most conventional bacteria.

Chlamydiae proliferate in embryonated eggs and in some types of tissue culture (McCoy cells) and animal tissues. They are not visible by Gram stain but are seen using either Kosters stain, a modified Ziehl–Neelsen stain, as bright red minute rods in clusters (Figure 21.2) or by fluorescent antibody stain. In Giemsa-stained material, they appear as blue or purple inclusions in the cytoplasm of cells. Antigen detection kits are available for rapid diagnosis from a swab in farm animals but PCR is the most effective means of laboratory diagnosis.

Chlamydia infections are notable for the balance between infection and host which usually leads to persistent infections. Many infections are subclinical because the organism is tightly host-adapted to parasitise the animal without engendering a strong inflammatory response. Like leptospirosis, more overt disease can result from infections that are in the non-natural host species. Thus, infections passed from persistently infected birds may cause overt disease in humans.

Animal Disease

Chlamydia abortus

Chlamydia abortus is the cause of ovine enzootic abortion. Sheep become infected and they harbour the organism – a latent infection. When ewes become pregnant, the *Chlamydia* already present in the body infect the placenta, causing abortion which occurs in late pregnancy, after day 90 of gestation. Irrespective of the timing of infection, pathology and growth of the organism are not apparent until this late stage when fetal growth is rapid. Subsequent fertility of ewes that have aborted their lambs is not impaired. It appears that the resistant elementary bodies may persist in faeces and then on pasture

Fundamentals of Veterinary Microbiology, First Edition. Andrew N. Rycroft.
© 2024 John Wiley & Sons Ltd. Published 2024 by John Wiley & Sons Ltd.
Companion website: www.wiley.com/go/veterinarymicrobiology

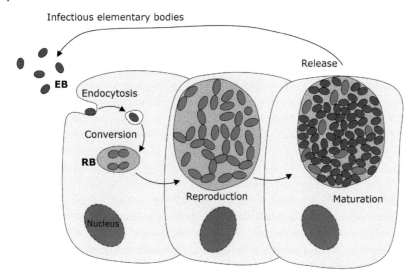

Figure 21.1 The growth and development cycle of *Chlamydia*. The infective form of *Chlamydia* is the elementary body (EB) of approximately 0.3 μm diameter. This is taken into the host cell by endocytosis and transforms into a larger reticulate body (RB) of approximately 1.0 μm diameter, which divides by binary fission to form many new *Chlamydia* cells. The progeny then mature into elementary bodies and are released from the dying host cell to infect further host cells.

Figure 21.2 *Chlamydia abortus* in sheep placenta stained by modified Ziehl–Neelsen stain. The elementary bodies (pink) appear as a cluster because they have matured inside the host cell which has then disintegrated.

contaminated with the products of an abortion from one lambing season to another. Perhaps more important is persistent carriage by infected animals who can harbour, and perhaps excrete, the pathogen for life. The immune response fails to clear the quiescent infection which persists in the liver and spleen. Venereal transmission from infected rams may also occur.

Abortion in ewes is thought to protect them from subsequent disease. The original vaccines were inactivated and conferred limited protection until the vaccine became ineffective, probably because the prevalent strain changed antigenicity. Vaccination against the disease using a live attenuated vaccine, derived by chemical mutagenesis, is now considered more effective as this is able to prevent reinfection and most of the shedding of the pathogen at lambing (Burall et al. 2009). Vaccination of young animals prevents disease and may also prevent infection but will not clear it from animals that are persistently infected from previous seasons. Therefore, it may take several seasons for the full effect of vaccinating a flock to appear. Failure to vaccinate animals will also leave them susceptible to infection and disease.

Chlamydia abortus is now recognised as a cause of infection in humans. This is particularly during the lambing season when infectious elementary bodies of *C. abortus* are shed in large quantities in the products of abortion. Infective aerosol can be inhaled by people who are exposed while caring for the animals. There are several reports of pregnant women suffering severe infections, including spontaneous abortion, stillbirth, flu-like illness and septicaemia, following exposure to animals infected with *C. abortus* (Essig and Longbottom 2015). Advice that pregnant women should avoid sheep and goats is now supported by strong evidence. This applies particularly during the time of lambing and when there are abortions among the animals.

Chlamydia felis

Chlamydia felis is the agent of feline upper respiratory tract infection, pneumonitis and conjunctivitis (Longbottom and Coulter 2003). It is common in the domestic cat population, particularly kittens, and spread between cats in households and centres where there is high population density. From an infection that typically begins in one eye and spreads to the second, if not treated the infection can spread to the respiratory tract, cause pneumonitis clinical deterioration and even death (Gruffydd-Jones et al. 2009).

Vaccination with a live, attenuated vaccine is used in the routine protection against conjunctivitis. This does not give complete protection and vaccinated animals can still shed chlamydiae.

While *C. felis* is host-adapted to the cat, there is both anecdotal and some clear evidence that it can occasionally cause chronic conjunctivitis in humans (Hartley et al. 2001). However, it seems rare as a cause of human disease.

Chlamydia psittaci

Chlamydia psittaci is the agent of psittacosis in birds: parrots, parakeets, budgerigars, macaws, cockatoos and lorries. Disease was originally thought to be associated only with psittacines but was subsequently shown to be common in other wild and domesticated birds, including poultry. The disease is known as ornithosis in non-psittacine birds but the term 'avian chlamydiosis' is now used for all avian infections with *C. psittaci*.

Eight serotypes are recognised based on the major outer membrane protein (OmpA). Serotypes A–F are associated with avian disease while the other two (known as M56 and WC) have been isolated from mammals (Longbottom and Coulter 2003). Most infections occur in psittacine birds and pigeons. Epidemics of avian chlamydiosis have also been reported in wild birds and major outbreaks of avian chlamydiosis have been seen in turkeys and ducks. In some cases, these have led to human infections. For this reason, avian chlamydiosis is a notifiable disease in the UK.

It is probable that most *C. psittaci* is spread between birds by inhalation of desiccated droppings and the oral and nasal secretions of infected birds. *C. psittaci* may cause acute, subacute, chronic or subclinical (inapparent) infections. Subclinical infections do not display clinical signs, but the birds can serve as carriers that shed the organism intermittently. Shedding can be reactivated by stress factors such as transport, poor nutrition, overcrowding and other factors. Disease can be mild, but acute avian chlamydiosis is a generalised infection affecting the major organs (Arzey et al. 1990). There is often pneumonia, respiratory distress, lethargy, anorexia, ruffled feathers, diarrhoea, ocular and nasal discharges, and reduced egg production. Mortality rates vary greatly.

Zoonotic infection is acquired through exposure of humans to infected pet birds and poultry that shed infectious elementary bodies in dried faeces, feather dust or respiratory secretions and aerosols. It can be mild but is potentially a life-threatening severe, atypical pneumonia with dyspnoea, high fever and muscle weakness.

Human *Chlamydia*

Apart from the zoonotic potential of *C. psittaci*, *C. abortus* and perhaps *C. felis*, some *Chlamydia* cause exclusively human disease. For clarity, these are briefly discussed below.

Chlamydia trachomatis

Strains of *Chlamydia trachomatis* are the cause of human infection. There are three biovars. The genital tract biovar of *C. trachomatis* is the most common cause of sexually transmitted bacterial infection. Many cases are asymptomatic but chronic infection can lead to pelvic inflammatory disease, infertility from fibrosis of the fallopian tubes and ectopic pregnancy. The trachoma biovar is the leading cause of a severe tropical, blinding eye infection, known as trachoma, affecting perhaps 400 million humans world-wide. Finally, a third biovar of *C. trachomatis* is the cause of an invasive urogenital infection called lymphogranuloma venereum, a tropical, sexually transmitted suppurative lymphadenitis (Elwell et al. 2016).

Another species, *C. pneumoniae*, is a cause of human respiratory disease and has also been implicated in the development of atherosclerosis.

References

Arzey, K.E., Arzey, G.G., and Reece, R.L. (1990). Chlamydiosis in commercial ducks. *Australian Veterinary Journal* 67: 333–334.

Burall, L.S., Rodolakis, A., Rekiki, A. et al. (2009). Genomic analysis of an attenuated *Chlamydia abortus* live vaccine strain reveals defects in central metabolism and surface proteins. *Infection & Immunity* 77: 4161–4167.

Elwell, C., Mirrashidi, K., and Engel, J. (2016). *Chlamydia* cell biology and pathogenesis. *Nature Reviews Microbiology* 14: 385–400.

Essig, A. and Longbottom, D. (2015). *Chlamydia abortus*: new aspects of infectious abortion in sheep and potential risk for pregnant women. *Current Clinical Microbiology Reports* 2: 22–34.

Gruffydd-Jones, T.J., Addie, D., Belák, S. et al. (2009). *Chlamydophila felis* infection. ABCD guidelines on prevention and management. *Journal of Feline Medicine and Surgery* 11: 605–609.

Hartley, J.C., Stevenson, S., Robinson, A.J. et al. (2001). Conjunctivitis due to *Chlamydophila felis* (*Chlamydia psittaci* feline pneumonitis agent) acquired from a cat: case report with molecular characterization of isolates from the patient and cat. *Journal of Infection* 43: 7–11.

Jacquier, N., Viollier, P.H., and Greub, G. (2015). The role of peptidoglycan in chlamydial cell division: towards resolving the chlamydial anomaly. *FEMS Microbiology Reviews* 39: 262–275.

Longbottom, D. and Coulter, L.J. (2003). Animal chlamydioses and zoonotic implications. *Journal of Comparative Pathology* 128: 217–244.

Wilkat, M., Herdoiza, E., Forsbach-Birk, V. et al. (2014). Electron tomography and cryo-SEM characterization reveals novel ultrastructural features of host-parasite interaction during *Chlamydia abortus* infection. *Histochemistry and Cell Biology* 142: 171–184.

22

Bovine Tuberculosis and Johne's Disease

Mycobacterium species are small, round-ended, Gram-positive rods. They are strict aerobes and those that are pathogenic are very slow growing. Some saprophytic mycobacteria will grow to form colonies in a few days, but the pathogenic species take at least 2–8 weeks to grow and are fastidious in their nutritional requirements. *Mycobacterium* species are the agents of bovine tuberculosis, avian tuberculosis, Johne's disease and, in humans, tuberculosis and leprosy. *M. tuberculosis* is the agent of human tuberculosis while *M. bovis* causes bovine tuberculosis. These are very closely related, with more than 99.9% similarity at the genomic level. These two, together with five other minor species of *Mycobacterium*, form the closely related *Mycobacterium tuberculosis* complex (Smith et al. 2006).

While *M. tuberculosis* is occasionally isolated from many other animals (such as dogs), it has not been shown to sustain a transmissible population in any species apart from humans. *M. bovis* is also isolated from other ruminants and other mammals and known to be capable of causing disease in a wide range of animals, but likewise, this mostly represents spillover from cattle into other animals, such as the badger.

Acid-fast Bacteria

Although they are Gram-positive in their cell wall structure, mycobacteria are difficult to stain and view using a Gram stain. They repel aqueous stains because their cell walls contain the component mycolic acid, a long-chain waxy molecule which is covalently attached through arabinogalactan to the peptidoglycan (Figure 22.1). Collectively, this is known as the mycolyl-arabinogalactan-peptidoglycan complex.

Instead of Gram staining, the Ziehl–Neelsen stain is used to view the mycobacteria in a smear of material or histological section. Traditionally, this involved heating a smear to drive the strong, red stain carbol fuchsin solution into the bacteria. The smear was then decolourised with 3% HCl in ethanol (known as acid/alcohol). Only mycobacteria, and particularly the pathogenic ones, would retain the red stain under these conditions. Background tissue and all other bacteria were counterstained with methylene blue to give contrast. The bacteria that retain the red stain are displaying the property known as 'acid fast' because they are not decolourised with acid/alcohol (Figure 22.2). This property reflects the fundamental structure, and consequential resistance properties, of these organisms.

Mycobacteria are distributed in soil, water and animals; many are saprophytic. The most important mycobacteria that are pathogenic include *M. bovis* and *M. avium* subsp. *paratuberculosis*. There are also mycobacteria that cause progressive tuberculosis-like disease in cold-blooded animals, such as *M. xenopi* and *M. piscium*.

Mycobacterium species are relatively resistant to drying. They can remain viable for years in the dry state in dust or dried faeces and also for some time, depending on physical factors, etc., in moist conditions. This is significant in the epidemiology of mycobacterial disease. They are also relatively resistant to antibiotics and chemical agents, and this is exploited in the methods used for their isolation from contaminated specimens. Before culture, it is common to pre-treat specimens with strong NaOH or oxalic acid to destroy normal contaminating bacteria while leaving the mycobacteria relatively unharmed.

Fundamentals of Veterinary Microbiology, First Edition. Andrew N. Rycroft.
© 2024 John Wiley & Sons Ltd. Published 2024 by John Wiley & Sons Ltd.
Companion website: www.wiley.com/go/veterinarymicrobiology

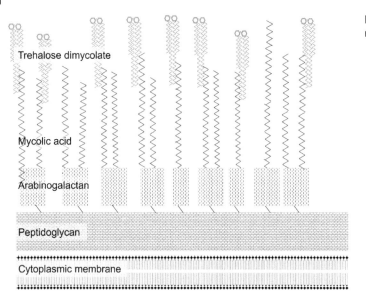

Figure 22.1 The cell envelope structure in pathogenic mycobacteria.

Trehalose dimycolate

Mycolic acid

Arabinogalactan

Peptidoglycan

Cytoplasmic membrane

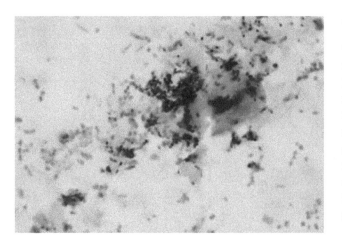

Figure 22.2 Many acid-fast bacilli (red) in the tissues of an animal with tuberculosis stained by Ziehl–Neelsen stain.

Culture

Culturing and identifying mycobacteria is a specialist task, not least because the pathogenic mycobacteria are category 3 pathogens and as such must be handled under strict containment. In addition, culture may take many weeks and growth media are different from those used for most bacteria. Dorset egg medium or Lowenstein-Jensen medium with malachite green as a selective agent are used and the cultures are held in bottles instead of plates. For this reason, PCR-based methods to detect mycobacterial DNA have become really valuable in detection of the pathogens. These are safer, highly sensitive, specific and very much more rapid than culture.

Animal Susceptibility to *Mycobacterium* Species

Different animal species are known to differ in their susceptibility to the different mycobacterial pathogens. Examples are given in Table 22.1.

Table 22.1 Susceptibility to different mycobacterial pathogens.

	M. tuberculosis	*M. bovis*	*M. avium* subsp. *paratuberculosis*
Horse	+	++	+
Cattle	+	+++	+
Dog	+++	+++	+
Cat	+	+++	+
Pig	++	+++	++
Sheep	+	++	++
Human	+++	+++	+/++

+++, ++ = degree of progressive tuberculosis; + = localised non-progressive but may easily elicit type IV hypersensitivity to tuberculin.

Bovine Tuberculosis

This is a chronic, eventually fatal wasting disease caused by *M. bovis*. It is particularly associated with intensive dairy production and the disease is most common in areas where dairying is concentrated. It has an insidious onset and a prolonged course, primarily seen as pneumonia and wasting, often with lesions elsewhere in the body. The disease is worldwide in occurrence but in many places, there have been substantial decreases in prevalence following campaigns for its eradication.

Pathogenesis of Bovine TB

The pathogenesis of tuberculosis and the bacterial components needed for survival in the host are both complex subjects (Smith 2003). Because of its worldwide distribution and its impact on global health, much of what we know has been derived from studies of *M. tuberculosis* rather than *M. bovis* (Vázquez et al. 2017), but the biochemical mechanisms involved appear to be largely the same (Pollock et al. 2006; Abdelaal et al. 2022).

Infection is acquired by the respiratory route (cattle more than six months of age), via the alimentary tract (postnatal, calf infection) and by the congenital route. Disease begins as a microscopic lesion. At first, the bacillus is not recognised by the body. The bacteria multiply slowly (doubling time 24 hours) and are ingested by macrophages. Inside the macrophages, phagosome-lysosome fusion is inhibited (Vázquez et al. 2017). In time, sensitisation through lymphocyte recognition leads to the ingress of more T-lymphocytes. An infectious granuloma (tubercle) then forms and grows to macroscopic size. This granuloma, in the presence of tumour necrosis factor (TNF)-α, is intended to restrict bacterial dissemination. If the infection is not destroyed by the cell-mediated immunity of the granuloma, the bacteria can persist indefinitely in walled-off lesions, or the lesion can release bacilli to spread and produce tubercles in other tissues and organs of the body such as the udder and uterus.

Damage to Host Tissues – Immunopathology

Mycobacterium bovis produces no known extracellular toxins. Instead, the growth of *Mycobacterium* elicits inflammatory host responses that are needed to control infections but can also cause extensive tissue damage. This tissue damage is caused by the excessive production of cytokines from host tissues in response to components of the pathogen such as lipoarabinomannan (LAM); this is known as an immunopathological effect (Smith 2003).

The cytokine response is a complex process of regulation and cross-regulation intended to suppress the development of the infection (van Crevel et al. 2002), but the pathogen successfully modifies the cytokine response. For example, proinflammatory cytokines are produced such as TNF-α. Systemic overproduction of TNF-α causes unwanted inflammatory effects such as fever and wasting. Similarly, interleukin (IL)-1 is also produced in excess at the site of disease. While these are helpful in controlling the spread of *M. bovis* in the tissues, they do have damaging effects on the host animal. Another proinflammatory cytokine is IL-12. This is protective because it induces interferon (IFN)-γ, a cytokine which induces a T-helper (Th) 1 immune response needed to clear intracellular pathogens and which itself is known to be protective against tuberculosis.

Anti-inflammatory cytokines are also induced in response to *M. bovis* infection. IL-10 is produced by macrophages after binding mycobacterial LAM (van Crevel et al. 2002). This molecule antagonises the proinflammatory cytokine response by downregulating TNF-α, IFN-γ and IL-12 and therefore interferes with the host defence. Transforming growth factor (TGF)-β is another cytokine that is overproduced at the site of a tuberculosis lesion in response to mycobacteria (Dahl et al. 1996). This also appears to counteract the protective immune response by supressing IFN-γ production. TGF-β may also be involved in tissue damage and fibrosis during tuberculosis.

Further subversion of the cytokine response by *Mycobacterium* infection is being recognised. It appears that the pathogen modulates the host cytokine network to promote the stable, long-term carriage of the pathogen in closed granulomas. This ensures that a latent reservoir of infection persists in animals for reactivation at a later time.

Control of Bovine Tuberculosis

Control of bovine tuberculosis has been through the policy of 'test and slaughter'. Where such eradication schemes are not practised, prevalence remains high. Transmission in cattle is through shedding, usually aerosol, by one animal into the environment of another. This occurs when an infected individual becomes an 'open case', i.e. there are lesions in the body from which the agent can be excreted to the exterior (such as tuberculosis of the udder). In this case, there is continuous shedding of the bacilli.

To control the spread of infection, it is necessary to recognise animals that are infected before they begin shedding the organism. Early detection of infected animals and the prevention of open cases are therefore crucial for control. The earliest and perhaps the most important method for preventing transmission of bovine TB to humans is pasteurisation: heat treatment of foods to kill pathogens without compromising the quality. Pasteurisation of milk kills *M. bovis* (and also *Brucella* species and others) and has been the primary barrier to the transmission of bovine tuberculosis from cattle to humans.

Single, Comparative, Intradermal Test in Cattle

This is the standard procedure for routine tuberculin testing of herds in UK. Similar tests (known as the Heaf test and Mantoux test) are used to detect tuberculosis in humans. Small volumes (0.1 ml) of mammalian and of avian purified protein derivative (PPD) tuberculin are separately injected intradermally into measured skinfolds in the mid-neck region of cattle. PPD is a sterile solution of protein precipitated with trichloroacetic acid from filtrates of steamed cultures of *M. bovis* strain AN5 grown on synthetic medium: 'mammalian' tuberculin (M). A culture of *M. avium* subsp. *paratuberculosis* is used to provide 'avian' tuberculin (A). These injection sites are re-examined after 72 hours using callipers to measure any swelling. An increase in skinfold thickness of 3 mm is considered doubtful; 4 mm or over is positive. Any degree of swelling accompanied by oedema is considered positive. Retesting, when necessary, is carried out not earlier than 30–60 days after the herd test. Animals reacting positively in the test are slaughtered to curtail the opportunity for transmission of *M. bovis*.

A comparative test is necessary because cattle are also susceptible to infection with *M. avium* subsp. *paratuberculosis* (MAP). Animals that have been exposed to MAP may show enough sensitisation for a degree of cross-reaction with mammalian PPD to occur. Hence, the use of mammalian PPD alone in the test would cause condemnation of animals suffering only from infection with MAP. Infection of cattle with MAP is common. It can occasionally cause tuberculosis-like disease, but it is not so alarming because this usually produces only localised lesions and it does not readily transmit between animals as does *M. bovis*.

The injected PPD stimulates sensitised CD4+ lymphocytes, otherwise known as T-helper cells, to secrete cytokines that recruit polymorphonuclear leucocytes and then macrophages to the site of injection. The cytokines also cause local inflammation leading to leakage of fluid through vessel walls, seen as redness and swelling. Interpretation of the result depends on the circumstances. Non-specific infection is assumed to exist if either Johne's disease or skin tuberculosis is known to exist in the herd, or if any avian[+]/mammalian[−] reactors are found during tests.

It should be noted that a positive skin test reaction is an immune response (a type IV hypersensitivity reaction) that indicates exposure to *M. bovis* or MAP. It does not correlate with a protective immune response. Indeed, infected cattle with a strongly positive response to PPD will usually go on to develop full-blown tuberculosis. Immunity does develop in animals but is often inadequate to halt developing infection. Testing and slaughter of reactors is the fastest, cheapest and most certain means of eradication. Vaccination of cattle is not currently practised because it would interfere with the standard tuberculin test results, causing false-positive results.

IFN-γ Stimulation Test

The IFN-γ stimulation test is an alternative to the comparative intradermal tuberculin test. It has the advantage that only a single farm visit is required. During the visit, blood samples are taken. Bloods are processed to separate and retrieve the lymphocytes, and these are cultured. The lymphocytes are then exposed to PPD and after a period of time, samples of the culture supernatant are taken for the concentration of IFN-γ to be measured using an ELISA. High levels of IFN-γ in a sample indicate that the animal has lymphocytes that are presensitised, and respond, to the PPD. This test has not replaced the intradermal test, but it appears to detect early cases that may be missed by the skin test. Conversely, the skin test may likewise detect cases which are missed by the IFN-γ test. Using both tests improves the overall sensitivity of the detection. A positive response in both tests gives higher specificity than each test used alone.

Other (Direct) Diagnostic Methods

Samples from the living animal or lesions seen at PM may be subject to ZN staining either as unfixed smears or fixed tissue sections for acid-fast bacilli by microscopy. Culture is possible but is rarely necessary since the advent of PCR for detection and identification, and whole-genome sequencing for detailed analyses.

Tuberculosis in Other Animals

Horses are naturally resistant and tuberculosis disease is rare. However, it does occur. Alimentary infection with *M. bovis* leads to progressive disease with tuberculous ulcers in the gut. The intradermal TB test is not considered reliable in horses.

In pigs, lesions of avian TB are not uncommon at slaughter. These occur through alimentary infection. The disease is non-progressive and localises in the lymph nodes of the head and neck.

In dogs, tuberculosis is occasionally acquired from human cases and in fact, dogs can act as a sentinel for the presence of human tuberculosis in a household. Lesions are seen in both the respiratory (tuberculous pneumonia) and alimentary tract (massive tuberculous lymphadenitis and gross exudative peritonitis).

Cats suffered from *M. bovis* infection at a time when unpasteurised milk was commonly consumed. More recently, *M. tuberculosis* is usually the cause, but this is considered to be less pathogenic than *M. bovis* in the cat.

Poultry suffer from avian tuberculosis. Wild birds and free-range domestic birds are similarly susceptible. This is usually a progressive alimentary infection; lesions in the intestinal wall eventually ulcerate to give an 'open case' after about 12 months. Nodular lesions are present in the liver, spleen, bone marrow and bones. Avian TB can be tested by injection of avian PPD into the wattle. This is considered very reliable.

Sheep and goats rarely suffer from tuberculosis disease.

In deer, TB due to *M. avium* is common. Disease due to *M. bovis* is increasing in prevalence and this is an important problem in deer farming.

The Badger Controversy

Badgers suffer from progressive, generalised tuberculosis following infection with *M. bovis*. It is transmitted between badgers by bites with saliva infected from heavily diseased lungs. It is a recognised problem in the West Country (Gloucestershire, Devon, Somerset) where the badger is a source of infection for cattle from faeces, urine and respiratory secretions.

In the UK, badgers carrying *M. bovis* have been blamed by some as the environmental reservoir of infection in dairy cattle. Certainly, a substantial proportion of badgers found dead by the roadside from 1971 onwards were shown to have demonstrable lesions of TB infection or culturable organisms present without overt signs of disease (Figure 22.3). Countering this argument, other people felt the badgers, a protected species, should not be harmed. To determine the impact of badgers as a cause of infection in dairy cattle, an experiment was set up. This was the Randomised Badger Culling Trial that took place over nine years. Badgers were (i) culled in designated areas, (ii) left alone in other areas and (iii) culled in response to herd infections with *M. bovis*. The trial was carefully designed to provide unambiguous evidence on the role of the badger in transmission of cattle TB. It was intended that it would provide a basis to resolve the controversy and determine appropriate policies for controlling bovine TB. Unfortunately, the experiment suffered from interference on both sides of the argument. Those against badger culling enabled badgers that had been caught to go free, while those who believed the badgers were responsible for transmission of disease were killing them in control areas where they should have been safe. The experiment was also subject to the disruption caused by the 2001 outbreak of foot and mouth disease in the UK.

Nevertheless, the results of the trial were sufficient to show that the contribution of badgers to TB in dairy cattle was somewhat limited. Rather unexpectedly, bovine TB was actually seen to increase in some areas that had undergone badger culling. This was interpreted as badgers moving into areas that had been culled, and this movement led to introduction of disease from outside. However, the results were contested and reinterpreted, and the two views (pro- and anti-culling of badgers) have only become more polarised.

While cattle can become infected by badgers, badgers can also become infected by cattle. It seems that cattle are themselves a primary reservoir of *M. bovis* for other cattle and movement of animals, even though they may have tested negative, makes a contribution to the spread of the

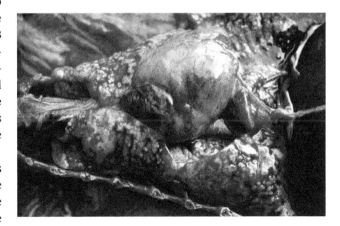

Figure 22.3 Disseminated tuberculosis in a badger.

disease. This was demonstrated when movements of dairy cattle during restocking after the foot and mouth disease outbreak of 2001 led to a very substantial dissemination of the disease in the UK.

Vaccination Against Bovine Tuberculosis

Killed bacterial vaccines are of no value as immunising agents in tuberculosis since they do not produce a cell-mediated response and antibody is of no value in protection. The live vaccine bacille Calmette–Guérin (BCG) is an undefined spontaneous avirulent mutant strain of *M. bovis*. It was originally produced by repeated cycles of culture of a virulent *M. bovis* on bile-potato medium. It has been used widely to immunise humans in the UK after they had been shown to be non-reactors in the tuberculin test (Heaf or Mantoux test). Evidence for protection in 80% of human vaccinees has been produced in the UK and US; other field trials have suggested little or no detectable protection.

Vaccines for future use in cattle may be based on BCG or on an acellular (subunit) vaccine, the response to which must be distinguishable from the response to disease. By using low-dose BCG vaccination, it may be possible to confer some protective immunity without compromising the established diagnostic tests currently in use (Nugent et al. 2018). Meanwhile, a project to vaccinate badgers using BCG is ongoing in the UK as a potential replacement for trapping and slaughter of healthy animals.

Treatment

Treatment of tuberculosis in animals is theoretically possible. However, in farm animals, treatment would be prohibitively expensive and require animals to be isolated for prolonged periods. Furthermore, the law currently requires that animals testing positive must be slaughtered to minimise further spread.

In companion animals, it is possible to use antimicrobials in treatment. However, *M. bovis* and *M. tuberculosis* are not susceptible to the common antimicrobials: penicillins, tetracyclines, cephalosporins, macrolides, etc. Streptomycin (an aminoglycoside) was the first anti-tuberculosis antibiotic (discovered in 1943), and rifampicin is also effective. But these and other drugs, such as isoniazid, must be given in combination and for a prolonged period of time (months) in order to be effective.

Johne's Disease

Mycobacterium avium subsp. *paratuberculosis* is the causative agent of Johne's disease or paratuberculosis. This is a chronic inflammatory disorder of the gastrointestinal tract of ruminants (Harris and Barletta 2001). It causes chronic diarrhoea and wasting in the later stages of the disease. Johne's disease is economically important as it is responsible for substantial production losses in the dairy industry through loss of milk production and disposal of animals (Arsenault et al. 2012; Orpin et al. 2020a).

Pathogenesis

As it colonises the host, MAP establishes persistent infections within host macrophages in the small intestine. Like *M. bovis*, MAP subverts the normal functions of the macrophage which would result in destruction of the internalised bacteria. In doing so, MAP is able to convert the cells which would normally be responsible for destruction of the invading pathogen into an environment protected from the host immune response. Maturation of the phagolysosome is blocked and the ability of the infected host to utilise IFN-γ in the protective Th1 immune response is also blocked because infected cells are unable to respond to IFN-γ.

Control

The organism is transmitted by the faecal–oral route. It is passed in faeces and survives well for many months in the environment. This is the primary source of the pathogen for transmission to further animals. Control of the disease is through a combination of hygiene, husbandry practice (Rossiter and Burhans 1996), testing and removal of infected animals and by vaccination (Orpin et al. 2020b).

Testing methods include serological tests (usually ELISA) seeking an antibody response associated with infection, and by detection of the DNA of the organism by PCR (Truyers and Jennings 2016). Culture is a slow process and less sensitive than modern PCR methods. Skin testing for paratuberculosis using extracts of MAP (referred to as johnin) has not been as successful as that used for *M. bovis* infection. This is probably because of the cross-reactivity with environmental MAP carried by birds. The skin test is no longer used for diagnosis, control or prepurchase testing of animals for Johne's disease.

Vaccination in conjunction with a management and/or testing approach may be an appropriate component in a Johne's disease control strategy for some herd situations. Both live, attenuated and killed vaccines are available. Vaccination of calves is carried out only when they are young (before 35 days of age) and has been shown to reduce subsequent shedding in vaccinates and delay the onset of clinical disease (Rossiter and Burhans 1996). Vaccination does not provide protection against infection and vaccinated animals will still become infected.

Treatment is also possible and is considered worthwhile in some cases (St Jean 1996) but takes many weeks and often fails to achieve a definitive cure.

References

Abdelaal, H.F.M., Thacker, T.C., Wadie, B. et al. (2022). Transcriptional profiling of early and late phases of bovine tuberculosis. *Infection and Immunity* 90: e00313–e00321.

Arsenault, R.J., Li, Y., Bell, K. et al. (2012). *Mycobacterium avium* subsp. *paratuberculosis* inhibits gamma interferon-induced signaling in bovine monocytes: insights into the cellular mechanisms of Johne's disease. *Infection and Immunity* 80: 3039–3048.

van Crevel, R., Ottenhoff, T.H., and van der Meer, J.W. (2002). Innate immunity to *Mycobacterium tuberculosis*. *Clinical Microbiology Reviews* 15: 294–309.

Dahl, K.E., Shiratsuchi, H., Hamilton, B.D. et al. (1996). Selective induction of transforming growth factor beta in human monocytes by lipoarabinomannan of *Mycobacterium tuberculosis*. *Infection and Immunity* 64: 399–405.

Harris, N.B. and Barletta, R.G. (2001). *Mycobacterium avium* subsp. *paratuberculosis* in veterinary medicine. *Clinical Microbiology Reviews* 14: 489–512.

Nugent, G., Yockney, I.J., Cross, M.L., and Buddle, B.M. (2018). Low-dose BCG vaccination protects free-ranging cattle against naturally-acquired bovine tuberculosis. *Vaccine* 36: 7338–7344.

Orpin, P., Sibley, R., and Bond, K. (2020a). Johne's disease in dairy herds 1. Understanding the disease. *In Practice* 42: 39–46.

Orpin, P., Sibley, R., and Bond, K. (2020b). Johne's disease in dairy herds 2. Effective control using the National Johne's Management Plan. *In Practice* 42: 159–168.

Pollock, J.M., Rodgers, J.D., Welsh, M.D., and McNair, J. (2006). Pathogenesis of bovine tuberculosis: the role of experimental models of infection. *Veterinary Microbiology* 112: 141–150.

Rossiter, C.A. and Burhans, W.S. (1996). Farm-specific approach to paratuberculosis (Johne's disease) control. *Veterinary Clinics of North America: Food Animal Practice* 12: 383–413.

Smith, I. (2003). *Mycobacterium tuberculosis* pathogenesis and molecular determinants of virulence. *Clinical Microbiology Reviews* 16: 463–496.

Smith, N.H., Gordon, S.V., de la Rua-Domenech, R. et al. (2006). Bottlenecks and broomsticks: the molecular evolution of *Mycobacterium bovis*. *Nature Reviews Microbiology* 4: 670–681.

St Jean, G. (1996). Treatment of clinical paratuberculosis in cattle. *Veterinary Clinics of North America: Food Animal Practice* 12: 417–430.

Truyers, I. and Jennings, A. (2016). Management and control of Johne's disease in beef suckler herds. *In Practice* 38: 347–354.

Vázquez, C.L., Bianco, M.V., Blanco, F.C. et al. (2017). *Mycobacterium bovis* requires P27 (LprG) to arrest phagosome maturation and replicate within bovine macrophages. *Infection and Immunity* 85: e00720–e00716.

23

Bacillus anthracis

Bacillus species are endospore-forming Gram-positive rods, most of which are naturally found in the soil. Very few are pathogens and only one species is a true pathogen of animals: *B. anthracis* (Beyer and Turnbull 2009). This is also a saprophyte in the soil but it possesses a capsule, enabling it to survive in the body by resisting phagocytosis, and it produces a powerful three-component exotoxin. Both the capsule and the toxin are required for pathogenicity. Both are encoded separately on plasmids: plasmid pXO1 directs synthesis of the toxin components and pXO2 carries the genes encoding the poly-D-glutamic acid capsule (Figure 23.1).

Capsule

The capsule is very unusual. It is composed of a homopolymer of the D-isomer of glutamic acid (Bruckner et al. 1953). This is useful in diagnosis of anthrax in a blood smear because it stains mauve or purple with polychrome methylene blue stain. This is known as M'Fadyean's reaction, devised by John M'Fadyean in 1903. This simple test has been the primary diagnostic test for anthrax in cattle and sheep for many decades. It is still the recognised method used to distinguish anthrax bacilli in a blood smear or tissue smear growing in the blood of ruminants that have died unexpectedly (Owen et al. 2013). The bacteria appear as chains of dark blue, square-ended rods surrounded (often asymmetrically) with the capsule (Figure 23.2). Animals that have died from other causes frequently show bacteria in the blood, but these do not have the characteristic capsule (Figure 23.3).

S-Layer

Beneath the capsule is an S-layer or surface array protein, BslA. This is a protein paracrystalline sheath completely covering the peptidoglycan surface (Missiakas and Schneewind 2017). It forms a porous mesh which functions as a protective barrier with selective permeability. The function of the S-layer in pathogenicity, if any, remains unclear but it promotes the invasion of host cells by *B. anthracis* and evasion of innate defences of the mammalian host.

Toxin

The extracellular toxin is only produced while *B. anthracis* is growing in the body (or growth conditions which mimic this, including CO_2 and 37 °C). Toxin was therefore first demonstrated in the filtered serum of guinea pigs. It comprises three components: oedema factor (EF), protective antigen (PA) and lethal factor (LF). Experimental use of the toxin components showed that separately, none of the three proteins is toxic. Instead, they come together in binary combinations to form lethal toxin and oedema toxin. Intravenous injection of PA and LF caused death of animals while intradermal injection of PA and EF caused oedema in the skin. PA is the common cell-binding component which is able to interact with the two separate enzyme components that are responsible for the cell damage. PA binds specifically to the cell surface receptor binding protein. EF or LF then binds to the PA, forming oedema toxin and lethal toxin respectively. These toxins are

Fundamentals of Veterinary Microbiology, First Edition. Andrew N. Rycroft.
© 2024 John Wiley & Sons Ltd. Published 2024 by John Wiley & Sons Ltd.
Companion website: www.wiley.com/go/veterinarymicrobiology

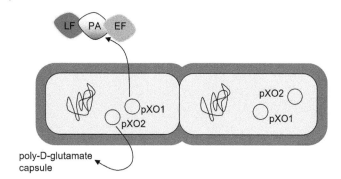

Figure 23.1 Two plasmids encode the genes for pathogenicity in *B. anthracis;* pXO1 directs toxin synthesis while pXO2 directs capsule synthesis.

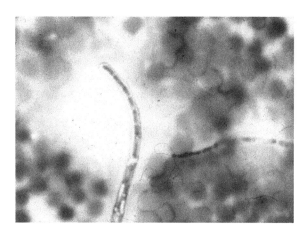

Figure 23.2 *Bacillus anthracis* in blood smear from a case of fatal bovine anthrax. The pink capsule surrounding the square-ended rods is diagnostic of anthrax. Not all the bacilli have a capsule and not all the bacteria in blood are *B. anthracis*.

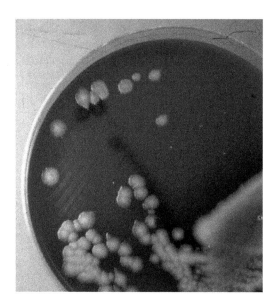

Figure 23.3 Colonies of *Bacillus anthracis* on blood agar.

internalised into the cell within a vacuole by receptor-mediated endocytosis. EF and LF are then released into the cytosol where their activity takes place (Figure 23.4).

The oedema factor is an adenylate cyclase which converts ATP to cyclic AMP (cAMP). The LF is a zinc metalloprotease (as are both tetanus toxin and botulinum toxin). Evidence is now strong that LF cleaves the amino terminus of a number of mitogen-activated protein kinase kinases (MAPKK) which relay environmental signals to the transcription system of the cell nucleus. However, there is also evidence that there are other, unknown targets of LF in the cell cytoplasm; proteolytic cleavage of MAPKK cannot explain why certain cell lines or mouse strains are resistant to LF action. Furthermore, although the MAPKK signalling pathways are involved in activation of macrophages and the production of cytokines (IL-1, IL-6

Figure 23.4 The action of the three-component anthrax toxin on the mammalian cell.

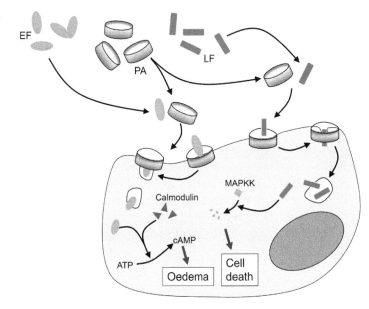

and TNF), the link between LF protease activity and the pathological outcome of anthrax is not well understood (Mock and Fouet 2001).

There is evidence for synergy between the actions of the two toxins. Indeed, it was originally considered that the toxin acted as a three-component toxin, known as the holotoxin, rather than the two binary combinations we now recognise. The combined effect of the toxins is to kill phagocytic cells (macrophages) and increase capillary permeability leading to systemic shock, through lowered blood pressure and circulatory collapse, haemorrhage and oedema. This toxin-induced vascular shock will kill the animal (Moayeri and Leppla 2009).

It is also now recognised that *B. anthracis* strains unable to produce anthrax toxin can still be virulent in animal models so long as the pXO1 plasmid is otherwise intact. AtxA is a global regulator of *B. anthracis*, located on pXO1. It is known to control the expression of virulence factors and is essential for pathogenicity in the absence of the toxin (Levy et al. 2014).

Anthrax

Anthrax is an acute disease which mainly affects herbivores (sheep, cattle and horses), but all mammals are susceptible (Moayeri et al. 2015). Anthrax spores are the dormant form which survives for decades or centuries. They are highly resistant to adverse environmental conditions and only destroyed by proper sterilising methods (autoclaving, 200 ppm hypochlorite solution or dry heating at 160 °C for two hours).

Spores normally enter the body from contaminated pasture, usually via the GI tract. When spiny or irritating vegetation is ingested simultaneously, the tissue damage allows the spores to access the tissues. At the site of entry, the spores are ingested by macrophages. The spores germinate in the phagolysosome of macrophages, probably triggered by intralysosomal signals. The vegetative form of the organism spreads via the lymphatics, eventually to the bloodstream, where they are able to multiply freely, and the toxins released will kill the animal. *B. anthracis* organisms which are shed from the carcass of a dead animal will form spores when they are in contact with air; spore formation requires the presence of gaseous oxygen.

Humans are also susceptible. Infection in humans is usually via injured skin or mucous membrane and occasionally by inhalation (known from the nineteenth century as wool sorter's disease). The main sources of infection in humans are contaminated animal carcasses and animal products, e.g. unsterilised bone meal fertiliser and leather hide.

While anthrax is a very severe disease, carrying a high mortality even with treatment, it is also controllable. For this reason, it is notifiable in the UK. Efforts to control the disease through diagnosis and vaccination have led to anthrax becoming rare in industrialised countries and much less frequent in developing countries. Occasional sporadic cases are reported in the UK every few years.

To reduce the incidence of disease, the live, Sterne spore vaccine was available for use in the UK until the 1980s. This vaccine, isolated in 1937, is an avirulent mutant because it lacks the pXO2 plasmid and cannot synthesise capsule. It is therefore unable to resist phagocytosis but produces toxin in the body for long enough to induce protective immunity. It has been used worldwide in livestock and has been very effective in prevention of the disease. Nevertheless, it does have some residual virulence in some animals and is not considered safe enough to use in humans. Instead, safer protection is offered by culture supernatant of *B. anthracis* containing PA protein and such vaccines, developed in the 1950s, are licensed and available if needed. However, there is evidence that spore-related antigens are required for a fuller and longer-lasting immunity, and research is continuing to utilise the Sterne strain which has been altered to genetically detoxify the EF and LF and to utilise a recombinant iron transporter for human vaccination (Balderas et al. 2016).

Treatment of the disease is not usually possible in herbivorous animals because cases are only identified postmortem. In humans, it is known that while the cutaneous form can be diagnosed and readily treated, once the disease enters the systemic form from gastrointestinal or inhalation entry, it resists antimicrobial treatment (ciprofloxacin and doxycycline) and is rapidly fatal. The same can be extrapolated to animals. However, the organism is extremely sensitive to penicillin G and this could be used prophylactically in the event of an anthrax outbreak.

Other *Bacillus* Species

There are very many *Bacillus* species that are found in the environment. The only other *Bacillus* species causing disease are *B. licheniformis* and *B. cereus*. *B. licheniformis* is a recognised cause of bovine abortion. *B. cereus* is occasionally a cause of food poisoning in humans and very rarely isolated from mastitis.

Notably, there is a very close relationship between *B. anthracis* and *B. cereus*. It can be difficult to distinguish the two with traditional bacteriological methods. While in the past, animals were used to demonstrate pathogenic capability, and therefore assign an isolate as *B. anthracis*, identification now uses PCR-based detection of plasmid genes for capsule and toxin (Turnbull 1999).

References

Balderas, M.A., Nguyen, C.T.Q., Terwilliger, A. et al. (2016). Progress toward the development of a NEAT protein vaccine for anthrax disease. *Infection and Immunity* 84: 3408–3422.

Beyer, W. and Turnbull, P.C.B. (2009). Anthrax in animals. *Molecular Aspects of Medicine* 30: 481–489.

Bruckner, V., Kovacs, J., and Denes, G. (1953). Structure of poly-D-glutamic acid isolated from capsulated strains of *B. anthracis*. *Nature* 172: 508.

Levy, H., Glinert, I., Weiss, S. et al. (2014). Toxin-independent virulence of *Bacillus anthracis* in rabbits. *PLoS ONE* 9: e84947.

Missiakas, D. and Schneewind, O. (2017). Assembly and function of the *Bacillus anthracis* S-layer. *Annual Review of Microbiology* 71: 79–98.

Moayeri, M. and Leppla, S.H. (2009). Cellular and systemic effects of anthrax lethal toxin and edema toxin. *Molecular Aspects of Medicine* 30: 439–455.

Moayeri, M., Leppla, S.H., Vrentas, C. et al. (2015). Anthrax pathogenesis. *Annual Review of Microbiology* 69: 185–208.

Mock, M. and Fouet, A. (2001). Anthrax. *Annual Review of Microbiology* 55: 647–671.

Owen, M.P., Schauwers, W., Hugh-Jones, M.E. et al. (2013). A simple, reliable M'Fadyean stain for visualizing the *Bacillus anthracis* capsule. *Journal of Microbiological Methods* 92: 264–269.

Turnbull, P.C. (1999). Definitive identification of *Bacillus anthracis* – a review. *Journal of Applied Microbiology* 87: 237–240.

24

Clostridium

The clostridia are all anaerobic, spore-forming, Gram-positive rods. They are primarily inhabitants of the intestinal tract and environment. Many species are therefore found in the soil and sewage. The clostridia are a group of bacteria which cause a number of different diseases of animals including enterotoxaemias, particularly in ruminants, but also in poultry and pigs. *Clostridium* species produce a variety of extracellular digestive enzymes and toxic substances known collectively as exotoxins. When in living tissues, these enzymes can have necrotising, haemolytic and lethal properties. This is consistent with them being rather primitive because they are simply attempting to digest their surroundings to supply small molecules that can be utilised as nutrients and a source of energy (Figure 24.1).

Clostridial Disease

The clostridial diseases are not spread from animal to animal. Instead, they are naturally present in the environment of the animals or in their gut. Disease occurs when there is some relevant change to the diet or other predisposing factor, or when wounds are contaminated with the organisms in soil or faeces.

Clostridium species also cause histotoxic infections (myonecrosis) which can arise from contaminated wounds or from spores dormant in the tissues. Two other specific diseases, botulism and tetanus, are caused by *Clostridium* species. Most clostridial diseases are effectively controlled by the use of toxoid vaccines.

If they are primitive, they are also ancient organisms which have never acquired the means of utilising oxygen. They can, however, respire anaerobically and use radicals such as nitrate as inorganic terminal electron acceptors. In so doing, they reduce NO_3 to NO_2 or even N_2 and are sometimes denitrifying bacteria in an anaerobic soil environment. Others, such as *Clostridium pasteurianum*, use N_2 as an electron acceptor and reduce this to ammonia, and so are free-living nitrogen fixers.

Enterotoxaemia

Some *C. perfringens* types and some other *Clostridium* species are responsible for a group of diseases, the enterotoxaemias, in sheep, goats and occasionally cattle. An enterotoxaemia is the transfer of bacterial exotoxin produced in the intestine into the blood. Sometimes, the absorption is facilitated by the toxin. The disease produced is related directly to the toxins produced and therefore the toxinotype responsible.

Clostridium perfringens

Clostridium perfringens is a major animal and human pathogen, previously known as *C. welchii* until the mid-1970s. In the early days of bacteriology (1920s), it was customary to distinguish different types of a particular micro-organism by the agglutination reactions (clumping) with serum raised in rabbits to the different antigen types on the bacterial surface. Although it was apparent that different types of *C. perfringens* existed, as recognised based on the toxins they produced, there was no value in using agglutination reactions in their classification or subtyping. For that reason, the species was

Fundamentals of Veterinary Microbiology, First Edition. Andrew N. Rycroft.
© 2024 John Wiley & Sons Ltd. Published 2024 by John Wiley & Sons Ltd.
Companion website: www.wiley.com/go/veterinarymicrobiology

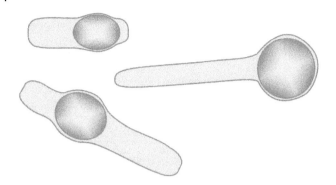

Figure 24.1 The endospores of *Clostridium* species form within the mother cell and often cause the bacteria to show a bulge. Different species show characteristic cell/spore morphology.

subtyped based on the profile of toxins they produced. These toxins are secreted into the growth medium during the exponential phase.

Toxinotypes

Five types (A–E) were recognised, and defined, by the production of four of the toxins: α toxin (CPA), β toxin (CPB), ε toxin (ETX) and ι toxin. This has recently been revised to seven toxinotypes with the addition of types F and G (Rood et al. 2018) (Table 24.1).

Although just six toxins are used to define the seven types, many more (at least 17) different toxins are produced by strains of *C. perfringens* but a particular strain will only produce a fraction of these.

Clostridium perfringens Type A

Clostridium perfringens type A is primarily a human pathogen causing gas gangrene (clostridial myonecrosis), a histotoxic infection in contaminated wounds. The primary exotoxins responsible are α toxin, which is a lecithinase C that hydrolyses phospholipids, and perfringolysin O (τ toxin), a cholesterol-dependent, pore-forming cytolysin. These toxins act synergistically in the development of gas gangrene (Awad et al. 2001).

The α toxin is cytolytic and haemolytic, and when injected into an experimental animal, it is dermonecrotic and lethal. It is produced by all strains of *C. perfringens* and its production is used to identify the species (Mehdizadeh Gohari et al. 2021). Clostridial myonecrosis is assisted when the wound has become contaminated with faeces or soil so that there is a mixed infection with facultative anaerobes such as *E. coli*. This organism will consume the local oxygen and provide the conditions necessary for the *Clostridium*, or other strict anaerobe, to flourish and produce potent toxins.

Clostridium perfringens Type B

Type B causes an enterotoxaemia in sheep known as lamb dysentery in the UK, where it can cause heavy losses in newborn lambs. The disease is prevalent in hill farms in southern Scotland, northern England and north Wales. It has not been found in North America.

Table 24.1 The toxin types of *Clostridium perfringens*.

Type	Toxins produced					
	Alpha α	Beta β	Epsilon ε	Iota *i*	CPE	NetB
A	++	−	−	−	−	−
B	+	+	+	−	−	−
C	+	+	−	−	−	−
D	+	−	+	−	−	−
E	+	−	−	+	−	−
F	+	−	−	−	+	−
G	+	−	−	−	−	+

The major toxin involved is β toxin but ε toxin is also produced. β Toxin is a membrane active, pore-forming toxin and has structural similarity to the α toxin of *Staphylococcus aureus*, known to be a potent toxin in that organism. It induces inflammation and necrosis of intestinal mucosa (Mehdizadeh Gohari et al. 2021).

Lambs of less than 14 days are affected. The *C. perfringens* type B is transferred to the lamb in trace quantities of faeces on the teat and in the environment. Colonisation is unhindered because the normal gut flora is just being established. It then multiplies in the gut contents after ingestion of large quantities of milk. β Toxin is highly sensitive to trypsin. However, it is likely that the trypsin activity is overwhelmed in these young lambs by the quantity of toxin so that the toxins damage the gut mucosa and are absorbed. The result is sudden death. Lambs are seen to stop feeding and suffer severe abdominal pain with bloody diarrhoea. Causing these signs are extensive haemorrhage and ulceration of the small intestine.

A chronic abdominal pain without the diarrhoea, seen in older lambs and known as pine, is due to *C. perfringens* type B. It may also be associated with haemorrhagic enteritis in goats, calves and foals.

Clostridium perfringens **Type C**

Type C produces mainly β toxin and has a different geographical distribution. It also affects a wider range of animals. In young ewes in the UK, it is responsible for an enterotoxaemia called struck. This is seen in Wales and southern Kent and is associated with animals overeating lush grass in the early spring, especially after poor-quality winter fodder. The dietary change seems to promote multiplication of type C in the abomasum and small intestine. β Toxin, which is usually inactivated by trypsin, causes necrosis of the mucosa. Perhaps this is due to insufficient pancreatic enzymes or simply the quantity of toxin produced. Due to the mucosal damage, the toxin is absorbed. There is little diarrhoea but the animals can die suddenly with fluid in the peritoneum and chest indicative of toxaemia.

Type C is also responsible for disease in newborn piglets. In an acute attack of necrotic enteritis, animals become depressed and develop bloody diarrhoea with necrotic material in the faeces. Within 24 hours they can be dead, with a fatality rate sometimes approaching 100%. As many as 10^9 *C. perfringens* per gram of faeces can be present. Again, the toxin produced causes damage to the intestinal mucosa and allows absorption of the toxin to the circulation. Similar peracute enterotoxaemia and necrotic enteritis are seen in young calves, lambs and goats.

Clostridium perfringens **Type D**

Type D also causes enterotoxaemia in lambs, known as pulpy kidney disease. The lambs affected are usually 3–10 weeks of age, occasionally older, rather than newborn. This is common in the UK if vaccination has been neglected. It is primarily due to the ε toxin produced in conditions of high nutrition: rich milk from ewes grazing a lush pasture or from excessive concentrates used to fatten older lambs. The diet leads to alterations in the gut flora, overgrowth of the *Clostridium* and production of the ε toxin (Garcia et al. 2013). This toxin is activated by the digestive enzymes. It leads to increased permeability of the small intestine, absorption of the toxin and enterotoxaemia. There is little or no intestinal ulceration or necrosis. The active ε toxin selectively damages the central nervous system, causing liquefactive necrosis of tissues and perivascular oedema. The oedema leads to raised intracranial pressure and further CNS damage.

Apart from the brain and meninges, another organ is damaged. The kidney shows a characteristic lesion in sheep due to rapid autolytic changes seen postmortem in the toxin-damaged tissue: the 'pulpy' kidney.

It is also recognised in calves, goats and sometimes in other animals. In young calves, the disease is similar but there is reported to be a haemorrhagic enterocolitis yet no kidney liquefaction.

Clostridium perfringens **Type E**

The role of *C. perfringens* type E in animal disease is quite unclear. It is certainly less important than other types. The primary toxin, ι toxin, is an ADP-ribosylating enzyme causing disruption of the actin cytoskeleton (Mehdizadeh Gohari et al. 2021). It has been implicated in necrotic enteritis of calves in Australia and in a colony of rabbits, but case reports have been rare.

Clostridium perfringens **Type F**

Strains producing the enterotoxin (CPE), which account for only a small proportion, are known to cause diarrhoea (food poisoning) in humans and also in foals and pigs. These have now been reassigned to toxinotype F.

Clostridium perfringens **Type G**

In chickens, *C. perfringens* type G causes necrotic enteritis (NE), a disease of substantial economic impact to the intensive poultry industry. NE in chickens is an acute or chronic enterotoxaemia (Songer 1996). The acute disease results in significant levels of mortality whereas the chronic disease leads to loss of productivity and welfare concerns.

The disease is believed to occur when several predisposing factors allow *C. perfringens* type G to multiply to high numbers in the small intestine. Original investigations suggested that the major virulence factor in the pathogenesis of necrotic enteritis was α toxin. However, studies using α-toxin-negative mutants have demonstrated that α toxin was not needed for necrotic enteritis. A new pore-forming toxin, necrotic enteritis toxin (NetB), was identified and shown to be the critical virulence determinant in this disease (Keyburn et al. 2008). *C. perfringens* NetB-deficient mutants were unable to induce disease in chickens. It is now thought that overgrowth of *C. perfringens* in the chicken intestine causes upregulation of NetB production and the resulting damage to the gut allows the ensuing enterotoxaemia.

The Histotoxic Clostridia

A number of *Clostridium* species cause myonecrosis or gangrene. The animal species affected, site of disease and development of lesions depend on the toxins produced by the species involved (Figure 24.2).

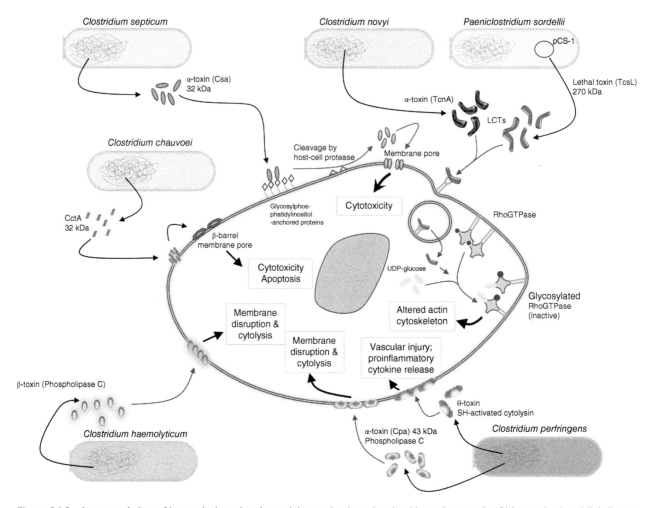

Figure 24.2 Integrated view of key toxin-based pathogenicity mechanisms involved in pathogenesis of histotoxic clostridial disease.

Clostridium chauvoei

Clostridium chauvoei causes blackleg in cattle and sheep. This is usually sporadic in occurrence but outbreaks with as many as 72 deaths in 12 days have been recently recorded. Blackleg, or blackquarter as it is sometimes known, is worldwide in distribution.

Spores of this organism, ingested from pasture or soil-contaminated silage, are deposited in the muscle and liver of cattle and other ruminants via the circulation and are thought to lie dormant. However, the occurrence of outbreaks supports the idea that the organism can access the tissues if animals are exposed to a substantial source of the pathogen. The spores may be activated by muscle trauma – perhaps a bruise caused by a kick. This may cause reduced blood supply to tissues, thus lowering the oxygen tension, and hence the redox potential, at the site of the damage. Spores then germinate and toxins are released from the organism which act locally to cause further damage to the muscle tissue (necrotising myositis or muscular gangrene) and allow spread of the vegetative (growing) form of the organism.

The primary toxin of blackleg, CctA, was only recently identified. It is a member of the leucocidin superfamily of bacterial toxins forming pores in host cells. It is now also recognised as the primary protective antigen in vaccines (Frey et al. 2012).

Clostridium septicum

Clostridium septicum is very closely related to *C. chauvoei*. It causes braxy: invasion of the abomasum of sheep leading to a fatal bacteraemia. It is also responsible for oedematous wound infections (myonecrosis) in cattle and other species after soil or faecal contamination of a traumatic wound, generally referred to as malignant oedema (Otter and Uzal 2020).

Braxy can cause significant deaths in a flock of lambs in the first year. It is recognised in the UK and Ireland, but also reported in the USA and Australia. The pathogenesis of braxy is not well understood but it seems to require predisposing damage to the abomasum. Ingesting cold or frozen feed or frosted pasture is a risk factor for the disease in both sheep and dairy calves. *C. septicum* increases vastly in numbers and invades the epithelial mucosa of the abomasum. The abomasal wall and small intestine become necrotic, haemorrhagic and oedematous. The organism then invades throughout the body, causing toxaemia.

Like other clostridia, *C. septicum* produces a number of different toxic products but evidence suggests that the primary toxin, which is responsible for the myonecrosis and oedema, is the haemolytic α toxin (Kennedy et al. 2005). This is a 46 kDa protein, of the same family as the ε toxin of *C. perfringens*, which is activated by enzymatic cleavage with trypsin to a 41 kDa form. This activated toxin then oligomerises to form pores in the cell membrane (Figure 24.2). Other proteases, such as cell membrane-bound furin, may actually be more important than trypsin in activating the toxin at the surface of target cells. Mutation of the *csa* gene, encoding the toxin in *C. septicum*, showed that the α toxin (Csa) is of primary importance and essential for virulence (Kennedy et al. 2005).

Clostridium novyi

Clostridium novyi is a very strictly anaerobic organism. The bacteria are highly sensitive to small quantities of oxygen and this sensitivity means they are considered fastidious and difficult to cultivate. *C. novyi* produces several toxins and is classified into three types based on the toxins produced. Types A and B are pathogenic while type C is considered non-pathogenic. A fourth type (D) is also named *C. haemolyticum*. Based on DNA evidence, types B and C and *C. haemolyticum* are the same organism, differing only in their toxin production (Table 24.2).

Clostridium novyi causes oedematous histotoxic wound infections such as 'big head' in rams. It is probably caused by young rams fighting. The damage to the skin allows the *C. novyi* into the damaged subcutaneous tissues where they are able

Table 24.2 *Clostridium novyi* and *C. haemolyticum* (C.h) toxin types.

Toxin	Activity	Type A	Type B	Type C	C. h
Alpha	Necrotising, lethal	+	+	−	−
Beta	Phospholipase C; necrotising, lethal; haemolytic	−	+	−	+
Gamma	Phospholipase; necrotising; haemolytic	+	−	−	−
Delta	Oxygen-labile haemolysin	+	−	−	−

to grow and cause a non-gaseous and non-haemorrhagic oedema. It is also responsible for infectious necrotic hepatitis in sheep, known as black disease, often following liver fluke (*Fasciola hepatica*) infestation. Spores of *C. novyi* type B germinate in the liver and produce toxins which result in tissue necrosis.

The α toxin is a 250 kDa protein which causes oedema in tissues and is a lethal toxin when injected. It is a member of the family of large clostridial cytotoxins (LCT) which are glucosyltransferases that inactivate members of the Rho and Ras small GTP-binding proteins (Orrell and Melnyk 2021). The effect of this is to interrupt signal transduction pathways in the host cell and break down the cytoskeletal structure (Figure 24.2).

Clostridium haemolyticum

Clostridium haemolyticum is very closely related to *C. novyi* and has been referred to as *C. novyi* type D. It causes bacillary haemoglobinuria (or red water disease) of cattle and occasionally sheep. The organism produces a phospholipase (lecithinase C) known as β toxin. This is lethal, necrotising, haemolytic and is released in the liver causing capillary damage and intravascular haemolysis (Navarro et al. 2017). Free circulating haemoglobin is then excreted in the urine.

The disease is largely sporadic but is associated with high levels of liver fluke (*F. hepatica*). Clinical signs are consistent with intravascular haemolysis: jaundice and haemoglobinuria.

Paeniclostridium sordellii

The organism previously known as *C. sordellii* was renamed *Paeniclostridium sordellii* in 2016 (Sasi Jyothsna et al. 2016). It is found in soil and the gastrointestinal tract of animals. It has been known for many decades but has been increasingly recognised as a pathogen of both animals and humans, causing severe and fatal infections in both. In animals, *P. sordellii* infection occurs particularly in sheep, cattle and foals. Many strains are relatively non-pathogenic but those expressing lethal toxin (TcsL) and in some strains the additional haemorrhagic toxin (TcsH) are particularly virulent. These toxins are encoded on a plasmid designated pCS1 (Couchman et al. 2015).

Paeniclostridium sordellii is a cause of sudden death in sheep. This is a rapidly fatal necrohaemorrhagic and emphysematous abomasitis (Otter and Uzal 2020). It primarily affects lambs aged between four and 10 weeks but older sheep can also become diseased. These show a partially distended and displaced abomasum. Infection by *P. sordellii* has also caused 'malignant oedema' (gas gangrene) through contaminated vaccinations, and infection of the genital tract of ewes associated with parturition. In cattle, a similar course is seen leading to sudden death. Infection takes place orally and calves primarily suffer gastrointestinal disease in the same manner as lambs.

In horses, *P. sordellii* causes enteric disease with necrotic, haemorrhagic and oedematous intestines. Disease is also seen in neonatal foals on colonisation of the internal umbilicus. In poultry, *P. sordellii* has been shown to be the cause of necrotic enteritis (Rimoldi et al. 2015).

Genome analysis shows that *P. sordellii* produces a range of known virulence determinants, including a cholesterol-dependent cytolysin sordellilysin (Sdl), neuraminidase (NanS) and a phospholipase C (Csp). However, the toxins responsible for disease appear to be the two LCT TcsH (300 kDa) and TcsL (270 kDa) that are present in only a small proportion of strains isolated (Just and Gerhard 2004). These are closely related to the TcdA and TcdB toxins respectively of the (primarily) human pathogen *C. difficile*.

TcsL and TcsH glycosylate Rho-GTPases, such as Ras, in mammalian cells. Rho-GTPases control the cell cycle, apoptosis, and the structural consequences of actin polymerisation such as cell morphology. Inactivation of the Rho proteins causes disruption of cell signalling leading to cell rounding and death (Figure 24.2). TcsL is a highly potent cytotoxin essential for the most aggressive actions of *P. sordellii* in natural disease (Carter et al. 2011).

The Neurotoxic Clostridia

Clostridium botulinum

Clostridium botulinum is a ubiquitous organism. Its spores are known to survive boiling for hours. Botulism is an intoxication due to ingestion of the potent neurotoxin produced by *C. botulinum*. Botulinum toxin is perhaps the most toxic substance known; 1.0 μg is the approximate lethal dose for a human being. Usually, the toxin is preformed before ingestion.

In infant children, the organism may multiply in the gut to release toxin. Occasionally, the organism may produce toxin directly in necrotic wounds on foals and horses.

The importance of botulism is as a severe human disease, a public health threat, preventable by careful heat treatment and canning procedures for the preservation of non-acid foods. If heat treatment (autoclaving) of canned foods is inadequate, the spores will survive and then anaerobic conditions favour germination of the spores and toxin production by any *C. botulinum* present.

Botulism is also a disease of animals: birds, mammals and fish. In cattle, it is encountered following consumption of big-bale silage feed that has become contaminated with a rotting rodent carcass or similar material. The fatality rate is very high. Another risk is associated with poultry litter that has been applied to pasture as fertiliser or used as bedding for cattle (Hogg et al. 2008). Decaying broiler carcasses are a major source of toxin, the organism being naturally present in the intestinal tract of the birds and rodents. The disease is seen in small animals which consume rotting carcasses and in waterfowl that have eaten decomposing crustaceans in anaerobic sediments.

Strains of *C. botulinum* produce one of seven antigenically distinct toxins: A–G. The neurotoxin is absorbed from the intestinal tract into the bloodstream and then carried to the peripheral nervous system where it binds to gangliosides at the neuromuscular junction. The toxin is cleaved before it is active and operates in three modules, one of which is a zinc metalloprotease. It exerts its neurotoxic effect by a complex, multistep process that ultimately blocks the release of the neurotransmitter acetylcholine at the synapse and neuromuscular junction (Figure 24.3). This causes a flaccid paralysis and death.

Antitoxin antibody (neutralising antibody) prepared in animals is available, but this is only useful for detoxifying free toxin in the early stages of the disease. Once fixed, the toxin cannot be removed and has a slow decay. Vaccination of

Stimulus at cholinergic synapse

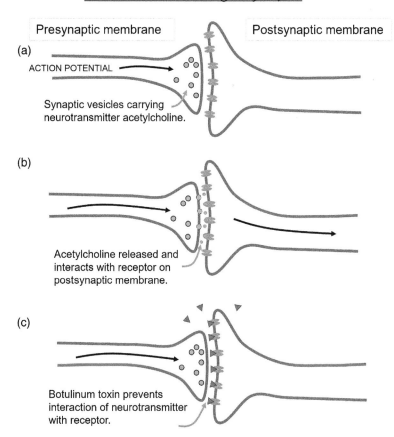

Figure 24.3 Action of botulinum toxin at the neuromuscular junction. (a) An action potential arrives at a resting synapse; (b) the action potential causes release of acetylcholine into the synaptic cleft and interacts with the receptor on the postsynaptic membrane; (c) when botulinum toxin is present, it blocks the receptor, preventing transfer of the action potential into the axon to stimulate the muscular contraction.

livestock with toxoid is practised in some parts of the world and to attempt to protect unaffected animals when an outbreak is under way.

Clostridium tetani

Clostridium tetani is also ubiquitous in soil and is found particularly in faeces of horses and other animals. It produces round, terminal spores which give it a drumstick appearance under the microscope.

   Clostridium tetani is not tissue invasive but grows superficially in deep anaerobic wounds. The wound may be the umbilicus, a surgical suture, a burn or accidental injury. It is usually contaminated with soil or faeces. Like *C. perfringens* infections, a low redox potential with concurrent infection and necrotic tissue assists the germination of spores and the production of disease.

   The organism produces tetanospasmin during the late exponential phase. This is a powerful neurotoxin. From the site of infection in tissues, the toxin binds to gangliosides at the neuromuscular junction. It is internalised and passes along the inside of peripheral nerve cells (axons) to reach the postsynaptic membrane of inhibitory neurons (Popoff 2020). Here, it is released to cross the synaptic cleft where it is then localised within synaptic vesicles of the presynaptic nerve terminal. Tetanospasmin acts by blocking the release of neurotransmitters for inhibitory synapses (glycine and γ-aminobutyric acid). It does this by cleaving synaptobrevin, a protein on the vesicle that is essential for fusion of small synaptic vesicles with the synaptic membrane (Figure 24.4). This causes the inhibitory neuron to fail and allows uncontrolled excitatory synaptic activity (paralysis by constant tensing of muscles – tetani).

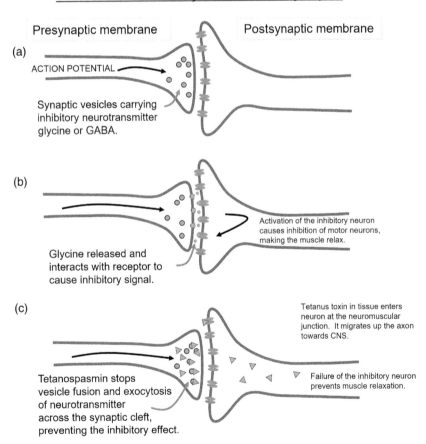

Stimulus at inhibitory interneuron synapse

Presynaptic membrane

Postsynaptic membrane

(a)

ACTION POTENTIAL

Synaptic vesicles carrying inhibitory neurotransmitter glycine or GABA.

(b)

Activation of the inhibitory neuron causes inhibition of motor neurons, making the muscle relax.

Glycine released and interacts with receptor to cause inhibitory signal.

(c)

Tetanus toxin in tissue enters neuron at the neuromuscular junction. It migrates up the axon towards CNS.

Tetanospasmin stops vesicle fusion and exocytosis of neurotransmitter across the synaptic cleft, preventing the inhibitory effect.

Failure of the inhibitory neuron prevents muscle relaxation.

Figure 24.4 Action of tetanus toxin at the neuromuscular junction of inhibitory synapses. (a) An action potential arrives at the synapse of an inhibitory neuron; (b) the action potential causes release of glycine (or GABA) into the synaptic cleft and this interacts with the receptor on the postsynaptic membrane; (c) when tetanus toxin arrives via the nerve cell and migrates to the inhibitory neuron, it arrives in the cytoplasm of the presynaptic inhibitory neuron and cleaves the protein necessary for vesicle fusion. This prevents transfer of the neurotransmitter and so prevents the inhibitory effect of the impulse on the muscle. Muscular contraction is not controlled.

While tetanus is difficult to treat (again the antitoxin is only effective in the early stages and will not alter fixed toxin), prevention is simple. Formalin-treated tetanospasmin (toxoid) is used as the vaccine to generate immunity in all species. Because the quantity of toxin reaching the bloodstream in natural disease is inadequate to generate antitoxic antibody, vaccination with tetanus toxoid is given to generate antibody in any cases of tetanus or where it is suspected or even a remote possibility.

Diagnosis of Clostridial Disease

Diagnosis of clostridial disease in animals is not straightforward. Clinical history, signs and postmortem appearance may match those expected, but this is not always the case and laboratory confirmation can be needed. Culturing *Clostridium* species from gut contents or faeces is not useful: clostridia will usually be present in the bowel and so finding them in the gut of a sick or dead animal has no diagnostic value. If a *Clostridium* is present in tissues in large numbers shortly after death, this is likely to be the cause, and samples can be examined directly by Gram staining and taken into transport medium for anaerobic culture. But postmortem invasion of clostridia into tissues from the gut can be rapid in animals that have died from other causes and if lesions are in the gut, it can be impossible to be clear whether organisms present are actually involved in disease or have invaded postmortem. Bacterial growth and metabolic activity do not stop on death of an animal. On the contrary, ideal anaerobic conditions are created for clostridia to flourish. For these reasons, alternative methods of diagnosis have been used over the years.

The most accurate diagnostic methods were animal protection tests to demonstrate and identify specific toxins. For ethical and financial reasons, these are rarely used now. If an animal died of suspected clostridial disease, blood plasma or gut contents could be taken, centrifuged and filtered to remove any debris and live or dead organisms, and the cell-free material injected into experimental animals, usually mice or guinea pigs. Toxicity for the experimental animals would indicate toxins in the sample. To identify the toxin, and confirm the micro-organism involved, the toxic effects could be neutralised with specific antiserum. Using known antiserum, previously raised by immunisation of horses or rabbits with known (inactivated) toxin preparations, test animals could be protected against specific toxins while control animals, not receiving the antiserum, died.

Tissue samples can be taken at postmortem investigation and subjected to fluorescent antibody tests. The tissue is processed for histopathology but in place of staining, specific antiserum is applied. After washing to remove unbound antibody, a second antibody, joined to a fluorescent label, is then applied so that the microorganisms, recognised by the primary antibody, can be clearly seen.

References

Awad, M.M., Ellemor, D.M., Boyd, R.L. et al. (2001). Synergistic effects of alpha-toxin and perfringolysin O in *Clostridium perfringens*-mediated gas gangrene. *Infection and Immunity* 69: 7904–7910.

Carter, G.P., Awad, M.M., Yibai Hao, Y. et al. (2011). TcsL is an essential virulence factor in *Clostridium sordellii* ATCC 9714. *Infection and Immunity* 79: 1025–1032.

Couchman, E.C., Browne, H.P., Dunn, M. et al. (2015). *Clostridium sordellii* genome analysis reveals plasmid localized toxin genes encoded within pathogenicity loci. *BMC Genomics* 16: 392.

Frey, J., Johansson, A., Bürkia, S. et al. (2012). Cytotoxin CctA, a major virulence factor of *Clostridium chauvoei* conferring protective immunity against myonecrosis. *Vaccine* 30: 5500–5505.

Garcia, J.P., Adams, V., Beingesser, J. et al. (2013). Epsilon toxin is essential for the virulence of *Clostridium perfringens* type D infection in sheep, goats, and mice. *Infection and Immunity* 81: 2405e2414.

Hogg, R., Livesey, C., and Payne, J. (2008). Diagnosis and implications of botulism. *In Practice* 30: 392–397.

Just, I. and Gerhard, R. (2004). Large clostridial cytotoxins. *Reviews of Physiology, Biochemistry and Pharmacology* 152: 23–47.

Kennedy, C.L., Krejany, E.O., Young, L.F. et al. (2005). The alpha-toxin of *Clostridium septicum* is essential for virulence. *Molecular Microbiology* 57: 1357–1366.

Keyburn, A.L., Boyce, J.D., Vaz, P. et al. (2008). NetB, a new toxin that is associated with avian necrotic enteritis caused by *Clostridium perfringens*. *PLoS Pathogens* 4: e26.

Mehdizadeh Gohari, I.M., Navarro, M.A., Li, J. et al. (2021). Pathogenicity and virulence of *Clostridium perfringens*. *Virulence* 12: 723–753.

Navarro, M.A., Dutra, F., Briano, C. et al. (2017). Pathology of naturally occurring bacillary hemoglobinuria in cattle. *Veterinary Pathology* 54: 457–466.

Orrell, K.E. and Melnyk, R.A. (2021). Large Clostridial toxins: mechanisms and roles in disease. *Microbiology and Molecular Biology Reviews* 85: e00064–e00021.

Otter, A. and Uzal, F.A. (2020). Clostridial diseases in farm animals: 2. Histotoxic and neurotoxic diseases. *In Practice* 42: 279–288.

Popoff, M.R. (2020). Tetanus in animals. *Journal of Veterinary Diagnostic Investigation* 32: 184–191.

Rimoldi, G., Uzal, F., Chin, R.P. et al. (2015). Necrotic enteritis in chickens associated with *Clostridium sordellii*. *Avian Diseases* 59: 447–451.

Rood, J.I., Adams, V., Lacey, J. et al. (2018). Expansion of the *Clostridium perfringens* toxin-based typing scheme. *Anaerobe* 53: 5–10.

Sasi Jyothsna, T.S., Tushar, L., Sasikala, C., and Ramana, C.V. (2016). *Paraclostridium benzoelyticum* gen. nov. sp. nov., isolated from marine sediment and reclassification of *Clostridium bifermentans* as *Paraclostridium bifermentans* comb. nov. proposal of a new genus *Paeniclostridium* gen. nov.to accommodate *Clostridium sordellii* and *Clostridium ghonii*. *International Journal of Systematic and Evolutionary Microbiology* 66: 2459–2459.

Songer, J.G. (1996). Clostridial enteric diseases of domestic animals. *Clinical Microbiology Reviews* 9: 216–234.

25

Staphylococcus – Skin and Soft Tissue Infection

Staphylococcus species are Gram-positive cocci that grow in bunches and are catalase positive (they decompose hydrogen peroxide to water and oxygen). They are facultative anaerobes and are metabolically quite active. They are also versatile – in the range of diseases they can cause, the numerous pathogenicity factors, the varied habitats they occupy and the way they have adapted to become resistant to many classes of antimicrobials.

Staphylococci are normal commensals of the skin and mucous membranes of the upper respiratory tract and intestinal tract of many animals. There are approximately 60 species of *Staphylococcus* and traditionally these have been divided into the pathogenic and the *relatively* non-pathogenic species on the production of coagulase, and this remains generally true.

Coagulase-positive Staphylococci

Coagulase-positive staphylococci were previously considered a single species, *S. aureus*, and this is largely still the case in human medicine. However, it was recognised that animals carried different biotypes of coagulase-positive staphylococci, associated with different animal species. Biotypes A, B, C and D were considered to be *S. aureus* while biotypes E and F, found on the skin and in the nares, mouth, pharynx and anus of dogs, cats and horses, were renamed *S. pseudintermedius* (Phillips and Kloos 1981; Devriese et al. 2005).

The pathogenic species (*S. aureus*, *S. pseudintermedius*) are aggressive pathogens when they gain access to a sterile site (body tissue without a resident microbial flora) or are otherwise able to overgrow due to reduced immunity or tissue damage. The relatively non-pathogenic species can still cause infections, but these are less aggressive and usually require a lowered immune status or presence of a foreign body to colonise soft tissues and invade.

Distinguishing the Pathogenic Staphylococci

Coagulase is a specific protein found almost exclusively in the pathogenic staphylococcal species: *S. aureus* and *S. pseudintermedius*. Free coagulase is an extracellular protein, elaborated by the bacteria, which causes a clot to form when the bacteria are mixed into a small quantity of citrated plasma. The protein has no enzyme activity. Instead, it binds to prothrombin in the plasma, causing it to become proteolytically active staphylothrombin. This thrombin–coagulase complex then converts the fibrinogen to fibrin to form a clot. Thus, prothrombin is activated without being converted to thrombin. Furthermore, coagulase can bind to fibrinogen as well as to prothrombin (Figure 25.1).

A separate component is clumping factor. This has been referred to as 'bound coagulase' and it is this that is usually detected by the simple routine clumping test. In this test, a suspension of bacteria from a plate culture is mixed on a glass slide with plasma. If the clumping factor is present, the bacteria avidly clump together, visibly and rapidly – usually within five seconds. Indeed, a fraction of coagulase is firmly attached to the cell. However, this effect is not due to a bound coagulase but primarily to an 87 kDa surface fibrinogen-binding protein, clumping factor (ClfA) (McDevitt et al. 1992).

While coagulase is closely correlated with pathogenicity of *S. aureus* and others, its presence was considered only to reflect the pathogenic make-up of the organism and was not in itself essential for virulence. Coagulase-negative mutants of *S. aureus* showed no reduction in virulence in a mouse model. However, in other studies it has been demonstrated that

Fundamentals of Veterinary Microbiology, First Edition. Andrew N. Rycroft.
© 2024 John Wiley & Sons Ltd. Published 2024 by John Wiley & Sons Ltd.
Companion website: www.wiley.com/go/veterinarymicrobiology

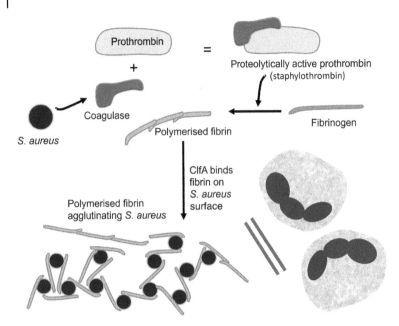

Figure 25.1 Coagulase causes proteolytic activation of prothrombin to then convert fibrinogen to fibrin.

coagulase embeds the staphylococci within a network of fibrin, protecting them from immune recognition and enabling the organisms to multiply as a bacterial community at the centre of lesions (Sewid et al. 2018).

Furthermore, *S. aureus* mutants deficient in the fibrinogen-binding protein ClfA have reduced virulence for a mouse model of arthritis and sepsis. It is probable that the bacterial cells become coated with fibrinogen *in vivo*, which inhibits deposition of C3b and prevents access of neutrophils to any opsonins that are there. Clumping factor has also been shown to bind and activate complement factor I. This is a regulatory factor which converts C3b to the inactive form iC3b and C3d. The increased concentration of factor I ultimately prevents formation of C3 convertase and activation of the later components of complement.

The coagulase activity of *S. pseudintermedius* has very similar properties to that from *S. aureus*. It binds prothrombin and facilitates the deposition of fibrinogen on the bacterial surface to provide protection from phagocytosis (Sewid et al. 2018).

Another secreted enzyme, closely correlated with pathogenicity and easily detected in the diagnostic laboratory, is deoxyribonuclease (DNase). Strains usually possess both coagulase and DNase, or neither of them.

Major Pathogenicity Factors

Coagulase-positive staphylococci (*S. aureus* and *S. pseudintermedius*) cause skin and other soft tissue infections. They are the most common cause of acute pyogenic (pus-producing) infections in companion animals. They are a principal cause of bovine mastitis, canine pyoderma, wound infections in all animals, abscesses and suppurative lesions, tick pyaemia in sheep, otitis externa in dogs, osteomyelitis following wound or surgical infection. The ability of *S. aureus* to cause such a diverse range of infections is due in part to cell surface-associated components and extracellular toxins. The pathogen encodes a remarkable repertoire of virulence factors. These molecules promote host colonisation, facilitate evasion of the human innate immune system, damage host cells and alter immune responses (DeLeo and Otto 2008).

α-Toxin

There are four recognised haemolysins produced in different combinations by strains of *S. aureus* and *S. pseudintermedius*. α-Toxin is a protein produced by most strains of *S. aureus* and *S. pseudintermedius*, including >94% of isolates from bovine mammary glands (Kenny et al. 1992). It produces a zone of clear haemolysis (confusingly termed β-haemolysis) around colonies on blood agar (see Chapter 26). The toxin is secreted as 34 kDa monomers which integrate into the membrane of a target cell. These bind to a wide range of mammalian cells where they form cylindrical heptamers creating pores which leak ions and may lyse the cells. The toxin causes cell necrosis and is lethal to animals when injected intravenously. Some target cells include mast cells and platelets whose contents have damaging consequences when released from the cell. Mutants of *S. aureus* unable to produce α-toxin are much less able to cause disease than their congenic parental strain in animal models of infection (Bubeck Wardenburg et al. 2007). Furthermore, the quantity of α-toxin produced by strains correlates in animal models to the severity of infection (Tong et al. 2015).

β-Toxin

β-Toxin is a 35 kDa exotoxin that causes a much wider zone around colonies on blood agar. However, the effect on RBCs is not lytic until the cultures are allowed to cool after incubation (Dinges et al. 2000). The β-toxin is a sphingomyelinase (a phosphorylase which converts sphingomyelin to ceramide). This causes the RBCs to become sensitised to the effects of other, weaker haemolysins (from other bacteria) which, when produced within the affected zone of β-toxin, causes complete lysis. It is produced by many animal strains but few human-derived strains. *In vivo*, the enzyme damages membranes and may cause cell leakage and contribute to necrosis but the role of the β-toxin in pathogenicity of *S. aureus* is not clearly determined.

The contribution of γ and δ toxins (both of which have haemolytic properties) to causation of disease is not clear.

Leucocidins

Relatively few strains of coagulase-positive staphylococci produce leucocidin. Panton-Valentine leucocidin (PVL) was discovered in 1932. It is a two-component toxin (F and S) which binds to macrophages and polymorphonuclear leucocytes and kills them. The two components act synergistically. However, pathogenic staphylococci are capable of surviving inside, and multiplying in, leucocytes, so the contribution to disease in those strains which produce it is unclear. This is reinforced by experiments that show mutants lacking PVL are still pathogenic while those lacking α-toxin are much reduced in virulence.

TSST-1

Toxic shock syndrome toxin (TSST-1) is a 22 kDa protein toxin. It is absorbed from the mucosal surface and acts as a superantigen. Superantigens are a group of microbial proteins which are very powerful immunomodulators. They induce massive T-cell proliferation; 5–40% of the cells become activated which can be compared to approximately 0.001% for a conventional antigen. The toxin binds to and cross-links the relatively invariable regions on major histocompatibility complex (MHC) class II antigens on host antigen-presenting cells (APC) and the T-cell receptor of the T-cells without prior internalisation and processing by the APC. Superantigens interact with the variable region of the T-cell receptor β chain and each superantigen has affinity for a set of Vβ elements. This results in a preferential expansion of all the T-cells bearing those Vβ elements, which is followed by a high production of cytokines. The superantigen-induced overproduction of cytokines (TNF-α) is believed to strongly influence the development of cardiovascular shock associated with microthrombus formation on the capillaries. Cells to which TSST-1 binds may be destroyed by certain cytotoxic T-cells. Immunomodulators (modulins) such as this may downregulate the immune response to staphylococcal infections, explaining the poor immune response in severe staphylococcal infections.

Enterotoxins

Certain strains of *S. aureus* (approx. 30%) produce potent enterotoxin. These are protein and heat stable and are known to be responsible for staphylococcal food poisoning in humans. At least eight separate staphylococcal enterotoxins are recognised. They appear to interact with mast cells to cause release of inflammatory mediators during staphylococcal food poisoning. They are also superantigens that bridge the Class II MHC and T-cell receptor without presentation of antigen. This triggers inappropriate release of cytokines from lymphocytes.

Staphylococcal food poisoning is caused when a toxin-producing strain of *S. aureus* grows on a foodstuff which is then consumed. Since *S. aureus* derives from an animal or human host rather than the environment, foods only become contaminated from the secretions or infected wounds of a human or animal. The organism must then incubate on the foodstuff which is a suitable substrate for growth before being eaten and the preformed toxin ingested. Even if the foodstuff is heated, the preformed enterotoxin is resistant to moderate heating. All the staphylococcal enterotoxins are emetic, and they also cause gastroenteritis and usually diarrhoea. While humans and primates are susceptible, it is not known whether companion animals carry the same, as yet unidentified, cellular receptors in the intestinal tract.

Proteases, Hyaluronidase and Lipases

Other digestive enzymes are produced by staphylococci. They facilitate nutrition of the bacteria and cause spread of the organisms and tissue destruction.

Exfoliative Toxins

These toxins are produced by some strains of *S. aureus*. They cause a blistering effect in humans, particularly young infants, known as ETA and ETB. Involvement in animal disease is not yet known.

Protein A

Protein A (Spa) is a cell wall-anchored component of almost all *S. aureus* strains. It is an IgG binding protein that binds to the Fc portion of IgG molecules except IgG3. It also binds IgM. In this way, it is known to inhibit opsonophagocytosis by binding IgG by the Fc region, which prevents classical complement fixation and recognition by the neutrophil Fc receptor. The Fab portion is free to bind to antigen, but the IgG is no longer capable of activating complement and causing deposition of C3b on the surface of the organism.

Fibronectin-Binding Proteins

FnBPs are present on the surface of the majority of isolates of *S. aureus*. Their role is probably to allow them to adhere to and colonise damaged tissue (wounds).

Capsule

Capsular polysaccharides are produced by approximately 90% of *S. aureus* strains. Although 12 capsular serotypes have been described, most clinical isolate strains carry capsule types 5 or 8 (Arbeit et al. 1984). Capsule expression reduces the uptake of bacteria by neutrophils in the presence of normal complement. That is, the capsular polysaccharide provides a poorly stabilising surface for C3 convertase and thereby inhibits complement activation by the alternative pathway. In turn, this prevents deposition of the major opsonin, C3b. However, the induction of specific antibody to *S. aureus* does not necessarily result in protection, and anticapsular antibodies are not inherently protective against *S. aureus* as they are against many other encapsulated pathogens (Spellberg and Daum 2012).

The role of the polysaccharide capsule is unclear but it almost certainly inhibits phagocytosis in the absence of specific antibody; that is, it provides a poorly stabilising surface for C3 convertase and thereby inhibits complement activation by the alternative pathway and so inhibits deposition of the major opsonin C3b. One reason for the lack of certainty over its role is that the capsule seems to be produced only under certain environmental conditions, particularly *in vivo*. Another is that 12 chemically different capsule polysaccharides are known and will differ in their functional ability.

Other Pathogenicity Characters

A large number of other bacterial components are now known to be involved in staphylococcal invasion by interference with neutrophil extravasation chemotaxis, complement action and neutrophil-mediated killing, by manipulating B-cell and T-cell responses, and by killing host cells (Thammavongsa et al. 2015).

Methicillin-resistant *Staphylococcus aureus*

Methicillin-resistant *Staphylococcus aureus* (MRSA) and *S. pseudintermedius* (MRSP) are simply lineages of these pathogens that have acquired a gene (*mecA*) that encodes a transpeptidase that is not inhibited by therapeutic concentrations of β-lactam drugs. The pathogen can therefore cross-link peptidoglycan, and survive, in the presence of penicillin group drugs such as amoxicillin and cloxacillin. It is referred to as methicillin resistant because this drug was used for treating staphylococcal infections at the time of discovery of MRSA in 1961. This has since been superseded by other β-lactamase stable drugs but the name remains. These strains are no more able to colonise, or cause disease, than other strains of *S. aureus* but when they do cause infection, they do not respond to penicillins or β-lactamase stable penicillins.

Coagulase-negative Staphylococci

Coagulase-negative/DNase-negative staphylococci are relatively non-pathogenic and are usually harmless commensals (Becker et al. 2014). There are a considerable number of species of coagulase-negative staphylococci; many are considered to be the same from a disease standpoint and are merely referred to as coagulase-negative staphylococci or sometimes *Staphylococcus epidermidis*. In human medicine, they are frequently termed *S. albus*. They are often isolated from clinical samples and can usually be regarded as secondary invaders of little importance. However, they can be quite adhesive, particularly to plastics, and are sometimes the cause of infections associated with indwelling catheters or similar plastic implants. This can be important when the animal is debilitated or immunocompromised through lymphosarcoma or steroid therapy, and particularly when the organism displays multiple antibiotic resistance.

Some coagulase-negative staphylococci are associated with specific disease in animals.

Staphylococcus schleiferi

Staphylococcus schleiferi is a leading cause of drug-resistant pyoderma and otitis in dogs (Misic et al. 2015). It was considered as coagulase variable but has been subdivided into those strains that do produce coagulase, *S. schleiferi* subsp. *coagulans,* and those that do not, *S. schleiferi* subsp. *schleiferi*. It is also reported to produce α-toxin. Without careful discrimination in the laboratory, it can be confused with *S. pseudintermedius* and coagulase-negative staphylococci. Many strains carry the *mecA* gene and are therefore methicillin-resistant staphylococci (Morris et al. 2006; May et al. 2012).

Staphylococcus hyicus

Staphylococcus hyicus is the cause of exudative epidermitis in pigs (greasy pig disease). This affects young pigs, particularly between one and seven weeks of age (Foster 2012). It is a generalised skin infection with greasy exudate, exfoliation and vesicle formation. It is highly contagious between groups of pigs and enters through breaks in the skin. The skin becomes thickened. Milder cases show wrinkling skin and dandruff-like scaling.

Staphylococcus hyicus has been used as a species name for many years and it was formally recognised in 1978. It is usually coagulase-negative although a few strains (~3%) are tube-coagulase positive. It is also usually DNase positive.

Pathogenicity

It has been demonstrated that closely similar lesions could be induced by injection of concentrated sterile culture filtrate. This led to the purification of an exfoliative toxin (Exh) which is distinct from ETA and ETB that are produced by some strains of *S. aureus*. The 30 kDa toxin is Cu dependent: removal of Cu ions by chelation removes toxin activity (Andresen et al. 1997). Subsequently, at least four antigenic types of the *S. hyicus* exfoliative toxin were demonstrated. These cleave desmoglein-1 in pig skin, causing loss of cell adhesion between cells of the epidermis. Exfoliative toxin is the key pathogenicity determinant in porcine exudative epidermitis and strains of *S. hyicus* not able to produce the Exh toxins are non-pathogenic (Leekitcharoenphona et al. 2016).

References

Andresen, L.O., Bille-Hansen, V., and Wegener, H.C. (1997). *Staphylococcus hyicus* exfoliative toxin: purification and demonstration of antigenic diversity among toxins from virulent strains. *Microbial Pathogenesis* 22: 113–122.

Arbeit, R.D., Karakawa, W.W., Vann, W.F., and Robbins, J.B. (1984). Predominance of two newly described capsular polysaccharide types among clinical isolates of *Staphylococcus aureus*. *Diagnostic Microbiology and Infectious Disease* 2: 85–91.

Becker, K., Heilmann, K., and Peters, G. (2014). Coagulase-negative staphylococci. *Clinical Microbiology Reviews* 27: 870–926.

Bubeck Wardenburg, J., Bae, T., Otto, M. et al. (2007). Poring over pores: α-hemolysin and Panton-Valentine leukocidin in *Staphylococcus aureus* pneumonia. *Nature Medicine* 13: 1405–1406.

DeLeo, F.R. and Otto, M. (2008). An antidote for *Staphylococcus aureus* pneumonia? *Journal of Experimental Medicine* 205: 271–274.

Devriese, L.A., Vancanneyt, M., Baele, M. et al. (2005). *Staphylococcus pseudintermedius* sp. nov., a coagulase-positive species from animals. *International Journal of Systematic and Evolutionary Microbiology* 55: 1569–1573.

Dinges, M.M., Orwin, P.M., and Schlievert, P.M. (2000). Exotoxins of *Staphylococcus aureus*. *Clinical Microbiology Reviews* 13: 16–34.

Foster, A.P. (2012). Staphylococcal skin disease in livestock. *Veterinary Dermatology* 23: 342–351.

Kenny, K., Bastida, F.D., and Norcross, N.L. (1992). Secretion of alpha-hemolysin by bovine mammary isolates of *Staphylococcus aureus*. *Canadian Journal of Veterinary Research* 56: 265–268.

Leekitcharoenphona, P., Pampa, S.J., Andresen, L.O., and Aarestrup, F.M. (2016). Comparative genomics of toxigenic and non-toxigenic *Staphylococcus hyicus*. *Veterinary Microbiology* 185: 34–40.

May, E.R., Kinyon, J.M., and Noxon, J.O. (2012). Nasal carriage of *Staphylococcus schleiferi* from healthy dogs and dogs with otitis, pyoderma or both. *Veterinary Microbiology* 160: 443–448.

McDevitt, D., Vaudaux, P., and Foster, T.J. (1992). Genetic evidence that bound coagulase of *Staphylococcus aureus* is not clumping factor. *Infection and Immunity* 60: 1514–1523.

Misic, A.M., Cain, C.L., Morris, D.O. et al. (2015). Complete genome sequence and methylome of *Staphylococcus schleiferi*, an important cause of skin and ear infections in veterinary medicine. *Genome Announcements* 3: e01011–e01015.

Morris, D.O., Rook, K.A., Shofer, F.S., and Rankin, S.C. (2006). Screening of *Staphylococcus aureus*, *Staphylococcus intermedius*, and *Staphylococcus schleiferi* isolates obtained from small companion animals for antimicrobial resistance: a retrospective review of 749 isolates (2003-04). *Veterinary Dermatology* 17: 332–337.

Phillips, W.E. and Kloos, W.E. (1981). Identification of coagulase-positive *Staphylococcus intermedius* and *Staphylococcus hyicus* subsp. *hyicus* isolates from veterinary clinical specimens. *Journal of Clinical Microbiology* 14: 671–673.

Sewid, A.H., Hassan, M.N., Ammar, A.M. et al. (2018). Identification, cloning, and characterization of *Staphylococcus pseudintermedius* coagulase. *Infection and Immunity* 86: e00027–e00018.

Spellberg, B. and Daum, R. (2012). Development of a vaccine against *Staphylococcus aureus*. *Seminars in Immunopathology* 34: 335–348.

Thammavongsa, V., Kim, H.W., Missiakas, D., and Schneewind, O. (2015). Staphylococcal manipulation of host immune responses. *Nature Reviews Microbiology* 13: 529–543.

Tong, S.Y.C., Davis, J.S., Eichenberger, E. et al. (2015). *Staphylococcus aureus* infections: epidemiology, pathophysiology, clinical manifestations, and management. *Clinical Microbiology Reviews* 28: 603–661.

26

Streptococcus

Streptococcus species are Gram-positive cocci which tend to grow in chains. That is, they divide in the same plane at each cell division and then do not immediately separate into individual daughter cells. Most appear to be aerotolerant, not benefiting from or being damaged by molecular O_2, but some streptococci (*Peptostreptococcus* species) are strict anaerobes. Biochemically, they differ from the other Gram-positive cocci in that they are always catalase negative: they do not produce the enzyme to split H_2O_2 with the release of oxygen.

Classifying Streptococci

Members of the genus *Streptococcus* are found in the normal flora of animals (mouth, upper respiratory tract and gut) and some species are able to cause disease. Streptococci are very diverse, with complex relationships between apparently different organisms, and have not been easy to classify (Facklam 2002). Originally, in medical bacteriology, streptococci were grouped on the basis of their haemolysis produced on blood agar: α, β or γ, and this method of description continues today.

- α Haemolysis is when the bacterial colony is surrounded by a narrow zone of partial haemolysis and a green discolouration of the medium.
- β Haemolysis describes the effect when the bacterial colony is surrounded by a clear zone of complete haemolysis that is sharply demarcated from the unaltered red cells in the surrounding medium.
- γ Haemolysis means non-haemolytic – no change in the medium surrounding the colony – but this term is rarely used in place of non-haemolytic.

On reports from clinical laboratories, it is still common to see streptococci described as β-haemolytic or α-haemolytic.

More usefully, the streptococci were recognised as falling into one of four broad groups (Sherman 1937) and this still fits with modern identification systems based on serogrouping.

- Pyogenic (pus-forming, often β-haemolytic)
- Viridans (greening around colonies on blood agar; usually α-haemolytic)
- Enterococci (faecal habitat; often non-haemolytic; grow on MacConkey medium)
- Lactic (found in milk), now known as *Lactococcus* species.

Lancefield Groups

In 1933, a serological scheme was developed for the subdivision of β-haemolytic streptococci. This is the Lancefield grouping scheme, which is based on an antigenic carbohydrate cell wall component (Lancefield 1933). There are 20 Lancefield groups, each designated by a letter of the alphabet, and these groups are related to the host and disease specificity of the *Streptococcus* isolate. Some α-haemolytic streptococci (groups B and D) also carry a Lancefield antigen. Some other streptococci, e.g. *S. pneumoniae* and *S. uberis*, do not carry a Lancefield antigen and are untypable.

Fundamentals of Veterinary Microbiology, First Edition. Andrew N. Rycroft.
© 2024 John Wiley & Sons Ltd. Published 2024 by John Wiley & Sons Ltd.
Companion website: www.wiley.com/go/veterinarymicrobiology

To test streptococci for the Lancefield group, the soluble antigen is first extracted by incubating the whole bacteria with either acid or (latterly) a proteolytic enzyme. Originally, this was used in an immunoprecipitation test with whole antiserum in capillary tubes but that has been superseded by a rapid co-agglutination test in which the antigen is mixed with antibody-coated latex particles. Visible clumping of the latex particles indicates that the antibody has bound to the antigen and brought the latex particles together.

Streptococci associated with specific diseases are usually found in specific sites in the body. For example:

- tonsil – *S. pyogenes*, *S. equi*, *S. suis*
- genital tract – *S. zooepidemicus*, *S. canis*, *S. dysgalactiae*
- bovine mammary gland – *S. agalactiae*
- intestine – faecal streptococci *S. faecium*, *Enterococcus faecalis*.

Similarly, some *Streptococcus* species are associated with particular animal species. For example:

- *S. pyogenes* (group A) – humans
- *S. canis* (group G) – dogs
- *S. equi* (group C) – horses.

Habitat and Pathogenicity

Survival of streptococci outside the body is poor. Most are fastidious organisms which are adapted to life on a host where complex nutrients are available. They are transmitted by direct contact or through aerosol and droplets.

Pathogenicity factors are found on pyogenic streptococci, i.e. those organisms of groups A, B, C, D, E and G which cause pus-forming infections: *S. pyogenes*, *S. agalactiae*, *S. dysgalactiae*, *S. equi*, *S. canis*, *S. uberis*, *S. suis* and *S. porcinus*. Some such pathogenicity-related traits may also be present in non-pyogenic streptococci.

Groups A and C produce a hyaluronic acid capsule. This is non-antigenic as it is chemically indistinguishable from the hyaluronic acid in ground substance of connective tissue. It is antiphagocytic. Streptococci which are phagocytosed are rapidly killed inside the phagocytic cell (Figure 26.1).

M protein is found on group A, and M-like proteins on groups C and G streptococci. This is associated with surface fibrillar structures and is instrumental in evading opsonophagocytosis by binding the complement regulatory proteins C4BP and factor H which destabilise the C3 convertase. This inhibits C3b deposition on the bacterial surface and vastly reduces the efficiency of phagocytosis. It is also a fibrinogen-binding protein which causes fibrinogen to coat the surface and hide surface structures that activate complement by the alternative pathway or are the target for immunoglobulins (Turner et al. 2019).

Toxins

Streptococci also produce many digestive enzymes, some of which are toxic to mammalian cells. Their purpose is to digest proteins and lipids in the environment of the bacteria to yield amino acids, etc. as a source of nutrition.

Streptolysin O is a haemolysin. It is a thiol-activated cytolysin that is inactivated by molecular oxygen. The molecule, of 57 kDa, requires cholesterol in the cell membrane in order to bind and so free cholesterol inactivates the ability to bind to the cell. It is produced by strains of group A and by many group B, C, F and G organisms.

Streptolysin S is an oxygen-stable haemolysin. It is of low molecular weight (2.7 kDa) and requires a carrier molecule such as RNA or albumin to retain its activity away from the bacterium. The cytolytic activity is permanently inactivated when the toxin is separated from the carrier molecule. It is a potent cytotoxin and may be important in killing phagocytic cells during infection (Molloy et al. 2011).

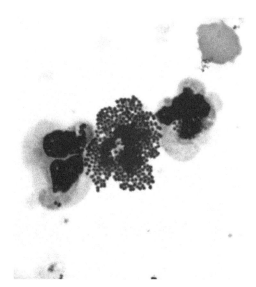

Figure 26.1 Phagocytic uptake of streptococci by neutrophils.

Hyaluronidase is found in groups A, B and C and *S. suis*. It hydrolyses the hyaluronic acid ground substance of connective tissue. It presumably digests the capsular material of the bacteria also but since this is in a dynamic state of turnover, it is constantly being replaced and loss of capsule does not represent lethal damage for the bacterium.

Streptokinase is produced by streptococci of groups A, C and G. The enzyme lyses fibrin clots, preventing the limitation of the spread of infection in the tissues by a fibrin barrier.

Streptococci Causing Animal Disease

Lancefield Group A

Lancefield group A has the single species *S. pyogenes*. Except in occasional instances, Lancefield group A streptococci never cause infection or disease in animals. They are invariably β-haemolytic and cause acute disease, scarlet fever, septic sore throat, puerperal fever, lymphadenitis and erysipelas in humans. Acute rheumatic fever and glomerulonephritis are sequelae. They possess all the above pathogenicity characters and sometimes an erythrogenic factor (scarlet fever).

Lancefield Group B

Lancefield group B has the single species, *Streptococcus agalactiae* (sometimes referred to as GBS). The colonies are usually weakly β-haemolytic. They have been a major problem in contagious, chronic bovine mastitis. This is because *S. agalactiae* lives in the bovine milk duct. It is considered host-adapted for colonising at that site; it provokes little inflammation and rarely penetrates the epithelial lining of the duct. Thus, it produces chronic bovine mastitis with clinical cases that are recurrent, leading to fibrosis in the udder and loss of milk production. On farms with a record of *S. agalactiae* mastitis, ultimate control has been through a programme of culling those animals known to carry the pathogen together with hygiene, treatment and other general measures for mastitis control. Such measures have greatly reduced the proportion of mastitis cases due to *S. agalactiae*.

Lancefield Group C

Lancefield group C includes four species. *S. equi* is classified into two subspecies, *equi* and *zooepidemicus*, based on early DNA-DNA hybridisation experiments. This is confusing because subspecies *equi* was almost certainly derived from an ancestral strain of *S. zooepidemicus*. For clarity, they will be considered as different species.

Streptococcus zooepidemicus is found in different species. In the horse, it is an opportunistic pathogen causing wound infections, rhinopharyngitis, arthritis, pneumonia, metritis and abortion. In cattle and goats, it is a cause of severe mastitis. In the dog, it can cause rapidly lethal pneumonia, particularly in some smaller breeds of dog, following kennel cough.

Equine Strangles

Streptococcus equi is the host-adapted agent of strangles in the horse. It is strongly β-haemolytic due to production of streptolysin S and often shows very mucoid colonies that coalesce into each other. *S. equi* is an obligate parasite of the horse and while infections have occasionally been reported in humans and other animals, these are very rare. It is therefore isolated almost exclusively from equids (Waller et al. 2011).

The organism is highly contagious and is spread from one animal to another in pus, by direct contact with mucous membrane, via fomites (such as wooden surfaces and grooming equipment) or by aerosol. Flies will also transfer infected pus from one animal to another. After an incubation of perhaps 3–6 days, the infection causes a high fever, with respiratory dyspnoea and abscessed lymph nodes of the head and neck. There is often a mucopurulent nasal discharge from the nose or from ruptured lymph nodes. The mortality is low (approximately 10%) but many animals that appear to make a full recovery will carry the organism, primarily in the guttural pouch, and remain a source of infection for other horses.

A variety of components contribute to the ability of *S. equi* to cause disease. Both *S. equi* and *S. zooepidemicus* use an adhesin (FimI) with an accessory protein to bind collagen. This is likely to play a major role in the binding of both pathogens to host tissue and is thought to enable *S. equi* to adhere to host tonsil epithelium. However, rather than remaining at the epithelial surface, *S. equi* rapidly invades the tonsil tissue and progresses to the lymph nodes of the head and neck. Once in the tissues, *S. equi* has several mechanisms for acquisition of iron. One that is unique to *S. equi* is equibactin. This is known to enhance the acquisition of iron *in vivo*. Toxins produced by *S. equi* include phospholipase, streptolysin S which is cytopathic for many types of host cells and a number of different superantigens that cause non-specific T-cell activation, disrupt the normal innate and adaptive immune response and cause huge and inappropriate release of proinflammatory cytokines. Evidence suggests that streptococcal superantigens contribute markedly to the pathogenicity of *S. equi* in equine lymph nodes.

Another component, designated Se18.9, is produced only by *S. equi*. This binds factor H of complement which regulates (inhibits) the formation of functional C3 convertase (C3bBb) and so C3b is not efficiently deposited on the bacterial surface. Furthermore, the hyaluronic acid capsule, that is overproduced in *S. equi* compared to *S. zooepidemicus*, contributes to the antiphagocytic properties of the organism. Hyaluronic acid appears identical to that in mammalian tissues and therefore causes the immune system to fail to recognise these pathogens as foreign.

Provisional diagnosis of strangles can be made on clinical signs but laboratory tests are needed to confirm a diagnosis. Isolation of β-haemolytic streptococci of Lancefield group C is tested by sugar fermentation and can also be confirmed by PCR using specific primers. Once the organism has been cultured and purified, colonies are inoculated into individual sugars in peptone water. These are incubated at 37 °C, usually with phenol red as an indicator. The sugars lactose, trehalose, sorbitol and ribose are not fermented but the β-glucoside salicin (which acts as a positive control) is fermented, causing acid production and yellowing of the indicator. Other Lancefield group C streptococci give a different fermentation pattern and, because of the severity of disease and rapid spread between horses, it is obviously crucial that a correct identification is made.

Matrix-assisted laser desorption/ionisation time-of-flight mass spectrometry (MALDI-TOF MS) has been examined for the discrimination of *S. equi* and *S. zooepidemicus* with less than complete identification of both organisms.

Efforts have also been made to use serological testing, particularly in the detection of 'silent' carrier animals and those that have recovered from the disease in which chondroids form in the guttural pouch. ELISA assays to measure antibody, using fragments of *S. equi* protein antigen, have been developed. These antigens are the N-terminus of the *S. equi* M protein (antigen C) and an N-terminal fragment of another protein (antigen A). However, it has been concluded that seronegativity in this ELISA was not a reliable indicator of the absence of guttural pouch carriage of *S. equi*.

Streptococcus equisimilis is isolated predominantly from suppurative arthritic joints of pigs aged between one and three weeks. Entry is via a skin wound, the tonsil or the umbilicus.

Streptococcus dysgalactiae causes acute bovine mastitis and joint-ill in lambs. In bovine mastitis, it does not cause herd outbreaks but cases occur sporadically. Strains are α-haemolytic (partial haemolysis on blood agar usually associated with a greening) or γ (non-haemolytic). They are carried on the skin of the udder, and in the mouth and vagina. In sheep, *S. dysgalactiae* causes outbreaks of polyarthritis, commonly known as joint-ill. This affects lambs less than four weeks old with development of disease at 10–14 days of age. Carriage by ewes and transmission to neonatal lambs via the umbilicus are thought to be the source of the pathogen, yet very large outbreaks of the infection can occur in some years, suggesting that additional predisposing factors, or particularly virulent strains, play a role in the spread or invasion of the pathogen.

While they can be the most aggressive pathogens, β-haemolytic streptococci of Lancefield groups A, C and G remain exquisitely sensitive to penicillin G and other similar penicillins; resistance is not known. However, treatment of animals with penicillin, and other antibiotics, can have negative and unexpected consequences and requires careful management (Brazil 2005).

Lancefield Group D

Lancefield group D streptococci are the enterococci, which are normal inhabitants of the large intestine of mammals and birds and so are always present in normal faeces. They are the only streptococci able to grow on MacConkey agar. They are not usually β-haemolytic. The two primary species are *Enterococcus faecalis* and *Streptococcus faecium*. Group D streptococci may cause UTI and wound infections.

Streptococcus bovis is also group D and a recognised cause of bovine mastitis. The taxonomy and relationships of *S. bovis* to other similar streptococci are not clear (Farrow et al. 1984). It has since been split into five species (Facklam 2002).

Streptococcus suis Disease

Perhaps one of the most important animal pathogens in group D is *S. suis*. It is a pig pathogen and was formerly assigned to Lancefield groups S and R, but is now recognised to be group D (Hommez et al. 1986). Thirty-five serotypes have now been defined based on capsular polysaccharide. Serotype 2 is a common serotype and may be carried by up to 90% of a group of pigs. Serotype 2 has a strong predilection for the meninges and is also zoonotic causing meningitis in humans.

This occurs occasionally in pig meat workers in developed nations from skin cuts and abrasions. Human disease is most commonly seen in South-East Asia among families living closely with backyard pigs, probably via the oral route from consumption of inadequately cooked pork products.

Pigs frequently harbour multiple strains of *S. suis* in the upper respiratory tract and crypts of the palatine tonsil without symptoms. When stress factors associated with intensive husbandry are present, disease outbreaks will occur. Sows carrying the organism can infect the piglets to cause either neonatal death from meningitis or the carrier state in the piglets. Serotype 1 is less severe than serotype 2 and will cause disease only in younger piglets and lead to arthritis and endocarditis rather than death. Whole-genome sequencing coupled with clear information about a large collection of isolates has shown clear genetic differences between systemic, respiratory and non-clinical (carriage) isolates of *S. suis* (Weinert et al. 2015).

There is strong evidence that *S. suis* gains entry to the body by being transported inside macrophages. Survival inside macrophages is probably crucial to the pathogenesis. This is unusual among the streptococci which are considered to be exclusively extracellular pathogens. The organism enters the bloodstream and spreads to the joints and meninges, etc. Considerable effort has been made to understand the pathogenicity of *S. suis*. Two proteins were strongly associated with virulence: 110 kDa extracellular factor (EF) and the 136 kDa muramidase released protein (MRP). More recently, using defined mutants, these have been shown to have no direct measurable effect on the pathogenicity of *S. suis*.

The components of *S. suis* responsible for disease in pigs or humans have not been adequately resolved. The capsular polysaccharide is clearly necessary and contributes to protection of the organism against opsonophagocytosis and killing. In experiments, removal of this capsule by mutation significantly increases phagocytosis, killing and clearance from the circulation. However, some encapsulated strains do not survive in blood while virulent encapsulated strains do persist. Therefore, capsular polysaccharide alone is not sufficient to confer resistance to opsonophagocytosis and killing; other factors must play a role. This phenomenon is indeed true of other, unrelated pathogens such as *E. coli*.

The haemolysin, known as suilysin, is a cholesterol-dependent, pore-forming toxin. Many virulent strains produce this toxin but many do not. Strains producing suilysin show a haemolytic effect that may be described as α-haemolysis or very weak β-haemolysis. It apparently plays a role in invasive disease in experiments with mice, while in the pig suilysin seems to confer little or no direct pathogenic property on the bacteria (Segura et al. 2017). However, it may enhance the virulence of invading strains through effects on the inflammatory response and by damage to respiratory epithelial cells in the early stages of infection (Meng et al. 2019).

Lancefield Group E

Streptococcus porcinus causes a severe cervical or mandibular lymphadenopathy (cervical lymphadenitis) in pigs (jowl abscesses) in the USA; this is not seen in the UK.

Lancefield Group F

Lancefield group F streptococci are not usually a recognised cause of animal disease but are considered important pathogens in humans. They were known as the '*S. milleri*' group but are now referred to as the *S. anginosus* group: *S. constellatus*, *S. intermedius* and *S. anginosus*. Instead of the group F antigen, these sometimes express either Lancefield group A or no Lancefield antigen. As tools for analysis and classification of strains improve, defining streptococci by the Lancefield grouping system is becoming less straightforward and boundaries for defining strains are often blurred.

Lancefield Group G

Lancefield group G streptococci is the small group, primarily isolated from canine infections but also from cattle and other species. Again, the Lancefield antigen is no longer always a clear indication of species and some strains typed as other streptococci, such as *S. dysgalactiae*, may carry the Lancefield group G antigen.

Non-groupable Streptococci

Some streptococci lack the Lancefield group antigen, e.g. *S. pneumoniae* (or pneumococci) which is a major cause of bacterial pneumonia in humans and occasional cases of animals disease such as respiratory disease causing poor performance in young thoroughbreds.

Streptococcus uberis has no Lancefield group antigen. It is non-haemolytic and ferments the carbohydrate aesculin – a biochemical feature used to recognise the organism on Edward's medium. It is responsible for an increasingly common form of environmental bovine mastitis in which only slight changes are seen in the udder tissue and the secretion. *S. uberis* is isolated from many sites including the skin, genital tract, faeces and udder teat and is thought to reside primarily within the gastrointestinal tract of cows, appearing as an opportunistic pathogen of the mammary gland (Sherwin et al. 2021).

Viridans group streptococci such as *S. salivarius* and *S. sanguis* are normal flora of the oral cavity of many mammals. They are relatively non-pathogenic although some are implicated in dental caries (*S. mutans*) and in bacterial endocarditis.

Lactic group streptococci include *S. lactis*, the milk-souring organism, and *S. thermophilus* in yoghurt. These are never implicated in disease.

References

Brazil, T. (2005). Strangles in the horse: management and complications. *In Practice* 27: 338–347.

Facklam, R. (2002). What happened to the streptococci: overview of taxonomic and nomenclature changes. *Clinical Microbiology Reviews* 15: 613–630.

Farrow, J.A.E., Kruze, J., Phillips, B.A. et al. (1984). Taxonomic studies on *Streptococcus bovis* and *Streptococcus equinus:* description of *Streptococcus alactolyticus* sp. nov. and *Streptococcus saccharolytics* sp. nov. *Systematic & Applied Microbiology* 5: 467–482.

Hommez, J., Devriese, L.A., Henrichsen, J., and Castryck, F. (1986). Identification and characterization of *Streptococcus suis*. *Veterinary Microbiology* 11: 349–355.

Lancefield, R.C. (1933). A serological differentiation of human and other groups of streptococci. *Journal of Experimental Medicine* 59: 441–158.

Meng, F., Tong, J., Vötsch, D. et al. (2019). Viral coinfection replaces effects of suilysin on *Streptococcus suis* adherence to and invasion of respiratory epithelial cells grown under air-liquid Interface conditions. *Infection and Immunity* 87: e00350–e00319.

Molloy, E.M., Cotter, P.D., Hill, C. et al. (2011). Streptolysin S-like virulence factors: the continuing *sagA*. *Nature Reviews Microbiology* 9: 670–681.

Segura, M., Fittipaldi, N., Calzas, C., and Gottschalk, M. (2017). Critical *Streptococcus suis* virulence factors: are they all really critical? *Trends in Microbiology* 25: 585–599.

Sherman, J.M. (1937). The streptococci. *Bacteriological Reviews* 1: 3–97.

Sherwin, V.E., Green, M.J., Leigh, J.A., and Egan, S.A. (2021). Assessment of the prevalence of *Streptococcus uberis* in dairy cow feces and implications for herd health. *Journal of Dairy Science* 104: 12042–12052.

Turner, C.E., Bubba, L., and Efstratiou, A. (2019). Pathogenicity factors in group C and G streptococci. *Microbiology Spectrum* 7: GPP3-0020-2018.

Waller, A.S., Paillot, R., and Timoney, J.F. (2011). *Streptococcus equi*: a pathogen restricted to one host. *Journal of Medical Microbiology* 60: 1231–1240.

Weinert, L.A., Chaudhuri, R.R., Wang, J. et al. (2015). Genomic signatures of human and animal disease in the zoonotic pathogen *Streptococcus suis*. *Nature Communications* 6: 6740.

27

Nocardia, Actinomyces and *Dermatophilus* – The Filamentous Pathogens

Nocardia

Nocardia species are strictly aerobic, Gram-positive, soil bacteria that form branching filamentous rods which are shorter than those of actinomycetes (Figure 27.1). These often fragment into coccoid forms that break off the filaments. *Nocardia* is a ubiquitous, saprophytic, soil organism. It is partially acid-fast because the cell walls contain mycolic acid (like mycobacteria) although these have a shorter chain length than those of *Mycobacterium* species. This enables it to resist decolourisation with acid/alcohol in the Ziehl–Neelsen stain but not as consistently or completely as mycobacteria.

The species name of this pathogen was previously *Nocardia asteroides*. However, like many other pathogens, *Nocardia* isolates from infections have been more accurately characterised by DNA analysis, and the taxonomy has been refined. The species *N. cyriacigeorgica*, *N. farcinica* and *N. abscessus* are now recognised (McHugh et al. 2017). Nevertheless, the clinical disease they are associated with is not dependent on the particular species.

Pathogenesis

Nocardia is able to cause granulomatous lesions in animals, particularly in the lung, brain and soft tissue. This is because it can survive, and grow, in macrophages. Infection usually begins by inhalation of the organism whose coccoid forms are present in the air. From mucosal surfaces, these are taken up by macrophages and if not destroyed, may form lesions and spread by the haematogenous route. *Nocardia* infections have a tendency to disseminate in the body while those due to actinomycetes tend to remain localised.

Actinomyces

Actinomyces species are branching and filamentous Gram-positive rods. They are often anaerobes but some are facultative anaerobes and they are never acid-fast. *Actinomyces* species reside on the mucous membranes of normal animals; they are common members of the normal microbial flora of the healthy oropharynx, gastrointestinal tract, upper respiratory tract and genital tract.

Pathogenesis

Infections with *Actinomyces* usually start with introduction of the organism into the host tissue. In cattle, *A. bovis* is the cause of lumpy jaw in which the organism gains access to soft tissue through a penetrating wound in the mucosal barrier of the oral cavity such as from a sharp thorn or piece of barbed wire (Figure 27.2). Infections can be mixed, involving the proliferation of different organisms in the lesion. In diagnostic imaging, the lesions may appear to be directly spreading through tissues, irrespective of physical barriers or tissue types, and may therefore be mistaken for malignant disease.

In the dog, the most common site of disease is the lower respiratory tract due to *A. viscosus*. This probably arises from aspiration of oral secretions or from bite wounds and can spread very widely. Normal immune clearance would be expected to remove such organisms and the reason why immunity fails, and bacteria proliferate, is not known. In the case of a bite

Fundamentals of Veterinary Microbiology, First Edition. Andrew N. Rycroft.
© 2024 John Wiley & Sons Ltd. Published 2024 by John Wiley & Sons Ltd.
Companion website: www.wiley.com/go/veterinarymicrobiology

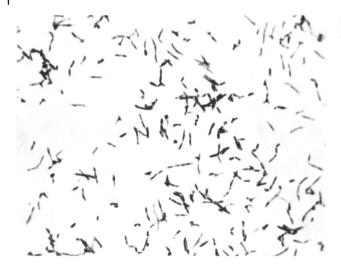

Figure 27.1 Microscopic appearance of a clinical isolate of *Nocardia* in culture, stained by Gram stain.

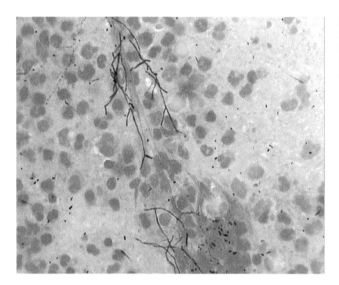

Figure 27.2 Microscopic appearance of pus aspirated from a case of lumpy jaw in a cow. The material has been stained by Gram stain. *Actinomyces bovis* is seen as branching, Gram-positive filaments that are fragmenting into 'beaded' filaments, short rods and coccoid forms.

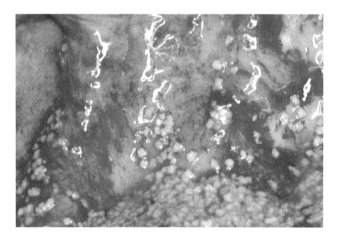

Figure 27.3 Dark yellow 'sulfur granules' seen macroscopically in the pleural surface of the chest cavity of a dog at postmortem examination. *Actinomyces viscosus* was recovered in pure culture.

wound, a localised granulomatous abscess of the skin develops. Respiratory inoculation can lead to a granulomatous thoracic lesion which may progress into the abdomen or cause a pyothorax. This is a slowly progressive, chronic inflammation. Characteristically, this infection generates large quantities of macroscopically visible 'sulfur granules' in the tissues (Figure 27.3). These are about 2 mm in diameter, often yellowish, and each is a tangled mass of branched bacterial filaments, encased in coagulated plasma (fibrin), pus cells and cellular debris. Infection with *A. viscosus* is sometimes confused with *Nocardia* infection.

Human infection can also occur. This is endogenous (host-derived) infection rather than zoonosis and is associated with failure of neutrophil function such as in chronic granulomatous disease (Reichenbach et al. 2009). As with *Nocardia*, there is an almost complete lack of understanding of the molecular mechanisms involved in the pathogenicity of *Actinomyces* sp.

Dermatophilus

Dermatophilus congolensis is a facultatively anaerobic, Gram-positive, filamentous rod. It is best known as the agent of 'mud fever', or dermatophilosis, a skin disease in horses associated with wet conditions. The same organism, perhaps host-adapted for different animal species, is the cause of streptothricosis in cattle, a serious, common problem in cattle in tropical sub-Saharan Africa that is closely associated with the wet season. Cattle become generally unwell and many show a severe, generalised form of the disease. It is also the agent of mycotic dermatitis and strawberry foot-rot in sheep.

Dermatophilus congolensis is part of the actinomycete group. It has a life cycle in which it forms filaments that undergo longitudinal division followed by transverse division to form highly motile coccoid forms, known as zoospores, which spread the infection across the skin (Figure 27.4). Apparently without the need for any injury, the organism then invades through the epidermis and forms skin lesions with thick fibrinous scabs (Figure 27.5). It is nevertheless suspected that ticks and biting flies may facilitate infection by the zoospores. When lifted, these scabs reveal yellow pus that may be placed on a slide, fixed and stained by Giemsa stain to show the typical 'snake-like' forms of the bacteria.

Mycotic dermatitis in sheep has a similar pathogenesis but the crusty lesions with pus cause matting of the wool. This can also become generalised and progressive and result in death, particularly in lambs.

Strawberry foot-rot in sheep begins with the appearance of dry scabs on the lower limbs after grazing on infected pasture. Infection may also be facilitated or enhanced by thorny plants that cause small abrasions in the skin. The lesions often heal, but in some cases spread around the leg and again the exudate forms hardened matting of the hair. When stripped off, this leaves granulation tissue with a bright red appearance, hence the name. These naturally heal but if the interdigital space is involved, the animal may become lame.

In the past there was confusion, because of the filamentous appearance, about whether causative agent was a fungus; hence names like mycotic dermatitis. This led to treatment with antifungals. *Dermatophilus* is a prokaryote and is susceptible to a range of antibacterial agents. Nevertheless, the notion that it is a fungus has persisted in some places and treatment with antifungals has continued to be given to animals. Drying of the skin surface and, if needed, use of penicillin, tetracycline or streptomycin is the treatment of choice for *Dermatophilus* infection in all animals.

Molecular characterisation of the *D. congolensis* genome showed a considerable number of potential virulence genes. However, none has been functionally studied and the bacterial components enabling pathogenicity are unknown (Branford et al. 2021).

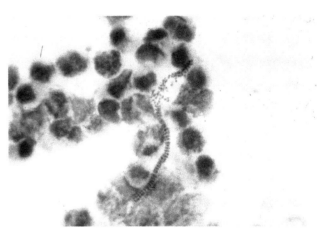

Figure 27.4 Microscopic appearance of *Dermatophilus congolensis* in a skin lesion, stained by Giemsa stain, showing both transverse and longitudinal cell divisions to release motile zoospores.

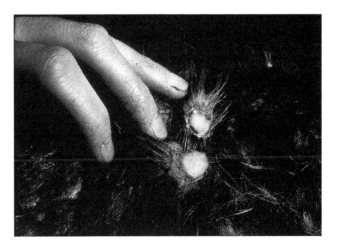

Figure 27.5 A lesion in the skin of a pony is lifted to reveal the pus beneath the scab.

References

Branford, I., Johnson, S., Chapwanya, A. et al. (2021). Comprehensive molecular dissection of *Dermatophilus congolensis* genome and first observation of *tet*(Z) tetracycline resistance. *International Journal of Molecular Sciences* 22: 7128.

McHugh, K.E., Sturgis, C.D., Procop, G.W., and Rhoads, D.D. (2017). The cytopathology of *Actinomyces*, *Nocardia*, and their mimickers. *Diagnostic Cytopathology* 45: 1105–1115.

Reichenbach, J., Lopatin, U., Mahlaoui, N. et al. (2009). *Actinomyces* in chronic granulomatous disease: an emerging and unanticipated pathogen. *Clinical Infectious Diseases* 49: 1703–1710.

28

Prescottella (Rhodococcus) equi

Prescottella equi (until recently *Rhodococcus equi*) is a small Gram-positive short rod related to the *Corynebacterium* group. It was first isolated from pneumonia in a foal in 1923 and was referred to as *Corynebacterium equi* until its name was changed in 1977 to the genus *Rhodococcus*. It sometimes grows in a coccoid morphology consistent with this previous name. Colonies have a characteristic salmon-pink colour which is seen best on non-blood medium (Figure 28.1). It is non-motile and otherwise resembles members of the *Corynebacterium* group. Based on phylogenomic analysis, it has now been renamed *P. equi* (Sangal et al. 2022).

Prescottella equi is naturally found in the soil and in the intestine of horses. It will persist in manure-contaminated soil for years and evidence suggests that, like other non-pathogenic former *Rhodococcus* species, it is a soil organism rather than an intestinal commensal. Consistent with this, *P. equi* is sensitive to bile salts, it prefers 30 °C for growth and is a strict aerobe.

This was also supported by the rather wide distribution of the organism in soil: it was isolated from 54% of a variety of soil samples. It was found to grow well in soil that had been enriched with dung. Growth in soil without herbivore faeces was comparatively poor and this was found to be because simple organic acids such as acetic and propionic acid were preferred nutrients. Therefore, in the natural environment, *P. equi* lives in soil but thrives in manured soil.

Pathogenesis

Prescottella equi is a pathogen of foals rather than older horses (Giguère et al. 2011). It affects the animals when they are less than five months old, causing a pyogranulomatous bronchopneumonia (Johns 2016). A proportion of foals with pulmonary infection will never show clinical signs and will eventually clear the infection. Other foals show a slowly progressive pneumonia in which large pulmonary abscesses develop in the lungs. There is sometimes an acute onset of severe respiratory distress. The disease is fatal in 40–80% of such cases (Cohen 2014). It also causes ulcerative enteritis.

In foals, the disease starts with inhalation of the organism very early in life. The younger the foal, the more susceptible to *P. equi* infection. Disease is first detected typically between five and seven weeks of age.

Pathogenicity

Strains of *P. equi* recovered from lesions in foals carry a large conjugative plasmid (80–90 kb). The plasmid carries genes, on a region of the plasmid known as a pathogenicity island, that are necessary for survival and multiplication inside macrophages. Without the plasmid, strains are unable to cause disease. Close analysis of the plasmid shows six genes known as the virulence-associated protein genes or *vap*. The most important of these appears to be *vapA* which encodes a temperature-inducible, surface-expressed lipoprotein, VapA. This is known to be essential for growth of the bacteria in macrophages *in vitro* and for persistent infection in mice (Figure 28.2).

VapA is expressed when the temperature is 37 °C and the pH slightly acid, consistent with the conditions inside a macrophage vacuole. It is not expressed when the temperature is lower and at an environmental pH of 8.0. VapA was previously thought to prevent the maturation of the phagosome and so inhibit fusion of the phagosome with lysosomes. However, the function of VapA lipoprotein is to generate a neutral pH intracellular environment. Once ingested into a vacuole of a

Fundamentals of Veterinary Microbiology, First Edition. Andrew N. Rycroft.
© 2024 John Wiley & Sons Ltd. Published 2024 by John Wiley & Sons Ltd.
Companion website: www.wiley.com/go/veterinarymicrobiology

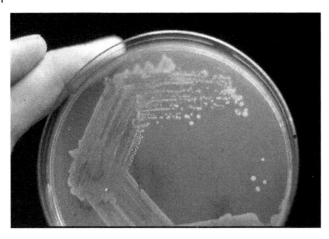

Figure 28.1 *Prescottella equi* showing the characteristic pink pigmentation.

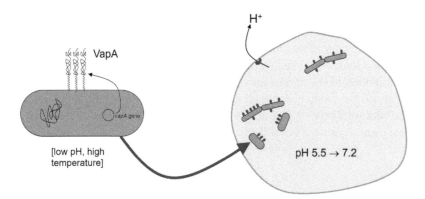

Figure 28.2 VapA is a surface-expressed, membrane-active lipoprotein encoded on a plasmid. It is essential for intracellular survival. When in the phagolysosome, it causes the H^+ gradient across the phagolysosomal membrane to be dissipated and consequently the loss of acidity, with pH increasing from the usual 5.0 to neutral.

macrophage, VapA is thought to damage the integrity of the vacuole membrane, allowing free flow of protons and dissipation of the H^+ gradient needed for acidification of the vacuole and thereby disarming the host defences (von Bargen et al. 2019).

Prescottella equi is taxonomically related to *Nocardia* and *Mycobacterium*. As such, it also produces mycolic acid and lipoarabinogalactan in the cell envelope. As with other mycolic acid-containing bacteria, this component may serve to protect the vulnerable components of the envelope from lysosomal enzymatic degradation and damage to the cytoplasmic membrane. However, experiments demonstrate that antibody to *P. equi* enhances the ability of macrophages and neutrophils to kill *P. equi*. This is probably because antibody interferes with the function of VapA or another essential component before uptake so that lysosome/phagosome fusion can take place and subject the bacteria to killing mechanisms.

Immune Response

Effective immunity to prevent disease is not present in young foals. It is unclear which of the components of the immune system is inadequate in the young foal, yet present in older foals when disease is rare. It is known that young foals lack cytotoxic T-lymphocytes. The suggestion that deficiency of IFN-γ induction, normally required to activate macrophage killing potential, has been shown to be unfounded. IFN-γ induction and antibody responses following *P. equi* challenge were very similar in foals to those of adult horses given the same infection challenge.

Investigations have now shown that foals generally have the ability to mount a protective immune response to *P. equi* infection. The reason that some foals are so susceptible to *P. equi* is probably complex rather than involving a simple explanation.

Human Disease

Prescottella equi is also responsible for pneumonia in humans immunocompromised with immunosuppressive drugs and came to prominence as a major secondary invader in people suffering from AIDS (Lin et al. 2019). Older horses are immune and immune-competent humans do not suffer from infections with *P. equi*. This suggests it is a pathogen that is only capable of causing disease as an opportunist, when the cell-mediated defences are damaged or undeveloped.

References

von Bargen, K., Scraba, M., Krämer, I. et al. (2019). Virulence-associated protein a from *Rhodococcus equi* is an intercompartmental pH-neutralising virulence factor. *Cellular Microbiology* 21: e12958.

Cohen, N.D. (2014). *Rhodococcus equi* foal pneumonia. *Veterinary Clinics of North America. Equine Practice* 30: 609–622.

Giguère, S., Cohen, N.D., Chaffin, M.K. et al. (2011). Diagnosis, treatment, control, and prevention of infections caused by *Rhodococcus equi* in foals. *Journal of Veterinary Internal Medicine* 25: 1209–1220.

Johns, I. (2016). Prevention and treatment of *Rhodococcus equi* infection in foals: an update. *In Practice* 38: 451–456.

Lin, W.V., Kruse, R.L., Yang, K., and Musher, D.M. (2019). Diagnosis and management of pulmonary infection due to *Rhodococcus equi*. *Clinical Microbiology and Infection* 25: 310e315.

Sangal, V., Goodfellow, M., Jones, A.L., and Sutcliffe, I.C. (2022). A stable home for an equine pathogen: valid publication of the binomial *Prescottella equi* gen. nov., comb. nov., and reclassification of four rhodococcal species into the genus *Prescottella*. *International Journal of Systematic and Evolutionary Microbiology* 72: 005551.

29

Corynebacterium – CLA

One of the few seven-syllable genus names in bacteriology, it is pronounced core-eye-knee-back-tier-i-um. *Corynebacterium* is a large genus of mostly harmless bacteria that reside on the skin and normal mucous membranes. They are taxonomically related to *Nocardia*, *Rhodococcus* and *Mycobacterium*.

Corynebacteria are small, tough, non-motile Gram-positive rods which form dry, opaque colonies in culture. They are usually quite innocuous. *Corynebacterium* species are frequently referred to by laboratory microbiologists as diphtheroids because they have the same basic morphology and characteristics as *Corynebacterium diphtheriae*, the causative organism of human diphtheria. However, *C. diphtheriae* is only pathogenic when it is infected with a temperate phage (a bacterial virus) which encodes a powerful toxin – diphtheria toxin – and this pathogen is not known to cause any disease in animals.

Corynebacterium pseudotuberculosis

Corynebacterium pseudotuberculosis causes caseous lymphadenitis (CLA), primarily in sheep and goats. It has worldwide distribution and is seen where sheep and goats are farmed. It was first observed in the UK in 1990 and appears to have been introduced from outside the country. It is non-motile and does not produce a polysaccharide capsule, but it does produce fimbriae. It is naturally carried on the skin of sheep and goats, and infects these animals through shearing wounds, ear tags and perhaps tick and fly bites, etc. This leads to the formation of abscesses containing dense, cheese-like pus, hence the Australian term for the disease: 'cheesy gland disease'. The abscesses form in subcutaneous tissues (Figure 29.1) and in lymph nodes. However, abscesses can also develop internally, in organs such as the lungs, kidneys, liver and mammary gland. This is visceral CLA. Internal abscesses may only be detected at postmortem examination but animals suffering with the infection will show reduced milk yield, poor condition and wasting (Baird 2003; Gascoigne et al. 2020).

Pathogenicity

Corynebacterium pseudotuberculosis is a facultative intracellular pathogen. It is reported to have a lipid cell wall that contains mycolic acid that may contribute to resistance to killing by phagocytic cells (Simmons et al. 1998). It also produces a potent phospholipase D enzyme exotoxin (PLD). This digests sphingomyelin and is crucial for pathogenicity.

The mechanism of contribution of PLD to virulence of *C. pseudotuberculosis* is not known. It is said to operate by allowing dissemination of the pathogen within the host by increasing local vascular permeability (Batey 1986). However, it may have a role in intracellular survival by damaging the phagolysosomal membrane. It has been suggested that PLD may impair the chemotaxis of neutrophils but this seems to contradict the massive accumulation of neutrophils and macrophages into the developing abscess lesions. Whatever its role, the essential contribution of PLD in the pathogenicity of *C. pseudotuberculosis* in sheep and goats has been clearly demonstrated by mutational studies.

Treatment and Control

Attempts at treatment are usually less than effective. Although the bacterium is susceptible to various antimicrobials, it is impossible for the drug to adequately penetrate the thick pus in established abscesses (Baird and Fontaine 2007).

Fundamentals of Veterinary Microbiology, First Edition. Andrew N. Rycroft.
© 2024 John Wiley & Sons Ltd. Published 2024 by John Wiley & Sons Ltd.
Companion website: www.wiley.com/go/veterinarymicrobiology

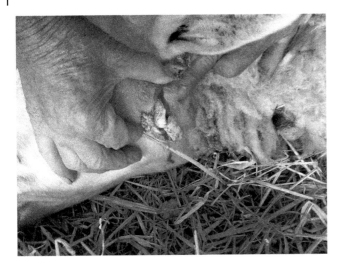

Figure 29.1 Thick pus from an abscess which is characteristic of caseous lymphadenitis.

Vaccination, on the other hand, can be effective in preventing the development of disease. Simple Al(OH)$_3$-adjuvanted, killed *C. pseudotuberculosis* bacteria can be quite effective in controlling the infection. Attempts at commercial vaccines for sheep and goats have also shown promise (Fontaine et al. 2006). Live vaccination using defined mutants deficient in the PLD has also been successful but awaits commercial use.

Corynebacterium pseudotuberculosis is also known to cause ulcerative lymphangitis in horses. This is seen as painful nodular abscesses on the underbelly and limbs.

References

Baird, G. (2003). Current perspectives on caseous lymphadenitis. *In Practice* 25: 62–68.

Baird, G.J. and Fontaine, M.C. (2007). *Corynebacterium pseudotuberculosis* and its role in ovine caseous lymphadenitis. *Journal of Comparative Pathology* 137: 179–210.

Batey, R.G. (1986). Pathogenesis of caseous lymphadenitis in sheep and goats. *Australian Veterinary Journal* 63: 269–272.

Fontaine, M.C., Baird, G., Connor, K.M. et al. (2006). Vaccination confers significant protection of sheep against infection with a virulent United Kingdom strain of *Corynebacterium pseudotuberculosis*. *Vaccine* 24: 5986–5996.

Gascoigne, E., Ogden, N., Lovatt, F., and Davies, P. (2020). Update on caseous lymphadenitis in sheep. *In Practice* 42: 105–114.

Simmons, C.P., Dunstan, S.J., Tachedjian, M. et al. (1998). Vaccine potential of attenuated mutants of *Corynebacterium pseudotuberculosis* in sheep. *Infection and Immunity* 66: 474–479.

30

Listeria – Growing in the Fridge

Listeria spp. are small, thin, facultatively anaerobic, Gram-positive rods (Figure 30.1). There are now eight species recognised but only two of these, *L. monocytogenes* and *L. ivanovii*, are pathogens, the others being harmless saprophytes. *Listeria* species are catalase positive, haemolytic and identified by the characteristic tumbling motility seen when they are grown at 18 °C. This is thought to be due to a reversal of the direction of rotation of the flagellae.

Listeriosis is most common in north and east Europe and North America. It has generally been thought of as a veterinary disease. In ruminants, it is seen as meningoencephalitis (circling disease); in monogastric animals (and young ruminants) it primarily causes sepsis. In pregnancy, the infection may cause inflammation in the placenta and fetus, and cause abortion. After abortion, the animal usually recovers but if the fetus is retained, septicaemia will usually occur. *Listeria* also causes gastroenteritis, conjunctivitis (surprisingly common in cattle), pneumonia, myocarditis and endocarditis (Schuchat et al. 1991).

Listeria organisms are widely distributed and naturally live as saprophytes in the environment, particularly the soil, decaying vegetation, silage, sewage and animal feed. Many healthy sheep and goats are carriers of the bacteria and shed the organisms intermittently in their faeces and milk – especially after periods of stress – and pasteurisation is an important control measure to prevent human infection from milk and cheese.

Listeria monocytogenes can proliferate in silage and this is a primary source of infection for some animals. Soil and sheep dung contaminate the grass and when this is cut, it is brought into the silo or silage bales. *Listeria* can then grow over a wide range of pH (5.0–9.0) and survive at pH as low as 4.0. It can then be ingested by ruminants, leading to outbreaks of disease involving several animals.

Listeriosis is also a potentially fatal food-borne infection of humans and may be considered a zoonotic disease (Farber and Peterkin 1991). While *L. monocytogenes* infects both humans and animals, *L. ivanovii* affects only cattle, sheep and goats. *L. ivanovii* has extremely rarely been shown to cause disease in humans (approximately one case per decade).

Transmission

The key to the epidemiology of *Listeria* as a food-borne pathogen of humans is its property of being able to grow at low temperature. The source of infection for humans is usually contaminated raw meat, unpasteurised milk or cheese made using unpasteurised milk, and foods containing raw vegetables (particularly organic vegetables, grown in well-manured soils) (Figure 30.2). This leads to human disease because the bacteria can grow at less than 10 °C. Legislation governs the numbers of *Listeria* organisms that may be present in foods for human consumption. However, even lightly contaminated food which is held in the fridge (especially when it is not working efficiently – perhaps 8–12 °C) will allow the *Listeria* to grow and heavily contaminate the food. If it is then eaten without further cooking, humans can be at risk. Those affected by *Listeria* are immunocompromised individuals, the young, the elderly and pregnant women. Normal adults are relatively resistant to disease.

Fundamentals of Veterinary Microbiology, First Edition. Andrew N. Rycroft.
© 2024 John Wiley & Sons Ltd. Published 2024 by John Wiley & Sons Ltd.
Companion website: www.wiley.com/go/veterinarymicrobiology

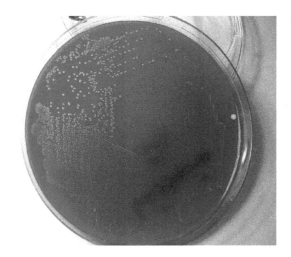

Figure 30.1 Colonies of *Listeria monocytogenes* are small and grey. In transmitted light, a weak haemolytic effect is apparent.

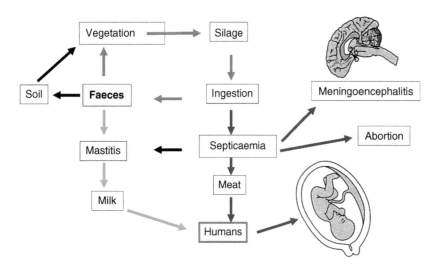

Figure 30.2 Transmission routes of *L. monocytogenes* between animals, the environment and humans.

Pathogenicity

Listeria monocytogenes is a facultative intracellular pathogen capable of invading epithelial cells and surviving and growing within them. When it is ingested by macrophages it evades killing by escaping into the cytoplasm (Figure 30.3).

The organisms produce listeriolysin (LLO) inside the phagosome. This 56 kDa cytolytic protein dissolves the phagosomal membrane so that the bacteria escape into the cytoplasm where they are relatively safe to proliferate (Hara et al. 2007). The bacteria then invade adjacent cells and so spread the infection laterally without ever becoming exposed to the humoral immune response. Listeriolysin, and other components involved in virulence, are encoded on a pathogenicity island (Listeria pathogenicity island-1). Two phospholipases C, PlcA and PlcB, co-operate with LLO to facilitate escape from phagocytic vacuoles and direct cell-to-cell spread. A metalloprotease is required for activation of PlcB and ActA mediates the actin-based intracellular motility of the bacteria which requires polymerisation of the cellular actin cytoskeleton. The expression of these virulence determinants is controlled by another gene, also present in the pathogenicity island. This is *prfA* encoding the positive regulatory factor PrfA (Scortti et al. 2007). PrfA is converted between the active and inactive form by environmental and host cell signals (de las Heras et al. 2011). Active PrfA is essential for expression of the other virulence-associated genes in the pathogenicity island and some outside it. Without this, the pathogen becomes avirulent (Vázquez-Boland et al. 2001).

Because of this intracellular location and spread, antibody against the *Listeria* is not protective and a cell-mediated immune response is required to overcome the infection and allow the animal to recover. It is currently thought that *Listeria*

Figure 30.3 *Listeria* enters host epithelial cells and escapes the intracellular vacuole into the cytoplasm where, through host cell actin polymerisation, it becomes motile and migrates to the adjacent cells.

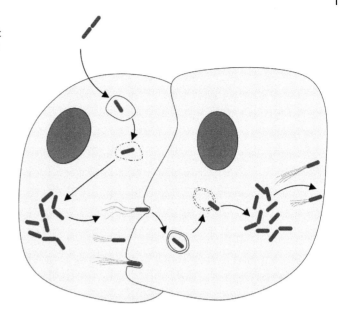

are released from infected cells by cytolytic T-cells that recognise and lyse infected cells. Neutrophils can kill *Listeria* when they are in the extracellular environment and there is strong evidence of a role for neutrophils in resistance to, and recovery from, infection. In addition, IFN-γ-stimulated macrophages may restrict intracellular multiplication of the bacteria.

References

Farber, J.M. and Peterkin, P.I. (1991). *Listeria monocytogenes*, a food-borne pathogen. *Microbiological Reviews* 55: 476–511.

Hara, H., Kawamura, I., Nomura, T. et al. (2007). Cytolysin-dependent escape of the bacterium from the phagosome is required but not sufficient for induction of the Th1 immune response against *Listeria monocytogenes* infection: distinct role of Listeriolysin O determined by cytolysin gene replacement. *Infection and Immunity* 75: 3791–3801.

de las Heras, A., Cain, R.J., Bielecka, M.K., and Vázquez-Boland, J.A. (2011). Regulation of *Listeria* virulence: PrfA master and commander. *Current Opinion in Microbiology* 14: 118–127.

Schuchat, A., Swaminathan, B., and Broome, C.V. (1991). Epidemiology of human Listeriosis. *Clinical Microbiology Reviews* 4: 169–183.

Scortti, M., Monzó, H.J., Lacharme-Lora, L. et al. (2007). The PrfA virulence regulon. *Microbes and Infection* 9: 1196–1207.

Vázquez-Boland, J.A., Kuhn, M., Berche, P. et al. (2001). *Listeria* pathogenesis and molecular virulence determinants. *Clinical Microbiology Reviews* 14: 584–640.

31

Erysipelothrix and *Trueperella*

Erysipelothrix rhusiopathiae

This microorganism is a slender Gram-positive rod which causes a variety of diseases in animals and humans. It grows as tiny colonies on blood agar and these are typically α-haemolytic. It is non-motile and catalase negative (unlike *Listeria* sp.). There are 23 serotypes based on heat-stable, peptidoglycan antigen extracted from the organisms. Serotypes 1a, 1b and 2 are most frequently implicated in disease. The organism is widespread in nature, being harboured in the lymphoid tissue (tonsils) and intestinal tract of carrier animals (Wood 1999).

Pathogenesis

Carrier animals shed the organism and contaminate the environment. Organisms then enter other animals by the oral or respiratory route or through a break in the skin. Once in the respiratory tract or intestine, they penetrate and gain access to the bloodstream. The pathogenesis involves swelling of endothelial cells of capillaries and venules, and thrombus formation. From the circulation, the organism localises in the joints and heart valves.

In pigs, *E. rhusiopathiae* may cause acute septicaemic disease. It is usually seen as rhomboidal (diamond-shaped) skin lesions. These are patches of ischaemic necrosis of the skin caused by thrombosis in the vessel supplying that region (Figure 31.1). It also causes chronic endocarditis and polyarthritis. The endocarditis in pigs usually involves the mitral valve, and there is a tendency for the vegetations to invade the endocardium. In turkeys, a similar picture involving acute septicaemia is produced. Sudden death of birds in a flock is common. Skin lesions, endocarditis and arthritis are also found. Disease occurs in many species, including fish (Reboli and Farrar 1989).

Pathogenicity

The mechanisms of pathogenicity and of immunity are not understood. Strains are known to differ greatly in virulence. The peripheral thrombosis and endocarditis suggest that blood-borne *Erysipelothrix* organisms are able to adhere to endothelium. *E. rhusiopathiae* is now known to be a facultative intracellular pathogen that can survive inside polymorphonuclear leucocytes and macrophages. It is also known that the possession of a capsule on its cell surface enables *E. rhusiopathiae* to resist phagocytosis by polymorphonuclear leucocytes and this correlates with virulence. This seems paradoxical for an intracellular organism, but capsule production is now regarded as the most important virulence factor of the organism (Ogawa et al. 2018). Neuraminidase production may be related to pathogenicity through enhanced penetration of tissues and damage to various tissues of the host, but no other toxins have been identified.

Vaccination

Vaccination of animals has been successful for many years. In the UK, adjuvanted, killed serotypes 1 and 2 are used. Attenuated live vaccine strains given orally have also been used to confer protection.

Fundamentals of Veterinary Microbiology, First Edition. Andrew N. Rycroft.
© 2024 John Wiley & Sons Ltd. Published 2024 by John Wiley & Sons Ltd.
Companion website: www.wiley.com/go/veterinarymicrobiology

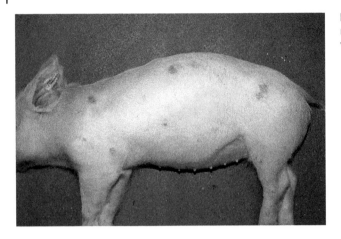

Figure 31.1 Characteristic red, rhomboidal skin lesions are the result of thrombotic vasculitis of end arterioles in a pig suffering with swine erysipelas.

Zoonosis

Erysipelothrix rhusiopathiae is also zoonotic. It causes local infection following puncture wounds in fish workers, farmers, meat processors and veterinary surgeons. The lesion usually occurs in the hands and fingers and shows inflammation, oedema and pain. Since there is already a human disease called erysipelas, caused by group A β-haemolytic streptococci, the infection from *E. rhusiopathiae* is known as erysipeloid. Notably, no immunity develops after a case of erysipeloid and so a relapse or reinfection of the individual can easily occur.

Trueperella pyogenes

Trueperella pyogenes is a small, Gram-positive rod which grows only slowly on blood agar to produce small, white colonies surrounded by a zone of β-haemolysis after 48 hours of incubation. Confusingly, until the 1980s it was known as *Corynebacterium pyogenes* and then *Actinomyces pyogenes*, then *Arcanobacterium pyogenes* and finally *Trueperella pyogenes*. It has a morphology typical of the corynebacteria group: Chinese characters in the arrangement of W, N and M. They may be curved and have slightly swollen ends.

Habitat

Trueperella pyogenes is a common inhabitant of the upper respiratory and genital tracts of domestic animals. Recent evidence suggests that it is also found associated with the ruminal wall of cattle. It is thought that the primary reservoir of *T. pyogenes* for infections is animals of various species. Little is known about the routes of transmission because the source of most infections is difficult to establish. In the absence of better evidence, it is assumed that most infections are endogenous or transmitted by vectors, or close contact, between animals.

Pathogenesis

Following initial injury or infection (virus, mycoplasma), *T. pyogenes* is one of the most common opportunistic pathogens of ruminants and pigs and is the cause of a wide variety of pus-forming infections in farm animals. It is usually seen as a mixed infection, typically alongside the strictly anaerobic, Gram-negative bacteria such as *Fusobacterium necrophorum* or *Prevotella* species (Rzewuska et al. 2019). Among these infections are liver abscesses, postpartum endometritis, pneumonia, kidney abscesses, endocarditis and abscesses at other sites and osteomyelitis in turkeys (Esmay et al. 2003). It is also a component of summer (dry cow) mastitis – probably spread to the udder teat, along with other bacterial pathogens, by *Hydrotaea* flies. It is a common component in ovine foot disease, and is a major component in pyometra, umbilical infections and pneumonia in sheep. Some infections with *T. pyogenes* can form truly dreadful chronic abscesses in farm animals. Depending on the location, these can contain litres of yellow pus (Figure 31.2). It is an occasional cause of disease in birds, horses and humans.

Figure 31.2 *Trueperella pyogenes* in pus from a lung abscess in a pig. The material is stained by Gram stain and shows microcolonies (clumps) of Gram-positive rods associated with degenerate neutrophils and other cell types.

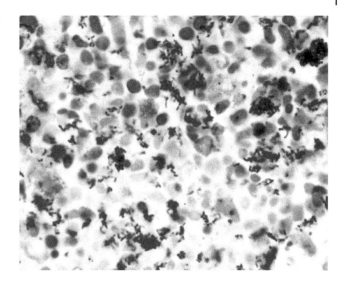

Pathogenicity

Pathogenicity depends on production of extracellular toxins: pyolysin, proteases, DNase and neuraminidases (NanH and NanP), together with fimbriae (Jost et al. 2002). The haemolytic exotoxin pyolysin is a member of the thiol-activated cytolysins, a family of pore-forming toxins found in other Gram-positive pathogens such as *Listeria monocytogenes* (listeriolysin), *Clostridium perfringens* (perfringolysin O), *Streptococcus suis* (suilysin) and *S. pneumoniae* (pneumolysin). It is a 55 kDa protein. Experiments suggest that pyolysin is cytotoxic for phagocytic cells. It also damages endometrial stromal cells, which are particularly sensitive to this toxin (Rzewuska et al. 2019). Pyolysin clearly contributes to the virulence of the organism and may be useful as a future vaccine component against *T. pyogenes* disease.

References

Esmay, P.A., Billington, S.J., Link, M.A. et al. (2003). The *Arcanobacterium pyogenes* collagen-binding protein, CbpA, promotes adhesion to host cells. *Infection and Immunity* 71: 4368–4374.

Jost, B.H., Songer, J.G., and Billington, S.J. (2002). Identification of a second *Arcanobacterium pyogenes* neuraminidase and involvement of neuraminidase activity in host cell adhesion. *Infection and Immunity* 70: 1106–1112.

Ogawa, Y., Shiraiwa, K., Nishikawa, S. et al. (2018). Identification of the chromosomal region essential for serovar specific antigen and virulence of serovar 1 and 2 strains of *Erysipelothrix rhusiopathiae*. *Infection and Immunity* 86: e00324–e00318.

Reboli, A.C. and Farrar, W.E. (1989). *Erysipelothrix rhusiopathiae*: an occupational pathogen. *Clinical Microbiology Reviews* 2: 354–359.

Rzewuska, M., Kwiecień, E., Chrobak-Chmiel, D. et al. (2019). Pathogenicity and virulence of *Trueperella pyogenes*: a review. *International Journal of Molecular Sciences* 20: 2737.

Wood, R.L. (1999). Erysipelas. In: *Diseases of Swine*, 8e (ed. A.D. Leman, B.E. Straw, W.L. Mengeling, et al.). Ames, IA: Iowa State University Press.

32

Mycoplasma – Cell-associated Pathogens

Mycoplasmas are part of a distinct group of prokaryotes called *Mollicutes* (Latin for soft skin). The mycoplasmas are free-living bacteria which possess no cell wall peptidoglycan. They require cholesterol in order to stabilise their plasma membrane but remain osmotically fragile. Because they have no peptidoglycan, they have no definite shape or size. For the same reason, they cannot be stained very well by Gram stain and appear, in stained smears under the microscope, as indistinct, pleomorphic blebs.

These bacteria carry a small genome (usually between 700 and 1000 kb). This presumably confers only a relatively small anabolic and catabolic ability compared to many bacteria. This may reflect the loss of genetic capacity (reductive evolution) as the organism has degenerated to rely on its close association with the host. It appears that *Mollicutes* are related to the Gram-positive bacteria (*Firmicutes*, Latin for firm skin). Evidence for this was first published by Woese et al. (1980) using 16S rRNA sequence analysis. This divergence apparently happened in a branch of Prokaryotes related to ancestors of *Clostridium* that led to the genera *Bacillus* and *Lactobacillus*.

Growth of these bacteria is very slow on artificial media (minimum three days to form a colony on blood agar) and many are very fastidious in their requirements and require specialised culture conditions. They usually form very small colonies, many of which have a central core, giving them a 'fried egg' appearance (Figure 32.1). Because they are metabolically simple, mycoplasmas are reliant on a close association with cells of higher organisms for some biological compounds. They are therefore highly adapted parasites which live on mucosal surfaces at different sites in different animals. In the body, they may become covered with host cell antigens. These antigens become incorporated into the mycoplasma membrane.

There are approximately 70 different species of *Mycoplasma* known to inhabit animals. Some are commensals of the respiratory and intestinal tract and udder, but many are pathogens of animals.

Pathogenicity of Mycoplasmas

The reason why *Mycoplasma* species cause disease is not known. There is a lack of those factors, such as toxins and components enabling survival in the face of innate immune defences, that are present in other bacterial pathogens.

Mycoplasmas usually have an intimate association with the cells of animals (and plants). They have evolved alongside their hosts to be 'quiet' intruders: living, like many commensal organisms, without prompting a response from the host nor causing it perceptible damage. Some, of course, do prompt an inflammatory response and these we see as the pathogens. The reason for those mycoplasmas causing a response may be to assist in their spread to other animals or it may be accidental as environmental changes or the genetics and physiology of the host alter in some way. It is the subtleties of this close association between host and *Mycoplasma*, and perturbation of the balance in that close relationship, that will be the key to understanding *Mycoplasma* pathogenicity in the future (Tryon and Baseman 1992).

Adhesion to mucosal surfaces is an important aspect of colonisation of host tissues and adhesion molecules are known to be required for colonisation. While no protein exotoxins have been demonstrated, the involvement of small molecules such as H_2O_2 in cellular damage has been proposed (Galvao Ferrarini et al. 2018). However, mutants of *M. gallisepticum* unable to produce H_2O_2 from glycerol were consistently virulent in the respiratory tracts of experimental chickens, implying that H_2O_2 is simply not required for mycoplasmas to cause disease, at least in some circumstances (Szczepanek et al. 2014).

Fundamentals of Veterinary Microbiology, First Edition. Andrew N. Rycroft.
© 2024 John Wiley & Sons Ltd. Published 2024 by John Wiley & Sons Ltd.
Companion website: www.wiley.com/go/veterinarymicrobiology

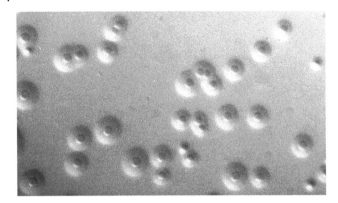

Figure 32.1 Colonies of *Mycoplasma bovis* growing on solid medium showing the characteristic central core (fried egg appearance).

What is clear is that mycoplasmas are stealthy. They are able to persist in the body of the host, either on the mucosal surface or even, it appears, in major organs, without alerting the innate immune system to their presence. Because mycoplasmas lack peptidoglycan or lipopolysaccharide, they lack at least some of the signals recognised by the Toll-like receptors of the innate immune system. Perhaps the immune system is alerted, but then suppressed or silenced by the mycoplasma. This is observed in the poor immunological responses to infection and in the relatively limited inflammatory response. Related to this is the antigenic variation displayed by many *Mycoplasma* species. The importance of altering surface antigens over time and the role this might play in evasion of the host immune defences remain to be investigated.

For many years, it was recognised that mycoplasmas bind immunoglobulin onto their surface. This was considered likely to be a passive means of coating the bacteria with 'self' antigen and thereby evading recognition by the innate immune system. More recently, a two-protein immunoglobulin (Ig) binding system was described by Arfi et al. (2016). This was originally found in the ruminant mycoplasma *Mycoplasma mycoides* subsp. *capri*. One protein, the mycoplasma immunoglobulin binding protein (MIB), captures antibody molecules with high affinity while the second, a serine protease known as mycoplasma Ig protease (MIP), cleaves the heavy chain of the Ig molecule. Analysis of genomes suggests that this system is widespread among the *Mycoplasma* pathogens and may contribute to avoidance of recognition and consequent immune evasion by mycoplasmas invading the body.

Identification of Mycoplasmas

Culturing and identifying mycoplasmas was a specialist task. Once an isolate had been grown, it was identified by a combination of techniques: biochemical tests, fluorescent antibody, growth inhibition tests using specific antiserum, rRNA sequencing and, more recently, denaturing gradient gel electrophoresis (DGGE). As PCR-based methods have been developed and MALDI-ToF analysis has become available, mycoplasmas can be identified as easily as other bacteria.

Bovine Mycoplasmas

Mycoplasma mycoides

The most severe mycoplasma pathogen is *Mycoplasma mycoides* subsp. *mycoides*. There are two subtypes: *Mycoplasma mycoides* subsp. *mycoides* (large colony type) and *Mycoplasma mycoides* subsp. *mycoides* (small colony type). Only the small colony type is the cause of contagious bovine pleuropneumonia (CBPP), a notifiable disease of cattle. It produces suppurative lesions in the lungs and pleura, and in the pericardium in cattle. It was eradicated from Europe at the end of the twentieth century and is now restricted to sub-Saharan Africa.

This pathogen was first isolated as the agent of bovine pleuropneumonia in 1891 and from then, other mycoplasmas were regularly referred to as pleuropneumonia-like organisms (PPLO). The large colony type never causes CBPP but does cause pneumonia, arthritis and mastitis in goats (often in CBPP-free countries) and has now been renamed *Mycoplasma mycoides* subsp. *capri* (Vilei et al. 2006).

Mycoplasma bovis

Mycoplasma bovis is frequently isolated from the nasal cavity of cattle but causes mastitis (Fox et al. 2005; Pfützner and Sachse 1996), pneumonia, polyarthritis, otitis media and keratoconjunctivitis (Caswell and Archambault 2008). *M. bovis* pneumonia often results from synergistic infection with bovine viral diarrhoea virus and infectious bovine rhinotracheitis virus, and the bacterial pathogens *M. haemolytica*, *P. multocida* and *H. somni*. Because of the relative ease of isolating these pathogens compared to the slow-growing *Mycoplasma* species, it is understandable that *M. bovis* has often been overlooked (Nicholas 2011). However, this has changed with the availability of molecular diagnostic methods such as PCR.

Avian Mycoplasmas

There are three important mycoplasmas affecting poultry globally: *M. gallisepticum*, *M. synoviae* and *M. meleagridis*.

Mycoplasma gallisepticum

This pathogen causes chronic respiratory disease in poultry. This is associated with reduced growth rate, reduction in egg production and decreased survival in chicks. It is transmitted by the respiratory route, and this is exacerbated by concurrent virus respiratory diseases. Infection may be common, yet clinical disease may be inapparent in most birds. The organism is now rare in most flocks in the UK through eradication in parent flocks using an effective live or inactivated vaccine (Feberwee et al. 2022).

Mycoplasma synoviae

Mycoplasma synoviae causes infectious synovitis in poultry. The infection results in lameness, lowered growth rate, upper respiratory tract disease, air sacculitis and breast blisters in chickens and turkeys. Infection is by the respiratory route, but the organism may get into the bloodstream and localise in the synovial tissue. The foot and hock joints, bursae and tendon sheaths develop thickening and oedema. The organism is even more fastidious than *M. gallisepticum*.

Mycoplasma meleagridis

Mycoplasma meleagridis causes air sacculitis in turkeys. Infection is by vertical (transovarian) transmission. There is some horizontal transmission by the respiratory route or venereally in breeding stock. The organism requires biotin for growth and infection causes the turkey poult to become deficient of biotin. This deficiency causes skeletal changes (known as turkey syndrome 65).

Porcine Mycoplasmas

There are three important mycoplasmas causing disease in pigs: *M. hyopneumoniae*, *M. hyorhinis* and *M. hyosynoviae*.

Mycoplasma hyopneumoniae

Mycoplasma hyopneumoniae causes enzootic pneumonia (EP) in pigs. This is one of the most important causes of disease-associated loss in the pig industry. *M. hyopneumoniae* is very slow growing and very fastidious. It is easily overtaken by other, non-pathogenic mycoplasmas in culture (Kobisch and Friis 1996).

The pathogenesis of EP is not understood and is likely to involve novel mechanisms in the host–pathogen interaction. The organism is transmitted by direct contact with respiratory secretions. It adheres to the respiratory epithelium and damages the cilia. This damage is associated with close interaction between the *M. hyopneumoniae* membrane and the epithelial cells of the trachea. A feature of EP, seen in histopathology, is the infiltration of lymphocytes that collect around the bronchioles in the lung. This is often termed a cuffing pneumonia. The organism also alters alveolar macrophage cell function in a subtle way so that the animal is immunosuppressed (Kuhnert and Jores 2020).

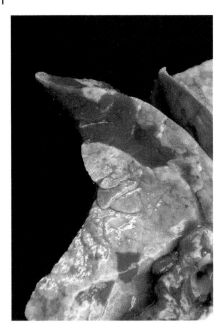

Figure 32.2 Lesions of enzootic pneumonia in the lungs of a 17-week-old pig following experimental infection with a pure culture of *M. hyopneumoniae*.

The onset of disease is gradual and often subclinical unless other, concurrent infection (e.g. with *P. multocida*) makes the condition deteriorate. Animals may show no signs or have a chronic cough, but secondary infection can allow invasive bacterial disease and death from pneumonia at about 4–6 months of age. The lesions, in the apical and cardiac lobes of the lung, show well-demarcated consolidation (Figure 32.2). Most cases of uncomplicated EP will begin to resolve after about 10 weeks.

Provisional diagnosis of EP is by recognition of typical lesions and clinical picture. Confirmation is by detection and localisation of the pathogen in tissues and by PCR. Culture is difficult and time consuming (Chae et al. 2020).

The immune response in a recovered animal is thought to be protective against EP. Vaccination with killed *M. hyopneumoniae* protects against experimental challenge. However, it may fail to protect against all naturally occurring cases of EP in the field.

Mycoplasma hyorhinis

Mycoplasma hyorhinis is often found in the lungs of pigs without any lesions from where it can be grown in 2–3 days to form visible colonies. It is not a primary cause of pneumonia but may be involved in the porcine respiratory disease complex along with other viral or bacterial pathogens. It occasionally causes polyserositis (serofibrinous lesions in the pericardial, pleural and peritoneal cavities) and arthritis in the pig, usually post weaning at 3–7 weeks of age (Friis and Feenstra 1994).

Mycoplasma hyosynoviae

Pigs are the natural and only host for *M. hyosynoviae*, and the organism has a particular affinity for joint tissue in the pig. It causes serious arthritis in growing and finishing pigs (Palzer et al. 2020).

The reservoir of the organism is tonsillar tissue. It descends through the respiratory tract to pneumonic lungs and then appears to spread haematogenously and localise in the joints, especially the hind legs. It causes difficulty in moving, stiffness, lameness, arched backs and an inability to rise. The disease may last for 7–10 days, but in some animals a chronic, protracted course may occur (Kobisch and Friis 1996).

Mycoplasma Infecting Other Species

Dog

Several *Mycoplasma* species have been isolated from dogs. However, relatively little is known of the role of mycoplasmas in canine disease (Chalker 2004). *M. cynos* is the only *Mycoplasma* species consistently associated with respiratory disease and experimental endobronchial infection has been shown to cause pneumonia and loss of cilia accompanied by alveolar infiltration with neutrophils and macrophages (Rosendal and Vinther 1977).

Horse

Mycoplasmas may be involved in respiratory tract infection causing poor performance in thoroughbreds. While this may have different causes or be a complex infection like kennel cough, viral, bacterial or mycoplasma agents have never consistently been shown to be the cause. Nevertheless, equine respiratory infection often responds to antibacterial antibiotics, suggesting a bacterial cause. In support of mycoplasma involvement, *M. felis* infection has been clearly associated with an outbreak of equine respiratory disease. Seroconversion to *M. felis* or high antibody titres were demonstrated in 100% of the diseased horses (Wood et al. 1997).

Haemotropic Mycoplasmas

Until approximately 20 years ago, the uncultivable agents of infectious anaemia in the dog and cat were considered to be *Haemobartonella* and *Eperythrozoon*, related to the Rickettsias (see Chapter 33). They are found in close association with mammalian erythrocyte membranes. Analysis of the sequence of 16S rRNA shows that these haemotropic bacteria are closely related to species in the genus *Mycoplasma* (Neimark et al. 2002). These bacterial pathogens have therefore been renamed as *Mycoplasma* species such as *Mycoplasma haemofelis*, the cause of an uncommon but moderate to severe, flea-transmitted haemolytic anaemia in cats (Barker 2019), and *Mycoplasma wenyonii*, the cause of pyrexia with hindlimb and udder oedema (Strugnell and McAuliffe 2012).

References

Barker, E.N. (2019). Update on feline Hemoplasmosis. *Veterinary Clinics of North America: Small Animal Practice* 49: 733–743.

Caswell, J.L. and Archambault, M. (2008). *Mycoplasma bovis* pneumonia in cattle. *Animal Health Research Reviews* 8: 161–186.

Chae, C., Gomes-Neto, J.C., Segalés, J., and Sibila, M. (2020). Diagnosis of *Mycoplasma hyopneumoniae* infection and associated diseases. In: *Mycoplasmas in Swine* (ed. D. Maes, M. Sibila, and M. Pieters (eds).). Leuven: ACCO.

Chalker, V.J. (2004). Canine mycoplasmas. *Research in Veterinary Science* 79: 1–8.

Feberwee, A., de Wit, S., and Dijkman, R. (2022). Clinical expression, epidemiology, and monitoring of *Mycoplasma gallisepticum* and *Mycoplasma synoviae*: an update. *Avian Pathology* 51: 2–18.

Fox, L.K., Kirk, J.H., and Britten, A. (2005). Mycoplasma mastitis: a review of transmission and control. *Journal of Veterinary Medicine Series B* 52: 153–160.

Friis, N.F. and Feenstra, A.A. (1994). *Mycoplasma hyorhinis* in the etiology of serositis among piglets. *Acta Veterinaria Scandinavica* 35: 93–98.

Galvao Ferrarini, M., Mucha, S.G., Parrot, D. et al. (2018). Hydrogen peroxide production and myo-inositol metabolism as important traits for virulence of *Mycoplasma hyopneumoniae*. *Molecular Microbiology* 108: 683–696.

Kobisch, M. and Friis, N.F. (1996). Swine mycoplasmoses. *Revue Scientifique et Technique* 15: 1569–1605.

Kuhnert, P. and Jores, J. (2020). *Mycoplasma hyopneumoniae* pathogenicity: the known and the unknown. In: *Mycoplasmas in Swine* (ed. D. Maes, M. Sibila, and M. Pieters (eds)). Leuven: ACCO.

Neimark, H., Johansson, K.-E., Rikihisa, Y., and Tully, J.G. (2002). Revision of haemotrophic *mycoplasma* species names. *International Journal of Systematic and Evolutionary Microbiology* 52: 683.

Nicholas, R.A.J. (2011). Bovine mycoplasmosis: silent and deadly. *Veterinary Record* 168: 459–462.

Palzer, A., Ritzmann, M., and Spergser, J. (2020). *Mycoplasma hyorhinis* and *Mycoplasma hyosynoviae* in pig herds. In: *Mycoplasmas in Swine* (ed. D. Maes, M. Sibila, and M. Pieters (eds)). Leuven: ACCO.

Pfützner, H. and Sachse, K. (1996). *Mycoplasma bovis* as an agent of mastitis, pneumonia, arthritis and genital disorders in cattle. *Revue Scientifique et Technique* 15: 1477–1494.

Rosendal, S. and Vinther, O. (1977). Experimental mycoplasmal pneumonia in dogs: electron microscopy of infected tissue. *Acta Pathologica et Microbiologica Scandinavica. Section B, Microbiology* 85: 462–465.

Strugnell, B. and McAuliffe, L. (2012). Mycoplasma wenyonii infection in cattle. *In Practice* 34: 146–154.

Szczepanek, S.M., Boccaccio, M., Pflaum, K. et al. (2014). Hydrogen peroxide production from glycerol metabolism is dispensable for virulence of *Mycoplasma gallisepticum* in the tracheas of chickens. *Infection and Immunity* 82: 4915–4920.

Tryon, V.V. and Baseman, J.B. (1992). Pathogenic determinants and mechanisms. In: *Mycoplasmas, Molecular Biology and Pathogenesis* (ed. J. Maniloff, R.N. McElhaney, L.R. Finch, and J.B. Baseman). Washington, D.C: American Society for Microbiology.

Vilei, E.M., Korczak, B.M., and Frey, J. (2006). *Mycoplasma mycoides* subsp. *capri* and *Mycoplasma mycoides* subsp. *mycoides* LC can be grouped into a single subspecies. *Veterinary Research* 37: 779–790.

Woese, C.R., Maniloff, J., and Zablen, L.B. (1980). Phylogenetic analysis of the mycoplasmas. *Proceedings of the National Academy of Sciences USA* 77: 494–498.

Wood, J.L., Chanter, N., Newton, J.R. et al. (1997). An outbreak of respiratory disease in horses associated with *Mycoplasma felis* infection. *Veterinary Record* 140: 388–391.

Arfi, Y., Minder, L., Di Primo, C. et al. (2016). MIB-MIP is a mycoplasma system that captures and cleaves immunoglobulin G. *Proceedings of the National Academy of Sciences USA* 113: 5406–5411.

33

Rickettsia – Arthropod Vector-borne Pathogens

Rickettsia microorganisms are obligate intracellular bacteria. They are Gram-negative and often transmitted between animals by arthropods such as ticks and fleas. Many are pathogens of animals, causing noteworthy diseases.

A *Rickettsia* organism was first described in 1909 as the cause of Rocky Mountain spotted fever in humans. It was shown that the agent (*Rickettsia rickettsii*) was transmitted by ticks and was actually a disease of ticks accidentally transmitted to humans. A few months afterwards, the discoverer, Ricketts, was studying a similar agent which caused human louse-borne typhus when he died of the disease. Shortly afterwards, another investigator, von Prowazek, also died of the disease. The agent of human typhus was named *Rickettsia prowazekii* and is the type species of this group of organisms.

Diagnosis of rickettsial disease is traditionally by microscopy of blood and tissues in which morulae (clumps of the tiny organisms in a vacuole) can be seen in the cytoplasm of cells (Figure 33.1). Since the advent of PCR-based diagnostics, the specificity and sensitivity of diagnosis have improved hugely.

There is a range of different rickettsial organisms, subdivided into Rickettsias and Anaplasmas. Among the Anaplasma family are *Ehrlichia* and *Anaplasma* species.

Ehrlichia ruminantium

Ehrlichia ruminantium is the agent of heartwater in cattle and goats in sub-Saharan Africa and the Caribbean. This is the most important tick-borne disease of domestic and wild ruminants in those regions (Allsopp 2015). The hard ticks transmitting infection are those of the genus *Amblyomma*. The clinical signs of disease result from increased vascular permeability. This leads to oedema and hypovolaemia and the name of the disease comes from the oedema fluid that may be seen in the pericardium.

Anaplasma phagocytophilum

Anaplasma phagocytophilum is the agent of tick-borne fever (pasture fever) in ruminants in Europe (primarily sheep and cattle in the UK, Ireland, Holland, Scandinavia and Spain). It is transmitted by the hard tick *Ixodes ricinus*. The pathogen infects eosinophils, monocytes and neutrophils leading to leucopaenia (Madison-Antenucci et al. 2020). It multiplies to form small colonies inside the cytoplasmic vacuoles of these cells (Figure 33.1). The pathogen is acquired by the ticks through biting infected animals; it is not transmitted vertically from adult females via the egg. The clinical signs are sudden fever in sheep and depression, respiratory signs, weight loss and decreased milk yield in cattle (Woldehiwet 1983).

When the tick bite also inoculates *Staphylococcus aureus* into the skin, this complicates the disease, with haematogenous spread leading to staphylococcal abscesses in joints and major organs of the body. This is known as tick pyaemia.

The pathogen was discovered in 1994 to cause disease in humans when it was referred to as human granulocytic ehrlichiosis (HGE), but now is more commonly referred to as anaplasmosis.

Fundamentals of Veterinary Microbiology, First Edition. Andrew N. Rycroft.
© 2024 John Wiley & Sons Ltd. Published 2024 by John Wiley & Sons Ltd.
Companion website: www.wiley.com/go/veterinarymicrobiology

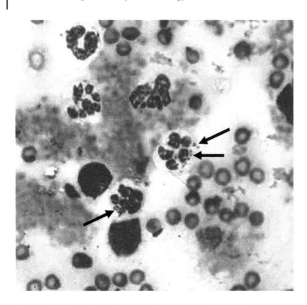

Figure 33.1 A blood smear of a sheep with tick-borne fever stained by Giemsa. The neutrophils show inclusions (arrows) due to intracellular colonies of *Anaplasma phagocytophilum*.

Anaplasma marginale

Anaplasma marginale infects cattle and sheep. It is transmitted by ticks of the genus *Boophilus*. They are rare causes of infection in the UK.

Neorickettsia risticii

Neorickettsia risticii (formerly *Ehrlichia risticii*) is the agent of equine monocytic ehrlichiosis or Potomac horse fever. First recognised in 1979 in Maryland, USA, it has since been found to be widely distributed in North and South America. *Neorickettsia* species are intracellular, Gram-negative bacteria associated with trematodes that parasitise aquatic insects (such as caddis flies and dragon flies) and snails (Taylor 2023). Horses become infected by ingestion of *N. risticii*-infected trematodes within aquatic insects or within free-living trematodes. Once inside the gastrointestinal tract, the bacteria escape the trematode and invade colonic and caecal epithelial cells and tissue macrophages. Bacterial translocation into the blood leads to infection of monocytes.

The most commonly reported clinical signs in horses with PHF include diarrhoea, fever, anorexia, lethargy and colic.

Coxiella burnetii

Coxiella burnetii is the agent of Q fever. The name 'Q fever' comes from query fever. It was used to describe a human febrile illness that broke out among abattoir workers in Brisbane, Australia in 1937. Since then, it has been recognised as a disease of many different animals.

It is an obligate intracellular organism but is now recognised as taxonomically distinct from the rickettsias. It is more closely related to *Legionella*, a human pathogen from a group of bacteria known to inhabit cells such as amoebae.

Coxiella burnetii grows primarily in cytoplasmic vacuoles. It is also surprisingly resistant to high temperature, disinfectants (including hypochlorite and formalin), low pH and environmental desiccation (Reimer 1993).

Cattle and other livestock become infected from tick bites, but infection usually goes unrecognised. That is because animals often show no clinical signs, and this allows infection to pass largely undiagnosed. However, it is considered to be enzootic in livestock and *Coxiella* may infect as many as 20% of dairy herds as judged from serological evidence of exposure (Paiba et al. 1999). It is a minor cause of abortion in pregnant cattle, sheep, goats, cats and other animals (Woldehiwet 2004). It also infects most other animals including fish, birds and reptiles (Cutler et al. 2007).

As in the 1937 outbreak, the infection is zoonotic. Q fever is acute or chronic in humans. It can be transmitted to humans by inhalation of aerosol of urine or faeces, or through unpasteurised milk or in the aerosol of the products of abortion or parturition. It may also be transmitted by inhalation of the dried dust of tick faeces. In mild form, it is a flu-like illness, but it can be a more severe zoonosis with endocarditis and can be fatal. Those at particular risk are farmers and meat workers although a high proportion of infections almost certainly go undiagnosed (Maurin and Raoult 1999).

Vaccination has been used, particularly in Australia, but the benefit of vaccination may not justify the widespread use of the vaccine in those at risk of exposure (Long 2021). Pasteurisation of milk is probably the most important measure for preventing widespread infection in the population.

A number of other rickettsial (e.g. *Rickettsia rickettsii*) and non-rickettsial (e.g. *Francisella tularensis*) tick-borne infections are recognised. Many of these do not cause disease in animals in Europe but are particularly important in the USA (Centers for Disease Control and Prevention 2022).

References

Allsopp, B.A. (2015). Heartwater – *Ehrlichia ruminantium* infection. *Revue Scientifique et Technique* 34: 557–568.

Centers for Disease Control and Prevention (2022). *Tickborne Diseases of The United States: A Reference Manual for Healthcare Providers*, 6e. Atlanta, GA: CDC.

Cutler, S., Bouzid, M., and Cutler, R. (2007). Q fever. *Journal of Infection* 54: 313–318.

Long, C.M. (2021). Q fever vaccine development: current strategies and future considerations. *Pathogens* 10: 1223.

Madison-Antenucci, S., Kramer, L.D., Gebhardt, L.L., and Kauffman, E. (2020). Emerging tick-borne diseases. *Clinical Microbiology Reviews* 33: e00083–e00018.

Maurin, M. and Raoult, D. (1999). Q fever. *Clinical Microbiology Reviews* 12: 518–553.

Paiba, G.A., Green, L.E., Lloyd, G. et al. (1999). Prevalence of antibodies to *Coxiella burnetii* (Q fever) in bulk tank milk in England and Wales. *Veterinary Record* 144: 519–522.

Taylor, S.D. (2023). Potomac horse fever. *Veterinary Clinics of North America. Equine Practice* 39 (1): 37–45.

Reimer, L.G. (1993). Q Fever. *Clinical Microbiology Reviews* 6: 193–198.

Woldehiwet, Z. (1983). Tick-borne fever: a review. *Veterinary Research Communications* 6: 163–175.

Woldehiwet, Z. (2004). Q fever (coxiellosis): epidemiology and pathogenesis. *Research in Veterinary Science* 77: 93–100.

34

Fungi as Agents of Disease

Veterinary mycology is concerned with the very few species of fungi which are pathogenic for animals or in some way cause disease. Fungi are primitive plants; they are eukaryotes. Because fungi lack chlorophyll, they are unable to utilise inorganic carbon and must therefore live as saprophytes, parasites or in a symbiotic association with other organisms (Czuprynski and Chengappa 2022).

Fungal Morphology

Depending on the species, the fungi can be divided into three morphological groups: yeasts, filamentous fungi and dimorphic fungi. Fungi reproduce by vegetative growth and by production of spores. These are not like bacterial endospores which are resistant. Fungal spores are stable and viable in the dry state but are killed by disinfectants and boiling.

Vegetative Spores

Arthrospores are formed by disarticulation of a septate hypha into separate cells. This type of spore is frequently produced by dermatophytes (ringworm fungi) when parasitising skin and hair (Figure 34.1).

Asexual Spores

Conidiospores are formed on the external surface of the conidiophore which may be simple or specialised, or they may arise directly from the mycelium or may be produced within a specialised structure. Conidiospores may be unicellular or multicellular. Some species of fungus (e.g. dermatophytes) produce two types of conidiospores differing in size and in the number of cells. In such cases, the small unicellular spores are known as microconidia and the large multicellular spores as macroconidia.

Other fungi produce asexual spores inside a specialised structure. These are sporangiospores such as are produced by *Mucor* species (Figure 34.2).

Sexual Spores

The taxonomy of fungi is determined largely by the sexual spores they produce. These require a sexual cycle (known as the perfect phase). Sexual spores are not usually produced during infection and are of little value in identifying a fungus from disease.

Fungal taxonomy has been revolutionised by the availability of DNA sequencing and molecular phylogenetic analyses. Reclassification of fungi, beyond the scope of this book, continues to take place (Hibbett et al. 2007). Nevertheless, the veterinary pathogens causing disease have not materially changed, and they largely retain their traditional names for the purposes of diagnosis and treatment.

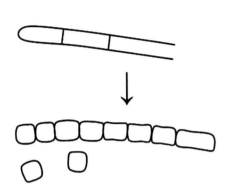

Figure 34.1 Formation of arthrospores from septate mycelium.

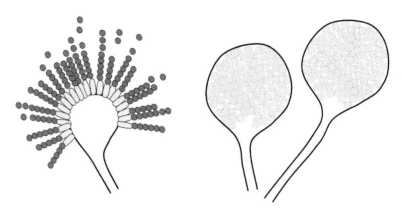

Figure 34.2 Asexual spores of fungi: conidiospores (left) are produced on the surface of the sporing head (the conidiophore); sporangiospores (right) are enclosed within the sporing head (the sporangiophore).

Fungal Pathogenicity

There are three main ways in which fungi can cause disease.

- By invading and growing in tissue: a mycosis.
- By producing toxigenic substances in themselves or in their growth substrates which when ingested cause disease: a mycotoxicosis.
- By producing sensitising substances: a fungal allergy.

Mycoses

Mycoses are diseased states caused by a fungus invading and growing in animal tissue *in vivo*. The fungi causing mycoses may be primary pathogens, i.e. capable of causing disease in a healthy host, e.g. dermatophytes, *Histoplasma*, *Coccidioides*. Alternatively, they may be opportunistic pathogens which cause disease only when the host is in some way abnormal, e.g. *Candida*, *Aspergillus*, Zygomycetes.

Depth of Infection

Mycoses may be described as superficial, subcutaneous or systemic. Superficial or cutaneous mycoses are those in which the skin and/or hair are involved, such as dermatophytosis (ringworm). A subcutaneous mycosis is one in which subcutaneous tissues are involved; cutaneous manifestations may also occur, e.g. sporotrichosis. A systemic mycosis is one in which internal organs are affected, e.g. aspergillosis.

The subcutaneous and systemic mycoses tend to resemble bacterial diseases such as tuberculosis in having a protracted incubation period, insidious onset of clinical signs which become increasingly severe, failing to respond to antibacterial antibiotics, and sometimes ending in death (Czuprynski and Chengappa 2022).

Source of Infection

Mycoses are also described as endogenous or exogenous according to the source of the fungus. A few species of fungi which are normally harmless commensals of the body can cause endogenous opportunistic infections when the host metabolism becomes in some way abnormal. This can include the use of immunosuppressive steroids, the use of antibiotics that damage or alter the normal balanced bacterial flora, pregnancy and in young animals.

Exogenous mycoses are those caused by fungi from an external source. Air-borne fungal spores (e.g. conidiospores) are the most important source of infections. These are produced in vast numbers; they are dry, easily detached and dispersed by air currents as seen in the epidemiology of systemic mycoses such as mycotic abortion in cattle. To cause disease, a fungus of exogenous origin must reach and enter the host, then germinate and grow. Most mycoses are non-contagious, and each case is contracted individually, from a fungus such as *Aspergillus*, which is present in the environment. Very few are contagious mycoses, transmitted from another infected animal by direct or indirect contact (dermatophytosis and epizootic lymphangitis).

Damage to Tissues

Compared to bacterial pathogenicity, little is known of the factors in fungal pathogens needed for invasion, survival and damage to the host. Few toxins are recognised and although many fungi are known to produce exotoxins and enzymes (such as mycotoxins produced on mouldy feedstuff), there is little conclusive evidence of toxin production within the body and toxins do not appear to be consistently needed for mycotic invasion and damage. One toxin, gliotoxin from *A. fumigatus*, apparently inhibits the mucociliary clearing function on mucosal surfaces and may play a significant role in establishment of the fungus in the animal body by damaging neutrophil function (Spikes et al. 2008).

However, once in animal tissues, fungi can damage the host in various ways. Mechanical damage is caused by penetration of tissues, nerves, walls of blood vessels and bone by fungal hyphae and by pressure. Zygomycetes have a predilection for blood vessels, penetrate into the lumen and cause thrombi.

The immunological reaction between host and fungus may lead to damage by inducing an intense inflammatory and immunological reaction, resulting in necrosis (immunopathology) and the formation of sinuses and fistulas. The immune process may also dissolve bone, causing osteitis and osteomyelitis.

References

Czuprynski, C. and Chengappa, M.M. (2022). Basic mycology. In: *Veterinary Microbiology*, 4e (ed. D.S. McVey, M. Kennedy, M.M. Chengappa, and R. Wilkes (eds).). Oxford: Wiley.

Hibbett, D.S., Binder, M., Bischoff, J. et al. (2007). A higher-level phylogenetic classification of the *Fungi. Mycological Research* 111: 509–547.

Spikes, S., Xu, R., Nguyen, C.K. et al. (2008). Gliotoxin production in *Aspergillus fumigatus* contributes to host-specific differences in virulence. *Journal of Infectious Diseases* 197: 479–486.

35

Aspergillus – Strength in Numbers

Aspergillus species are worldwide in distribution and are ubiquitous due to their ability to colonise many different natural substrates under a wide range of environmental conditions. The main growth substrates are rotting plant and animal material and aspergilli are particularly abundant in hay, straw and grain which have been inadequately dried, and which may become heated during storage. Aspergilli produce enormous numbers of dry, light asexual spores (conidiospores) which easily become air-borne (Figure 35.1). The route of infection is mainly respiratory but occasionally by ingestion or through wounds. For farm animals, hay which has been baled wet is a primary source of infection.

Aspergillosis is a non-contagious, mainly respiratory mycosis. The disease may be benign, acute or chronic and infection may be primary (infection of a healthy, susceptible organ) or secondary (growth in active or arrested lesions or after antibiotic, corticosteroid or immunosuppressive therapy for other diseases). The main pathogenic species is *Aspergillus fumigatus* but *A. nidulans*, *A. flavus*, *A. niger* and others also cause disease.

Avian Aspergillosis

Avian aspergillosis affects birds of all ages and both domestic and wild birds. The acute form is usually found in young birds and can cause considerable losses (Hauck et al. 2020). Affected birds often die within 24–28 hours from the onset of clinical signs: increased respiration, rise in temperature, listlessness, diarrhoea, loss of appetite and condition. The chronic form usually occurs in adult birds and tends to be of sporadic occurrence. *Aspergillus fumigatus* is the most common species involved (Neumann 2016). Pathological changes include granulomas in the lungs and fungal plaques in the air sacs (Girma et al. 2016) (Figure 35.2).

Mammalian Aspergillosis

Acute aspergillosis occurs when susceptible hosts are exposed to heavy concentrations of conidiospores and is characterised by numerous small miliary lesions. Cases have been recorded in young animals – calves and lambs. In chronic aspergillosis, the lesions are granulomatous and may be calcified.

Canine Nasal Aspergillosis

Infection of the posterior nasal turbinates in the dog by *A. fumigatus* is being increasingly recognised. The fungus causes necrosis and erosion of the turbinate bones and also affects the epithelium, submucosa and blood vessels.

Microscopy of nasal washings may show fragments of hyphae and spores and colonies of the mould may be obtained by culture. However, as *A. fumigatus* is such a common mould, diagnosis should not be made only on these criteria. Clinical signs, diagnostic imaging and serology should be taken into consideration (Benitah 2006). Serological methods have always been problematical because of the ubiquity of *Aspergillus* in the environment and the consequent prevalence of antibody

Fundamentals of Veterinary Microbiology, First Edition. Andrew N. Rycroft.
© 2024 John Wiley & Sons Ltd. Published 2024 by John Wiley & Sons Ltd.
Companion website: www.wiley.com/go/veterinarymicrobiology

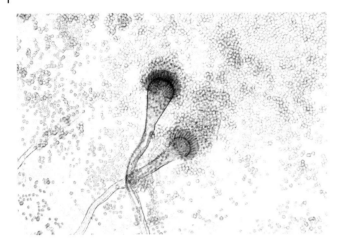

Figure 35.1 Microscopic appearance of *Aspergillus fumigatus* sporing heads producing huge numbers of conidiospores.

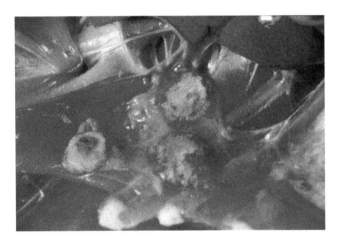

Figure 35.2 Fungal plaque of *Aspergillus fumigatus* growing on the surface of the air sac in a swan.

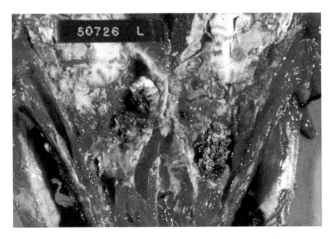

Figure 35.3 Nasal aspergillosis; fungus and cellular debris in the nasal cavity of a dog at postmortem.

to *Aspergillus* in many normal animals. Nevertheless, both ELISA and agar gel double immunodiffusion (AGID) are currently used as adjuncts to diagnosis (Barrs et al. 2015) (Figure 35.3).

A differential diagnosis has to be made with other clinical entities with similar effects, such as neoplasia or foreign body (Cohn 2014).

Equine Guttural Pouch Mycosis

The guttural pouch (GP) is a diverticulum of the Eustachian tubes in horses. It is a site that can become infected with fungi, particularly *Aspergillus* sp. The most likely source of infection is fungal spores from hay and straw: *Aspergillus fumigatus*, *A. nidulans*, *Penicillium* sp. and others. There appears to be no correlation between incidence of the disease and age, sex or breed of horse.

The initial lesion is found on the dorsal surface of the medial compartment of the GP. In this area, the internal carotid artery and the glossopharyngeal, vagus and spinal accessory nerves are in close apposition to the pouch (Lepage et al. 2004). This apposition is highly significant with regard to the clinical manifestations of the disease, the main clinical signs of which are potentially fatal epistaxis or paralysis of various cranial nerves leading to dysphagia or pharyngeal paralysis (Freeman 2015). Death may be due to epistaxis from the carotid artery or vein or from aspiration pneumonia resulting from pharyngeal paralysis.

Bovine Mycotic Abortion

Mycotic abortion is a non-contagious mycosis which affects only the gravid uterus. The main lesion is a mycotic placentitis. About 20 species of fungus have been implicated, of which *Aspergillus fumigatus* and *Absidia corymbifera* are most frequently encountered.

In cattle, the cotyledons of an infected placenta retain much of their maternal portion, are very thickened, especially at the margins, and the central area is often necrotic. Skin lesions have been observed on the fetus but only in a low proportion of cases. The cow shows no symptoms before aborting. After abortion, the placenta may be retained and fungal elements may be present in the uterine discharge (Figure 35.4).

The disease is not contagious and each infection is contracted from the environment. The most likely source of infection is fungal spores in mouldy hay and straw. Evidence suggests that infection takes place via the respiratory route. The spores of the fungal species implicated in mycotic abortion are less than 5 μm in diameter. They will therefore penetrate to, and be retained in, the alveolar ducts and the alveoli where phagocytosis takes place. Infection of the placenta is believed to follow haematogenous spread of the fungus.

The disease is markedly seasonal; in Britain, 70% of cases occur in the winter when animals are housed.

The gravid bovine uterus is a target organ due to physiological change. Mycotic abortion accounts for approximately 10% of bovine abortions investigated in the UK. Fungal abortion is also recognised in ewes, mares and sows (Elad and Segal 2018).

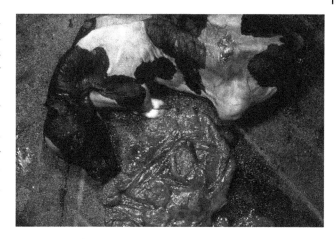

Figure 35.4 Bovine mycotic abortion.

References

Barrs, V.R., Ujvari, B., Dhand, N.K. et al. (2015). Detection of *Aspergillus*-specific antibodies by agar gel double immunodiffusion and IgG ELISA in feline upper respiratory tract aspergillosis. *Veterinary Journal* 203: 285–289.

Benitah, N. (2006). Canine nasal aspergillosis. *Clinical Techniques in Small Animal Practice* 21: 82–88.

Cohn, L.A. (2014). Canine nasal disease. *Veterinary Clinics of North America: Small Animal Practice* 4: 75–89.

Elad, D. and Segal, E. (2018). Diagnostic aspects of veterinary and human aspergillosis. *Frontiers in Microbiology* 9: 1303.

Freeman, D.E. (2015). Update on disorders and treatment of the guttural pouch. *Veterinary Clinics of North America: Equine Practice* 31: 63–89.

Girma, G., Abebaw, M., Zemene, M. et al. (2016). A review on aspergillosis in poultry. *Journal of Veterinary Science & Technology* 7: 382.

Hauck, R., Cray, C., and França, M. (2020). Spotlight on avian pathology: aspergillosis. *Avian Pathology* 49: 115–118.

Lepage, O.M., Perron, M.-F., and Cador, J.-L. (2004). The mystery of fungal infection in the guttural pouches. *Veterinary Journal* 168: 60–64.

Neumann (2016). Aspergillosis in domesticated birds. *Journal of Comparative Pathology* 155: 102–104.

36

Dermatophytes – Keratinolytic Fungi

The dermatophytes are filamentous fungi which can utilise keratin, the fibrous protein which is the main component of skin and its appendages (hair, nails, feathers), as their sole source of nutrition. Although molecular analysis shows that several new genera are justified, there remains wide acceptance of three genera covering all dermatophytes. About 30 species are recognised, classified into the genera: *Epidermophyton*, *Microsporum* and *Trichophyton* (de Hoog et al. 2017).

With the exception of a few species capable of saprophytic existence in soil, the main reservoir of dermatophytes is infective debris shed from an animal. Dermatophytes remain viable in dry skin scales for several weeks and for up to three years in dry hair.

The division of the dermatophytes into the categories anthropophilic, zoophilic and geophilic is a useful aid to epidemiology. Zoophilic species are animal pathogens. Certain zoophilic species are associated with certain animals which are probably the natural host and serve as a reservoir of infection; other species affect many different types of animals. All zoophilic dermatophytes can infect humans and animal ringworm is therefore of importance in public health (Pasquetti et al. 2017). Anthropophilic species are normally human pathogens only. However, a few anthropophilic species have been recovered from animals. The term 'geophilic' is used for dermatophytes capable of saprophytic existence in soil. Currently, all dermatophytes known to be geophilic are also zoophilic.

Dermatophytosis

Dermatophytosis (often known as ringworm from the ring-shaped lesions) is a contagious mycosis involving the upper layers of the skin and its appendages. It affects animals, birds and humans. Reaction to the fungus can vary from mild scaling to boggy painful swellings (kerion) in which the primary fungal lesion is complicated by secondary bacterial infection. Scutula, yellowish cup-shaped crusts composed of a dense mass of mycelium, arthrospores and inflammatory cells may be formed when animals are infected with *T. quinckeanum* or, rarely, *M. gypseum*; this type of ringworm is known as favus.

Dermatophytes Causing Animal Disease

The dermatophytes are differentiated by their appearance in culture (pigmentation and texture) and by their microscopic appearance (shape and abundance of macroconidia, microconidia and other features seen in culture).

Different species of dermatophytes are associated with infection of different animal species. Some are host-adapted and may cause little irritation or inflammation in the host to which they are adapted. For example, *M. canis* may cause very little pathological effect in the cat, particularly long-haired breeds. The single species of *Epidermophyton*, *E. floccosum*, is a human pathogen not known to cause disease in animals.

The most important dermatophyte in small animal dermatophytosis is *M. canis*. This is responsible for approximately 98% of ringworm in cats and about 85% of ringworm in dogs (Figure 36.1). Other species of *Microsporum* causing animal disease are *M. gypseum* from soil and *M. persicolor* from voles.

Fundamentals of Veterinary Microbiology, First Edition. Andrew N. Rycroft.
© 2024 John Wiley & Sons Ltd. Published 2024 by John Wiley & Sons Ltd.
Companion website: www.wiley.com/go/veterinarymicrobiology

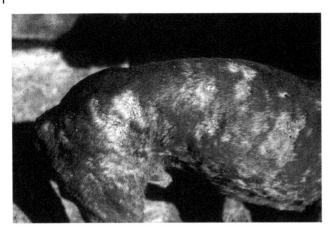

Figure 36.1 Severe lesions of dermatophytosis in a dog.

There are many species of *Trichophyton* and there is considerable variation among the members of the group. *T. verrucosum* is the agent of cattle ringworm seen as thick scaly lesions around the head and neck. *T. equinum* is seen in equids and *T. mentagrophytes* is commonly carried by rodents and transferred to dogs and other animals from rats and mice. *T. gallinae* is seen in poultry while *T. erinaceae* is common in hedgehogs and again transferred to domestic dogs.

Pathogenesis of Dermatophytosis

Dermatophyte infection is transmitted between animals or humans by arthrospores and hyphal fragments. When the environment is suitable, the arthrospores germinate to produce hyphae that grow into the skin and reach a hair follicle. The hyphae grow downwards into the follicle and can penetrate the hair shaft, releasing keratinolytic enzymes (Tsuboi et al. 1989). As the hyphae age, arthrospores form from the hyphae around the now brittle hair. The hair breaks and falls away to infect the environment. Hyphae will not penetrate living tissue.

Apart from the keratinolytic enzyme activity, little is known of the products or components of dermatophytes that contribute to their ability to survive in and invade host epidermis.

Diagnostic Methods

Because ringworm lesions are very variable and because many other skin conditions produce similar clinical signs, it is not advisable to diagnose the disease purely on the appearance. Demonstration of fungal elements in the specimen is necessary and, to identify the species of fungus causing an infection, it must be obtained in pure culture.

Polymerase chain reaction is increasingly available to give a sensitive and rapid confirmation of dermatophyte infection. However, standard methods of microscopy, Wood's lamp and identification by culture are still used.

Samples for investigation are best held in folded paper rather than in screw-topped plastic bottles which cause moisture to be retained and can create strong static, causing minute fragments of skin and hair to fly out unexpectedly.

Wood's Light

In ringworm caused by certain species of dermatophytes, infected hair will fluoresce a bright green under Wood's light. This is a long-wave ultraviolet light which allows maximum radiation at about 366 nm. Even minimal infection in which only a few hairs are involved may be detected in this way. However, it is important to remember that fluorescence of infected hairs only occurs when a limited range of species of *Microsporum* are involved. A negative result does not eliminate the possibility of ringworm.

Microscopic Examination

Small fragments of skin scrapings and hairs, including the hair bulb, are placed in a drop of 20% KOH solution, or paraffin oil, on a microscope slide, covered and allowed to clear before examination. In skin, all dermatophytes present the same picture: branching septate hyphae which may be divided into arthrospores (Figure 36.2). In hair, the method of spore formation and the size and arrangement of the spores can give a clue to the genus of dermatophyte involved. In the early stages of infection, before the spore sheath has developed, septate hyphae may be seen within the hair.

Culture

It is advisable to culture specimens from suspected cases of ringworm because some positives will be missed on microscopic examination. Also, knowledge of the infecting species is important in epidemiology and in tracking down the source of an

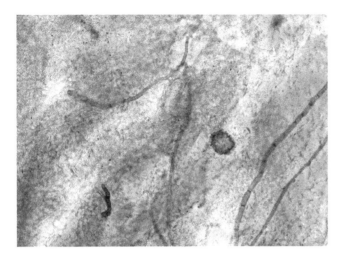

Figure 36.2 Septate mycelium of *Microsporum canis* in canine skin scales after clearing with potassium hydroxide solution and staining with blue-black ink.

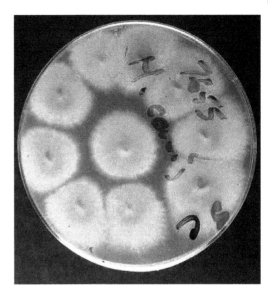

Figure 36.3 *Microsporum canis* in culture after 10 days at 28 °C on Sabouraud medium. The characteristic yellow pigmentation is seen from underneath the fungal colonies.

infection. For example, if a child had ringworm caused by *M. audouinii* (an anthropophilic dermatophyte), the source would be other children. *T. mentagrophytes* ringworm would probably have a source in mice while *M. canis* ringworm can usually be traced to a cat or dog.

Dermatophytes grow well on any nutrient medium which provides organic carbon and nitrogen, such as 4% malt extract agar or Sabouraud glucose agar. The medium is usually supplemented with antibacterial antibiotics and also cyclohex-imide which reduces contamination by saprophytic moulds. A minimum of 12 placings of hair or skin are inoculated to the surface of the medium and incubated at room temperature or 28 °C (Figure 36.3). Culture plates should be retained for three weeks before being considered negative. Dermatophytes are identified on a combination of gross colony characteristics and microscopic morphology. There are simple techniques for encouraging the production of characteristic structures such as micro- and macroconidia.

References

de Hoog, G.S., Dukik, K., Monod, M. et al. (2017). Toward a novel multilocus phylogenetic taxonomy for the dermatophytes. *Mycopathologia* 182: 5–31.

Pasquetti, M., Min, A.R.M., Scacchetti, S. et al. (2017). Infection by *Microsporum canis* in paediatric patients: a veterinary perspective. *Veterinary Sciences* 4: 46.

Tsuboi, R., Ko, I.-J., Takamori, K., and Ogawa, H. (1989). Isolation of a keratinolytic proteinase from *Trichophyton mentagrophytes* with enzymatic activity at acidic pH. *Infection & Immunity* 57: 3479–3483.

37

Yeasts: *Malassezia, Candida* and *Cryptococcus*

Yeasts are single-celled fungi. They may be spherical or oval or elongated depending on the species. Asexual reproduction is by budding so that daughter cells are produced as small versions of the mother cell. These buds are sometimes released early, resulting in a variety of sizes as the daughter cells grow, or late such that the daughter cell is full size when separated from the mother.

Traditionally, yeasts were identified by cultural characteristics, microscopic appearance and biochemical tests such as the ability to assimilate specific carbohydrates. These tests have been formulated as kits such as the BioMerieux API* Yeast Identification System.

Although there are always oddities and exceptions, animals suffer disease from only three yeasts: *Malassezia pachydermatis* and related species, *Candida albicans* and similar yeasts and *Cryptococcus neoformans*.

Malassezia pachydermatis

Malassezia pachydermatis is a non-mycelial, lipophilic yeast that is oval in shape and produces buds on a broad base so that it appears like an acorn as the bud emerges from the mother cell. It is considered to be a commensal organism that is normally present in low numbers in the external ear canal and normal skin in dogs and other animals. However, pathological changes such as atopic dermatitis or flea allergy may cause inflammation and lead to favourable conditions for the yeast to proliferate (Forsythe 2016). This leads to overgrowth of *Malassezia* in the skin or external ear and then to infection (Figure 37.1). It is also encouraged to overgrow when there is increased humidity of the skin (such as in skinfolds), corticosteroid therapy, endocrine disease such as hypothyroidism or changes in the normal bacterial flora from antimicrobial therapy (Guillot and Bond 2020). Furthermore, a proportion of dogs with dermatitis associated with *Malassezia* also have staphylococcal pyoderma. It is suggested that such dual infections may be synergistic, with each of the two organisms facilitating the overgrowth of the other (Bajwa 2017).

Candida albicans

Candida albicans is a normal commensal yeast of humans and animals, living on the skin and mucosal surfaces of the oral cavity, genital tract, intestine and urinary tract. The normal source of infection is therefore endogenous, and disease occurs when there is a predisposing condition. This can be immunosuppression from corticosteroids, antimicrobial therapy, cytotoxic drugs, diabetes mellitus, pregnancy, trauma or other circumstance which allows overgrowth of *C. albicans* (Pfaller and Diekema 2007).

When conditions are favourable, *C. albicans* will switch phase to form hyphae and this form invades epithelium of the mucous membrane (Figure 37.2). The hyphal form has been shown to be more invasive than the yeast form and mutants that are unable to form hyphae under *in vitro* conditions are generally attenuated in virulence (Mayer et al. 2013). These invasive hyphae are also known as 'germ tubes' and the ability to form hyphae from yeast cells when incubated in a sample of animal plasma at 37 °C in the laboratory is characteristic of the species *C. albicans*. In this pathogenic state, *C. albicans* is able to evade macrophages, adhere to host cells and develop biofilm (Dadar et al. 2018).

Fundamentals of Veterinary Microbiology, First Edition. Andrew N. Rycroft.
© 2024 John Wiley & Sons Ltd. Published 2024 by John Wiley & Sons Ltd.
Companion website: www.wiley.com/go/veterinarymicrobiology

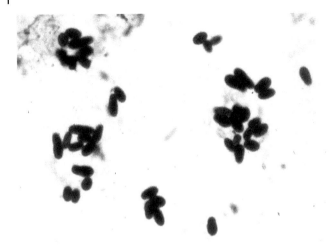

Figure 37.1 Microscopic appearance of yeast cells of *Malassezia pachydermatis* from the ear canal of a dog, stained by Gram stain.

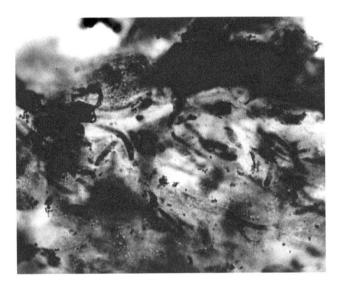

Figure 37.2 Hyphae of *Candida albicans* in mucosal tissue, stained by Diff-Quik®.

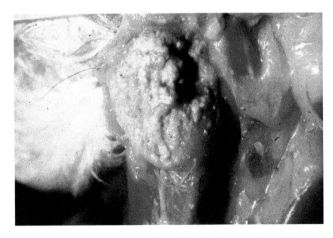

Figure 37.3 *Candida albicans* infection in the crop of a chicken – 'sour crop'.

The damage associated with *C. albicans* infections mainly depends on the associated host immune responses. The opportunistic infection usually remains superficial; it is known as thrush. In severely immunocompromised individuals, *Candida* can invade into deep organs and cause systemic disease.

There are relatively few reports of *Candida* infection in animals. In domestic poultry, wild birds and waterfowl, the disease affects the upper alimentary tract, particularly the crop ('sour crop'). Lesions may also be found in the mouth. In acute cases, the grey-white lesions adhere loosely to the mucous membrane. In chronic cases, the crop wall may be thickened and covered by a corrugated mass of yellow-white necrotic material. The underlying tissue is usually inflamed (Figure 37.3).

Mastitis is the most frequent *Candida* infection in cattle but mycotic abortion and rumenal infections have also been reported. In young pigs, candidsis is usually seen as lesions in mouth, oesophagus and stomach and in older animals, colonisation of stomach ulcers. Oral thrush occurs in young animals of various species. Cutaneous candidosis has been recorded in the dog and intestinal candidosis in dog and cat (Dadar et al. 2018).

While the most frequently isolated pathogen of the *Candida* genus is *C. albicans*, other species causing similar infections include *C. tropicalis*, *C. krusei*, *C. pelliculosa*, *C. glabrata* and others.

Cryptococcus neoformans

Cryptococcus neoformans is an encapsulated yeast of worldwide distribution (O'Meara and Alspaugh 2012). It has been isolated from fruit, milk and soil but many recent publications confirm that the main source of the fungus is accumulations of pigeon droppings in which there is a high concentration of creatinine (Sirag et al. 2021). As many as 5×10^7 viable cells of the yeast may be recovered per gram of droppings.

The epidemiology of the disease is typical of a non-contagious exogenous mycosis. Cases occur sporadically and each is contracted from the environment. The exception is bovine mastitis which appears to spread within a herd. The primary route of infection is usually respiratory, occasionally by skin penetration or rarely by ingestion.

Pathogenesis

Cryptococcosis is an acute, subacute or chronic exogenous mycosis with no clearly defined clinical pattern. The disease may affect the respiratory system or the central nervous system or be systemic. In humans, the CNS is most frequently affected, resulting in meningitis. There are

180 000 annual deaths worldwide from cryptococcosis (Rajasingham et al. 2017). While the yeast is usually opportunistic in immunocompromised individuals, it is also known to act as a primary pathogen (Kronstad et al. 2011).

Cryptococcus neoformans infection is usually controlled and eliminated by the immune system in the lung. Serological evidence of infection is therefore much more common than clinical disease. However, in some individuals the fungi are not controlled and disseminate to infect the central nervous system, where they cause meningoencephalitis (Nolan et al. 2017).

In animals, cryptococcosis takes different forms. The most important form of the disease in cattle is mastitis. In the horse, myxoma-like lesions of the lung and lip are most frequently encountered. Dogs and cats may show oral, pulmonary or cutaneous lesions and involvement of the CNS. In cats, respiratory tract infection is often accompanied by proliferative lesions of the nasal cavity. The tip of the nose is a common site of infection in the cat (Figure 37.4).

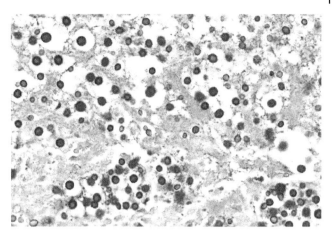

Figure 37.4 Yeast cells of *Cryptococcus neoformans* in nasal tissue from a cat. The dark red spherical yeast cells are surrounded by large clear areas of polysaccharide capsule. The stain is periodic acid–Schiff to show the fungal elements as dark red.

Serological Tests

Serological tests can be used in the diagnosis of cryptococcosis. In active systemic disease, any antibody formed is soon overwhelmed and apparently neutralised by the abundant polysaccharide antigen from the capsule. It is therefore necessary to test serum for both antibody and antigen. An antigen titre indicates active infection; antibody titre reappears as antigen disappears. Serological investigations are used to monitor treatment and to follow the course of the disease. In localised chronic infections, antibody is present. Agglutination tests using sensitised latex or whole cells are most frequently used in human medicine. Counter-immunoelectrophoresis has proven useful in the veterinary field. When interpreting the results of serological tests, it should be remembered that low levels of antibody are present in a proportion of normal dogs and cats.

References

Bajwa, J. (2017). Canine *Malassezia* dermatitis. *Canadian Veterinary Journal* 58: 1119–1121.

Dadar, M., Tiwari, R., Karthik, K. et al. (2018). *Candida albicans* – biology, molecular characterization, pathogenicity, and advances in diagnosis and control – an update. *Microbial Pathogenesis* 117: 128–138.

Forsythe, P.J. (2016). Acute otitis externa: the successful first-opinion ear consultation. *In Practice* 38: 2–6.

Guillot, J. and Bond, R. (2020). *Malassezia* yeasts in veterinary dermatology: an updated overview. *Frontiers in Cellular and Infection Microbiology* 10: 79.

Kronstad, J., Attarian, R., Cadieux, B. et al. (2011). Expanding fungal pathogenesis: *Cryptococcus* breaks out of the opportunistic box. *Nature Reviews Microbiology* 9: 193–203.

Mayer, F.L., Wilson, D., and Hube, B. (2013). *Candida albicans* pathogenicity mechanisms. *Virulence* 4: 119–128.

Nolan, S.J., Fu, M.S., Coppens, I., and Casadevall, A. (2017). Lipids affect the *Cryptococcus neoformans*–macrophage interaction and promote nonlytic exocytosis. *Infection and Immunity* 85: e00564–e00517.

O'Meara, T.R. and Alspaugh, J.A. (2012). The *Cryptococcus neoformans* capsule: a sword and a shield. *Clinical Microbiology Reviews* 25: 387–408.

Pfaller, M.A. and Diekema, D.J. (2007). Epidemiology of invasive candidiasis: a persistent public health problem. *Clinical Microbiology Reviews* 20: 133–163.

Rajasingham, R., Smith, R.M., Park, B.J. et al. (2017). Global burden of disease of HIV-associated cryptococcal meningitis: an updated analysis. *Lancet Infectious Disease* 17: 873–881.

Sirag, B., Khidir, E.-S., Dumyati, M. et al. (2021). *Cryptococcus neoformans* and other opportunistic *Cryptococcus* species in pigeon dropping in Saudi Arabia: identification and characterization by DNA sequencing. *Frontiers in Microbiology* 12: 726203.

38

Dimorphic Fungal Infections

There are a number of relatively rare fungal infections of animals that can be life-threatening. The agents of these infections are dimorphic: they exist as mycelial (filamentous) fungi in the natural environment but transform to a yeast phase when invading living animals. The environmental conditions that result in phase change vary with the fungal pathogen, but body temperature and nutritional factors are known to cause the mycelial form to transform to the yeast form. Discussed below are the most important of the dimorphic fungal infections in terms of animal disease.

Blastomycosis

Blastomycosis is one of the principal endemic systemic mycotic infections of dogs and humans in North America where it is an important veterinary problem. The disease is caused by the dimorphic fungus *Blastomyces dermatitidis*, which exists in the mycelial form in nature and converts to a yeast form at 37 °C in mammalian hosts. The risk of blastomycosis in dogs seems to be 10 times higher than in humans and dogs act as a sentinel for disease in humans. In dogs, mortality can be as high as 90% if prompt treatment is not initiated.

Pathogenesis

Infection with *B. dermatitidis* is usually acquired by the inhalation of aerosolised conidiospores, which are deposited in the alveoli and then produce an asymptomatic infection. This is often cleared without clinical signs and serological evidence confirms that many more individuals are infected than develop disease. *B. dermatitidis* is a facultative intracellular pathogen and unless destroyed by macrophages, infections will develop into a mild or progressive pneumonia with granulomas. This can disseminate outside the lung to produce granulomatous lesions elsewhere, particularly visible in the skin.

If left untreated, blastomycosis can present as a fulminant, progressive pneumonia and can be fatal. A substantial proportion of pulmonary infections spread by the lymphohaematogenous route and develop into secondary systemic disease. Most infections occur in immunocompetent hosts, and yet *B. dermatitidis* can also produce an opportunistic infection in immunocompromised hosts, particularly in humans (Pfister et al. 2011).

Distribution

The disease is reported to be endemic in a large region of North America, Africa and India. In North America, it is known to be endemic in regions that border the Great Lakes and the St Lawrence River, New York and southern Canada, as well as in the Mississippi, Missouri and Ohio River basins, south-eastern USA and the Eastern Seaboard. Most cases in the USA are reported in Arkansas, Kentucky, Mississippi, Tennessee and Wisconsin which appear to be hyperendemic areas for the disease.

Fundamentals of Veterinary Microbiology, First Edition. Andrew N. Rycroft.
© 2024 John Wiley & Sons Ltd. Published 2024 by John Wiley & Sons Ltd.
Companion website: www.wiley.com/go/veterinarymicrobiology

Epidemiology

The source of infection is the environment. Direct animal-to-animal or animal-to-person transmission is very rare. The yeast form is considered non-infectious and the dog is a dead-end host.

The epidemiology of *B. dermatitidis* is unclear because the precise ecological niche of the organism is not known for certain. A number of host and environmental risk factors have been identified but findings of important risk factors have not been consistent in all studies. Risk of infection is higher in areas with wet, sandy, acidic soils and high organic matter content. High humidity and fog have also been reported to increase infection risk by aerosolising and carrying spores to susceptible hosts. Increased incidence of the disease during late summer and early autumn may suggest the importance of suitable temperatures for the development and transmission of the organism.

Diagnostic Methods

Blastomycosis mimics other diseases. Cutaneous blastomycosis can resemble malignancy, and mass-like lung opacities due to *B. dermatitidis* in radiographs are sometimes confused with neoplasia. Blastomycosis may be clinically indistinguishable from tuberculosis. Cytological investigations of material from a skin lesion or tracheal wash may show round, multinucleated yeast forms that produce daughter cells from a single broad-based bud. Definitive diagnosis is now based on PCR detection of the pathogen but specimens for analysis may require invasive biopsy (Sidamonidze et al. 2012). There is no useful skin test (type IV hypersensitivity test).

Serological tests (immunodiffusion and complement fixation test) have been considered to have low sensitivity and widespread exposure to the organism may leave detectable antibody without establishment of disease (Turner et al. 1986). However, serological tests using ELISA have sought to improve the sensitivity of antibody testing for blastomycosis (Richer et al. 2014). There are also antigen detection tests with limited potential to assist in diagnosis (Durkin et al. 2004).

Histoplasmosis

Histoplasmosis is a non-contagious systemic mycosis caused by the dimorphic fungus *Histoplasma capsulatum*. The disease is endemic in the USA. It is most common in the Ohio and Mississippi River valleys, particularly the south and central part of the country, and also south Ontario and Quebec. Isolated cases have been recorded in Europe.

Histoplasma capsulatum is found in soil contaminated with the droppings of birds and in caves inhabited by bats. The saprophytic phase consists of fine, septate, branching hyphae bearing smooth-walled pyriform to spherical microconidia and large spherical, thick-walled tuberculate macroconidia borne on simple conidiophores (Figure 38.1).

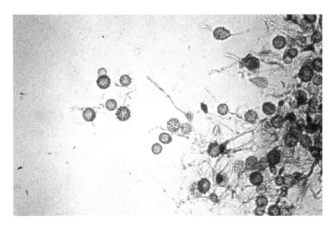

Figure 38.1 The infective, mycelial phase and tuberculate conidia (macroconidia) of *Histoplasma capsulatum* in culture.

Pathogenesis

The route of infection is respiratory. When *H. capsulatum*-contaminated soil is disturbed, the mycelium fragments and conidia may be inhaled. The small size of the microconidia enables them to enter the lower respiratory tract where they are phagocytosed by macrophages. The temperature of the living host causes the *H. capsulatum* to activate a transcriptional programme causing the switch to the yeast phase and expression of factors needed for pathogenicity (Webster and Sil 2008). Macrophage cells carry the fungus via the lymphatics to the reticuloendothelial system where the pathogen survives and replicates in macrophages (Figure 38.2). As with blastomycosis, most infections are inapparent (Garfoot and Rappleye 2016).

The innate immune response is not adequate to control *H. capsulatum* infection. A cell-mediated immune response develops and proinflammatory cytokines, produced primarily by CD4+ T-cells, potentiate the antifungal properties of tissue macrophages to allow resolution of the infection (Kauffman 2007). However, if an adequate T-cell response does not develop or there is a high burden of *H. capsulatum*, the infection will progress towards a fatal wasting disease (Coady and Sil 2015).

The disease most commonly affects the dog, but cats, cattle, horses and humans are also infected. The primary focus of infection is pulmonary but other organs are often involved. This is seen as a chronic cough, hepatomegaly and chronic debilitating digestive disturbances.

In tissues, *H. capsulatum* is present mainly intracellularly in macrophages as oval yeast cells with few buds.

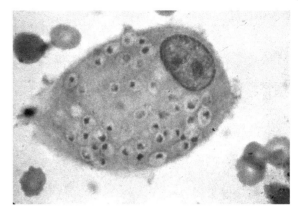

Figure 38.2 A macrophage with yeast phase cells of *H. capsulatum.*

Diagnostic Methods

There is a range of diagnostic methods used in the detection of histoplasmosis. Culture of *H. capsulatum* at 25 °C on Sabouraud medium is practicable but, depending on the jurisdiction, usually requires containment level 3 for operator safety. After 3–4 weeks, a positive culture will show the characteristic pale tan mould. Microscopy will show mycelium with the characteristic macroconidia (Figure 38.1).

Finding the distinctive 2–4 µm, oval, narrow-based budding yeasts by histopathology of tissue biopsy material or cytological examination of a smear allows a tentative diagnosis of histoplasmosis (Figure 38.2). Special stains, such as periodic acid–Schiff or Grocott, are helpful in recognition of fungi.

Other diagnostic techniques have been developed originally for use in humans. Detection of circulating or urinary polysaccharide antigen using an antibody-linked enzyme (ELISA) is used. While this detects antigen of *H. capsulatum*, it fails to discriminate when there is other dimorphic fungal disease.

Antibody detection, using the complement fixation test and immunoprecipitation test, is limited because antibody can persist for years after infection. The detection of a low antibody complement fixation (CF) titre means little other than that the patient has been exposed to *H. capsulatum* at some time.

Polymerase chain reaction-based detection of *H. capsulatum* is available but has not taken over from the accepted combination of serological, cytological and culture-based methods.

The histoplasmin skin test, to detect type IV hypersensitivity to *Histoplasma* antigen, was considered very important for recognising asymptomatic infection and for defining the geographical area where *H. capsulatum* is endemic. It was not a useful diagnostic test because of cross-reactivity with other fungi, especially *Blastomyces dermatitidis*. It also caused interference with subsequent complement fixation antibody testing and the skin test reagents are therefore no longer available (Kauffman 2007).

Epizootic Lymphangitis

Histoplasma capsulatum var. *farciminosum* causes epizootic lymphangitis in horses. It affects all equids and is endemic in Asia, East Africa and India but has been eradicated from Europe (Scantlebury et al. 2016). The disease was brought to the UK in horses returning from the South African war at the end of the nineteenth century. It was then eradicated from the British Isles at the beginning of the twentieth century but remains notifiable under the Diseases of Animals Act.

Epizootic lymphangitis is a contagious subcutaneous mycosis involving mainly the lymphatic system. The disease is characterised by suppurative lesions of the exposed surface of the skin associated with lymphatic vessels. Infected lymphatic vessels become dilated at intervals and form lines of hard abscesses. These often rupture to give ulcers from which blood-stained pus is discharged for several weeks. Lesions may also be found on the mucous membranes of the nostrils, pharynx and trachea. Involvement of the eye has been reported as another form of the disease.

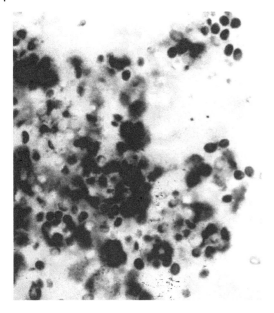

Figure 38.3 Yeast phase cells of *Histoplasma capsulatum* var. *farciminosum* in pus from a lesion in the leg of a horse with epizootic lymphangitis.

The route of infection is by penetration through minor wounds in the skin and the disease is spread by direct contact or by contact with infected grooming equipment, saddlery, etc. and by biting flies.

Diagnostic methods are limited in areas where the disease is present. The disease is diagnosed on clinical evidence and microscopic examination for yeast cells within pus (Figure 38.3). There is the potential for confusion with other diseases such as sporotrichosis, ulcerative lymphangitis and the cutaneous form of glanders. Culture of *H. capsulatum* var. *farciminosum* from clinical lesions can be definitive but it is rarely attempted when facilities are so limited (Scantlebury et al. 2016).

Coccidioidomycosis

Coccidioidomycosis is a non-contagious systemic mycosis mainly affecting the lungs of cattle, dogs, sheep and humans. *Coccidioides immitis* occurs in alkaline soil in certain arid regions of south-western USA and Mexico: it is a reportable disease in Arizona and California. The saprophytic phase consists of septate, branching hyphae which fragment into thick-walled barrel-shaped arthrospores.

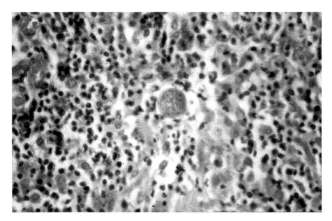

Figure 38.4 Microscopic appearance of a spherule of *Coccidioides immitis* in tissue.

Pathogenesis

The route of infection is respiratory and infections are most frequent in the summer following dust storms. Under conditions of increased CO_2 and body temperature, arthrospores undergo a complex metamorphosis into the form of a thick-walled spherule (15–90 µm) which, when mature, contains many nucleated, round spores known as endospores (Figure 38.4). This is a unique parasitic form that is pathognomonic of coccidioidomycosis (Viriyakosol et al. 2018). When spherules rupture, they release their endospores, which can mature into spherules by expansion.

From the initial lung infection, dogs can develop disease in bone, the eye, the central nervous system and other internal organs (Graupmann-Kuzma et al. 2008).

Diagnosis

Detection of spherules in tissues can only realistically be carried out at postmortem. Biopsy, antigen tests, PCR, etc. are therefore of little or no value. The current test is an agar gel immunodiffusion (AGID) assay for IgG and IgM antibodies. This is specific but relatively insensitive so some infected animals will not be detected. Furthermore, the test has not been fully characterised using animal serum. An ELISA to detect IgM and IgG and a latex particle agglutination (LA) test for IgM are also used. False-positive results are known to occur with both (Graupmann-Kuzma et al. 2008).

Sporotrichosis

Sporotrichosis is a dimorphic fungal infection that occurs sporadically and is acquired from the environment. *Sporothrix schenckii* grows saprophytically on many types of decaying and healthy plants, on wood and in soil and is worldwide in distribution (Mesa-Arango et al. 2002). It is said to be associated with sphagnum moss (Dixon et al. 1991). Genome sequencing has shown that the genus should be subdivided into six species rather than the single species.

The route of infection is by direct inoculation into tissue by trauma and the primary lesion can often be traced to a minor puncture wound. When inoculated into tissues, the mycelial-saprophytic form of *S. schenckii* changes to the yeast-parasitic form. These are distinctive, elongated (cigar shaped) yeast cells although they are often sparse in material recovered from lesions (Figure 38.5).

Sporotrichosis is a chronic non-contagious subcutaneous mycosis of horses and other animals characterised by subcutaneous nodule formation involving the lymphatics; the nodules eventually ulcerate and discharge pus. Less frequently, there is involvement of internal organs. A few cases of infection by the yeast phase have been recorded, such as a bite from an infected rat.

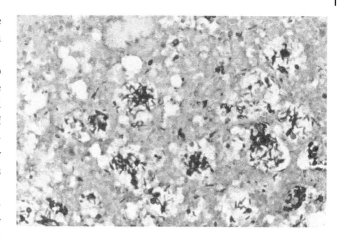

Figure 38.5 The characteristic cigar-shaped appearance of yeast cells of *S. schenckii* in pus, stained by periodic acid–Schiff.

The subcutaneous form of the disease in horses may, in endemic areas, be confused with epizootic lymphangitis. In the dog, involvement of bones and internal organs is more frequent. Other species in which the disease has been recorded include cattle, camels, rodents and humans.

Definitive diagnosis of sporotrichosis is based on fungal detection in culture although PCR-based methods are now a useful means of detecting the pathogen in pathological samples (Hu et al. 2003).

References

Coady, A. and Sil, A. (2015). MyD88-dependent signaling drives host survival and early cytokine production during *Histoplasma capsulatum* infection. *Infection and Immunity* 83: 1265–1275.

Dixon, D.M., Salkin, I.F., Duncan, R.A. et al. (1991). Isolation and characterization of *Sporothrix schenckii* from clinical and environmental sources associated with the largest U.S. epidemic of sporotrichosis. *Journal of Clinical Microbiology* 29: 1106–1113.

Durkin, M., Witt, J., LeMonte, A. et al. (2004). Antigen assay with the potential to aid in diagnosis of blastomycosis. *Journal of Clinical Microbiology* 42: 4873–4875.

Garfoot, A.L. and Rappleye, C.A. (2016). *Histoplasma capsulatum* surmounts obstacles to intracellular pathogenesis. *FEBS Journal* 283: 619–633.

Graupmann-Kuzma, A., Valentine, B.A., Shubitz, L.F. et al. (2008). Coccidioidomycosis in dogs and cats: a review. *Journal of the American Animal Hospital Association* 44: 226–235.

Hu, S., Chung, W.-H., Hung, S.-I. et al. (2003). Detection of *Sporothrix schenckii* in clinical samples by a nested PCR assay. *Journal of Clinical Microbiology* 41: 1414–1418.

Kauffman, C.A. (2007). Histoplasmosis: a clinical and laboratory update. *Clinical Microbiology Reviews* 20: 115–132.

Mesa-Arango, A.C., Del Rocío Reyes-Montes, M., Pérez-Mejía, A. et al. (2002). Phenotyping and genotyping of *Sporothrix schenckii* isolates according to geographic origin and clinical form of sporotrichosis. *Journal of Clinical Microbiology* 40: 3004–3011.

Pfister, J.R., Archer, J.R., Hersil, S. et al. (2011). Non-rural point source blastomycosis outbreak near a yard waste collection site. *Clinical Medicine & Research* 9: 57–65.

Richer, S.M., Smedema, M.L., Durkin, M.M. et al. (2014). Development of a highly sensitive and specific blastomycosis antibody enzyme immunoassay using *Blastomyces dermatitidis* surface protein BAD-1. *Clinical and Vaccine Immunology* 21: 143–146.

Scantlebury, C.E., Pinchbeck, G.L., Loughnane, P. et al. (2016). Development and evaluation of a molecular diagnostic method for rapid detection of *Histoplasma capsulatum* var. *farciminosum*, the causative agent of epizootic lymphangitis, in equine clinical samples. *Journal of Clinical Microbiology* 54: 2990–2999.

Sidamonidze, K., Peck, M.K., Perez, M. et al. (2012). Real-time PCR assay for identification of *Blastomyces dermatitidis* in culture and in tissue. *Journal of Clinical Microbiology* 50: 1783–1786.

Turner, S., Kaufman, L., and Jalbert, M. (1986). Diagnostic assessment of an enzyme-linked immunosorbent assay for human and canine blastomycosis. *Journal of Clinical Microbiology* 23: 294–297.

Viriyakosol, S., Walls, L., Okamoto, S. et al. (2018). Myeloid differentiation factor 88 and interleukin-1R1 signaling contribute to resistance to *Coccidioides immitis*. *Infection and Immunity* 86: e00028–e00018.

Webster, R.H. and Sil, A. (2008). Conserved factors Ryp2 and Ryp3 control cell morphology and infectious spore formation in the fungal pathogen *Histoplasma capsulatum*. *Proceedings of the National Academy of Sciences USA* 105: 14573–14578.

Index